WOMEN'S HEALTH CARE
A GUIDE TO ALTERNATIVES

WOMEN'S HEALTH CARE

A GUIDE TO ALTERNATIVES

Reston Publishing Company, Inc.
A Prentice-Hall Company
Reston, Virginia

Kay Weiss

Editor

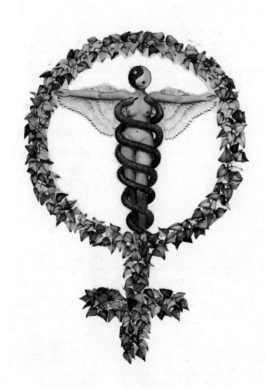

THE PENNSYLVANIA STATE UNIVERSITY
COMMONWEALTH CAMPUS LIBRARIES
ALTOONA

To Richard and Kristin

Illustrations by Linda Ruiz

Library of Congress Cataloging in Publication Data
Main entry under title:

Women's health care.

   Includes bibliographies and index.
   1. Therapeutic systems.   2. Gynecology—Popular works.
3. Obstetrics—Popular works.   4. Women's health
services.   I. Weiss, Kay. [DNLM: 1. Gynecology—Popular
works.   2. Obstetrics—Popular works.   3. Therapeutic
cults—Populars works.   WP 120 W872]
RG121.W85 1983   618   83-3167
ISBN 0-8359-8781-7
ISBN 0-8359-8780-9 (pbk.)

RG121
.W85
1984
(1)

10 9 8 7 6 5 4 3 2 1

Printed in the United States of America

Contents

Preface   *xiii*

About the Contributors   *xv*

Part One

CURRENT CRISES AND CONTROVERSIES IN WOMEN'S HEALTH CARE

by Kay Weiss   2

Inadequate Scientific Testing, Especially in Women's Health Care, 3; Scientific Medicine's View of Women's Ailments, 4; *References*, 5; *Listing of U.S. Women's Health Organizations*, 5.

Chapter One

CONTRACEPTION—1984

by Barbara Seaman   8

The Pill and the IUD—Increasing Disenchantment, 9; Sterilization—Not as Safe and Simple as it Sounds, 10; Back to the Barriers?, 11; Methods of Natural Birth Control, 18; Adverse Effects of Artificial Birth Control Methods, 21; The IUD—Problems and Medical Complications, 26; *Summary*, 28; *References*, 29.

Chapter Two

PREGNANCY AND BIRTH: CURRENT TREATMENT

by Doris Haire   34

Examples of Questionable Drug Use and Obstetrical Interventions, 35; Research Findings and Government Inaction, 38; Impact of Drugs on Unborn Infant, 38; Continued

Use of Drugs and Other Obstetrical Interventions Despite Potential Dangers, 41; Prevalence of Brain Damage Among the General Population, 43; Improper Commercial Labeling of Drugs, 44; *References, 45; Suggested Readings, 47; Listing of Organizations for Pregnancy and Birth, 47.*

Chapter Three

TREATMENT OF MENSTRUAL AND MENOPAUSAL PROBLEMS

by Kay Weiss   **50**

Extent of the Problem, 51; Menopause, 52; Menstruation, 54; Conclusion, 58; *References, 59.*

Chapter Four

ESTROGEN HORMONE DRUGS: THEIR USE AND ABUSE

by Kay Weiss   **60**

Sex Hormone Drugs—Major Public Health Problem, 61; Widespread Use of Estrogen Drugs, 62; Safety and Efficacy of Estrogens, 62; Early Evidence of the Carcinogenicity of Estrogens, 66; Menopausal Uses of Estrogen, 66; A Proposal to Make Estrogen Replacement Therapy (ERT) Safer, 68; Types of Estrogen, 68; The "Pill," 69: DES: A Case Study in Hormone Abuse, 70; Social, Political, and Economic Factors in Estrogen Promotion, 74; Conclusion, 77; *References, 78; Suggested Readings, 81.*

Chapter Five

WOMEN, DRUGS, AND PHYSICIANS

by Linda S. Fidell   **82**

Misprescribing of Drugs: Special Impact on Women, 83; Frequency and Seriousness of Adverse Drug Reactions, 83; Types of Drugs Implicated, 84; Continued Prescription Drug Abuse Despite Adverse Publicity, 85; Segments of Population Most Affected, 86; Recommendations for Continuing Physician Education in Pharmacology, 87; Sex Differences in Psychotropic Drug Use, 87; *References, 91; Suggested Readings, 93.*

Chapter Six

BREAST SURGERY: CURRENT TREATMENT

by Kay Weiss   **94**

Unnecessary Radical Surgery, 95; Alternative Procedures and Survival Rates, 97; Stage of Disease Should Determine Treatment, 97; Misdiagnosis and Unnecessary Surgery, 98; Early Detection, 98; Review of Treatment Options, 99; Conclusion, 99; *References, 100; Suggested Readings, 100.*

Chapter Seven

HYSTERECTOMY: CURRENT TREATMENT

by Susanne Morgan   **102**

Hysterectomy—Common Major Operation, 103; Rates of Unnecessary Hysterectomy, 104; Reasons For and Against Surgery, 105; Morbidity and Mortality, 106; Other Considerations: Mental and Physical, 106; Alternatives to Hysterectomy, 107; Sociological and Economic Factors That Contribute to Hysterectomy Rates, 107; Recommendations, 108; *References, 108; Suggested Readings, 110.*

Chapter Eight

CAESAREAN SURGERY: CURRENT TREATMENT

by Helen Marieskind   **112**

Types of Caesareans, 113; Morbidity and Mortality Considerations, 114; Psychological Costs and Other Complications, 115; Financial Costs, 115; Rationale for Caesarean Delivery, 115; Economic Incentives, 116; Conditions Believed to Warrant Caesarean Surgery, 116; Conclusion, 120; *References, 121.*

Part Two

HOLISTIC HEALTH AND ORTHODOX MEDICINE: CHANGING CONCEPTS OF HEALTH AND DISEASE

by Richard B. Miles   **124**

Growing Opposition to Orthodox Medicine, 125; Two Ways to See the World, 127; Historical Views of the Origin of Disease, 128; Four Stages in the Evolution of Thought, 129; Rational, Objective View Being Questioned Today, 130; Four Approaches to Health Disorders, 130; Definition of "Holistic," 133; Factors That Improve and Protect Body Self-Regulation, 134; Factors That Distort Body Self-Regulation, 134; New Directions in Health Care, 138; A Comparison of Views, 140; Summary, 141; *References, 142; Suggested Readings, 143; Listing of Holistic Health Organizations, 144.*

Part Three

SELF-HEALING IN THE NINETEENTH CENTURY: A WOMEN'S MOVEMENT

by Regina Markell Morantz   **146**

Growing Criticism of Established Medical Practice, 147; Health Reform Movement—Emphasis on Prevention and Self-Healing, 148; Women Assuming New Leadership Role, 149; Health Reform—A Source for Social Change, 152; Conclusion, 153; *References, 154; Suggesting Readings, 155.*

Part Four

ALTERNATIVE VERSUS ORTHODOX APPROACHES TO WOMEN'S HEALTH

by Kay Weiss **156**

Disadvantages of Western Orthodox Approach, 157; Comparison of Treatment Modalities, 158; Modern Alternative Modes of Medical Care, 158.

Chapter Nine

CHINESE MEDICINE AND WOMEN'S HEALTH

by Angela Longo and Sandy Newhouse **162**

Theories of Yin and Yang and the Five Elements, 163; Application to Women's Health Problems, 164; Father, Mother, and Child "Organs": Etiology of Disease, 165; Traditional Chinese Medicine, 166; Herbal Medicine, 169; Treatment of Specific Female Conditions, 170; Conclusion, 176; *References, 180; Suggested Readings, 181.*

Chapter Ten

ACUPUNCTURE FOR WOMEN'S HEALTH

by Louise Wensel **182**

Theoretical Background, 183; Scientific Basis, 184; Why Not Recommended by More American Physicians, 185; Indications and Contraindications, 185; Situations That May Be Helped by Acupuncture, 186; Other Conditions Amenable to Acupuncture, 193; Specific Points for Specific Conditions, 193; *References, 193; Suggested Readings, 194; Listing of Organizations for Acupuncture, 195.*

Chapter Eleven

HOMEOPATHY AND WOMEN'S HEALTH

by Jennifer Jacobs **196**

The Principle of Similars, 197; Homeopathic Remedies, 198; How Does Homeopathy Work?, 199; The Natural Healing Process, 199; Integrated Approach Beneficial for Women's Health, 200; Homeopathy in Pregnancy and Childbirth, 200; First-Aid, Acute, and Chronic Prescribing, 201; Limitations of Homeopathy, 202; A Case Study, 203; Responsibilities of the Homeopathic Patient, 204; *References, 204; Suggested Readings, 205; Listing of Organizations for Homeopathy, 205.*

Chapter Twelve

NUTRITION AS PREVENTION AND THERAPY FOR WOMEN'S DISEASES

by Suza Francina **208**

Dietary Factors in the Prevention of Disease, 209; Menstrual Problems and Nutritional Remedies, 211; Menopausal Problems and Nutritional Remedies, 214; Pregnancy,

Childbirth, and Lactation, 215; Nutritional Problems of the Oral Contraceptive, 217; Breast Diseases and Nutrition, 218; Female Cancer, Estrogen Production, and Diet, 219; The Relationship between Macrobiotic Diet and Consciousness, 224; *References, 224; Suggested Readings, 225; Listing of Organizations for Nutrition, 227.*

Chapter Thirteen

MEGAVITAMIN THERAPY AND PREGNANCY

by Linus Pauling   **228**

Importance of Extra Vitamin C for Good Health, 229; *References, 231; Listing of Organizations for Megavitamin Therapy, 232.*

Chapter Fourteen

HERBAL TREATMENTS FOR WOMEN

by Jeanne Rose   **234**

Herbs—Earliest Form of Medicine, 235; New Emphasis on the Use of Herbs for Medicinal Purposes, 236; Herbal Formulas for Late Menses, 237; Menstrual Regulation Formulations, 238; Formulas for Premenstrual Tension, Acne, and Water Retention, 239; Vaginal Infections, 240; Bladder and Kidney Infections, 241; Pregnancy and Childbirth, 242; Menopause, 243; Appendix—Definitions of Some Simple Herbal Terms, 243; *References, 244; Listing of Organizations for Herbology, 245.*

Chapter Fifteen

MASSAGE: THE ROOTS OF WOMEN'S HEALING

by Mirka Knaster   **246**

Early History, 274; Factors Contributing to the Decrease of Massage, 249; Nineteenth and Twentieth Centuries—Increased Recognition of the Value of Massage, 250; Place of Women in the Profession of Massage, 251; Rationale for the Use of Massage, 252; Neglect by American Medical Profession, 252; Rebirth of Massage as a Precious and Vital Talent, 253; *References, 255; Suggested Readings, 257; Listing of Organizations for Massage, 257.*

Chapter Sixteen

MASSAGE, REFLEXOLOGY, AND WOMEN

by Frances M. Tappan   **258**

Physiological Effects of Massage, 258; Types of Massage, 260; Massage of Premature and Newborn Babies, 261; Zone Therapy and Energy Flow, 265; Creating Positive Attitudes Toward Healing, 317; *References, 267; Suggested Readings, 268.*

Chapter Seventeen

ACUPRESSURE FOR WOMEN'S HEALTH

by Ann Patterson   **270**

History, 271; How It Works, 272; Underlying Principles: East Meets West, 273; Treatment Techniques, 275; Acupressure for Specific Problems, 276; Conclusions, 281; *References, 282; Suggested Readings, 283.*

Chapter Eighteen

ROLFING THE FEMALE BODY

by Angwyn St. Just   **284**

Advantages of Rolfing for Pregnancy—Improved Body Alignment, 285; Definition of Rolfing, 287; Checking Your Own Alignment, 288; Postpartum Realignment, 290; *References, 291; Suggested Readings, 291; Listing of Organizations for Rolfing, 292.*

Chapter Nineteen

HATHA YOGA FOR WOMEN'S HEALTH

by Judith Lasater   **294**

Definition and Purpose of Yoga, 295; Yoga as a Therapeutic Modality, 296; Yoga Poses for Female Discomforts, 297; Conclusion, 307; Appendix—Pose Descriptions, 307; *References, 309.*

Chapter Twenty

AEROBIC EXERCISE AND WOMEN

by Joan Ullyot   **310**

Principles of Aerobic Exercise, 311; Training Program, 311; Results, 312; Medical Aspects, 313; Conclusion, 317; *References, 317; Suggested Readings, 318.*

Chapter Twenty-One

HEAT THERAPY AND WOMEN—SWEAT BATHING

by Mikkel Aaland   **320**

Historical Significance and Widespread Practice of Sweat Bathing, 321; Medical Research on Physiological Benefits of Sweat Baths, 325; Heat Destroys Bacteria, Viruses, and Cancer Cells, 326; Positive Effects of Negative Ions, 328; Significance of Sweat Bathing for Women's Health, 329; *References, 331.*

Chapter Twenty-Two

BIOFEEDBACK: AN ALTERNATIVE HEALING TECHNIQUE

by Alyce M. Green   **334**

Definition, 335; Rationale, 336; Psychophysiologic Therapy, 338; Health Problems Specific to Women, 340; A Time of Challenge, 346; *References, 346; Suggested Readings, 348; Listing of Organizations for Biofeedback, 349.*

Chapter Twenty-Three

MEDITATION AS THERAPY FOR WOMEN

by Frances E. Vaughan   **350**

Introduction, 351; History, 352; How to Meditate, 352; Types of Meditation, 353; Medical Research, 355; Psychological Effects, 355; Effects on Pregnancy and Menopause, 358; Diagnostic Efficiency, 359; *Conclusions, 359; References, 360; Suggested Readings, 362.*

Chapter Twenty-Four

SELF-HYPNOSIS WITH APPLICATIONS TO WOMEN'S HEALTH

by Freda Morris   **364**

Case Study, 365; Who's in Charge of Me?, 366; Communication Modes, 367; Self-Control through Programming, 368; Female Health Problems Helped by Hypnosis, 369; The Mind Affects Body Chemistry, 371; Self-Hypnosis and Hypnotic Suggestion, 373; Mutual Hypnosis, 375; Women as Natural Hypnotists, 375; *References, 376; Suggested Readings, 377; Listing of Organizations for Hypnosis, 377.*

Chapter Twenty-Five

SELF-HEALING IN THE TWENTIETH CENTURY: SELF-HELP AND VAGINAL DISEASES

by Carol Downer   **378**

Growth of Women's Health Movement, 379; Early Opposition by Medical Profession, 380; Major Accomplishment of Women's Health Movement—The Treatment of Vaginal Infection, 381; Types of Vaginal Infections and Recommended Treatment, 382; *Conclusion, 385; References, 385.*

Chapter Twenty-Six

SELF-DIAGNOSTIC TESTS

by David Sobel   **388**

Home Pregnancy Tests, 389; Home Throat Cultures, 390; Urinary Tract Infections, 391; Diabetic Self-Monitoring, 392; Bowel Cancer Screening, 393; Home Blood Pressure Monitoring, 393; Resources, 394; *Suggested Readings, 396.*

Chapter Twenty-Seven

THE ROLE OF PSYCHOACTIVE DRUGS
IN MEDICAL SELF-HELP

by Andrew T. Weil   **398**

Introduction, 399; Advantages and Disadvantages of Psychoactive Drugs, 399; Historical Use of Drugs—Promoted by Medical Profession, 401; Dangers of Drug Addiction, 401; Beneficial Short-Term Use of Psychoactive Drugs—for Specific Situations, 402; Indications for the Use of Common Psychoactive Drugs, 402; Suggestions for Home Use, 404; Conclusion, 405; *References, 405; Appendix—Rx Marijuana, 406; Suggested Readings, 408.*

Appendix

SUGGESTED READINGS IN WOMEN'S HEALTH

by Mara Klempner   **410**

Name and Subject Index   *417*

Preface

This book was written in response to the need of women to have a forum in which to express their concerns about the dangers of currently accepted medical treatment, and to present safer alternatives to the often painful and perilous technological medicine.

The "new medicine" presented here is a collection of alternative practices that emerged during the 1960s and 1970s in response to the women's movement and the consumer movement. These practices are based on ancient forms of medicine which have been the medicine of most of the people on earth throughout most of human history. They are effective, safe, free, and patient-controlled. They deserve to be scientifically researched and made available in response to the needs of people everywhere.

The chapters presented here are not meant to imply a rejection of scientific medicine. They do suggest that orthodox medicine is not yet scientific enough because it neglects the environmental and emotional factors that affect us in health and disease.

Western medical science is based on analyzing the smallest elements of disease entities. It subdivides each physiological function, anatomical structure, and biochemical process into smaller and smaller subunits in order to study each of them in greater and greater detail. The study of physical diseases is reduced to molecular biology; psychological diseases are analyzed by their behavioral and biochemical components.

Traditional Chinese medicine in contrast is concerned with the interaction among the biological systems rather than with the description of their individual components. For example, it studies the way in which the liver relates to the other functions of the body rather than the anatomical or physiological characteristics of the liver as an isolated organ. It studies the relationships between the individual and the environment—the place, seasons, weather, time of day, and social milieu. All systems of medicine except those based on modern Western science are based on a holistic concept integrating body, mind, spirit and total environment.

Western medicine achieved great triumphs in the treatment of acute, infectious, and traumatic diseases. It fails us both in the prevention and the treatment of the chronic diseases that plague our population today—hypertension, diabetes, arthritis, cancer, many diseases of major organ systems, alcoholism, and mental illness. To effect cures of these diseases, patients must change from passive recipients of medical care to active self-responsible participants in their own cure.

Part One of this book explains why the American medical system is not adequate to meet the routine health needs of women. Part Four presents a sampling of the directions we might pursue to improve our health: techniques such as diet, exercise, touch, and introspection that can help us help ourselves. Linking those sections are essays which provide the rationale—the scientific, political and social reasons—why women are turning away from western scientific medicine to the "new medicine"—eastern, ancient, and holistic systems of self-treatment.

There is no specific holistic therapy for arthritis or breast cancer or migraine headaches or depression. Rather, the holistic approach in medicine is to achieve balance and integration of our body, mind, and spirit with our total environment. Techniques are presented which can be used with or without orthodox physicians—and, in fact, are always used when a lasting cure is effected.

KAY WEISS

About the Contributors

Mikkel Aaland is the author of *Sweat* (Santa Barbara, Ca: Capra Press, 1978), for which he spent three years traveling, consulting medical doctors, and researching the worldwide phenomena of sweat bathing and heat therapy. He is chairperson of the International Sweat Bath committee, under the International Sauna Society, Helsinki, Finland. He now lives in San Francisco.

Michael Castleman is managing editor of *Medical Self-Care* magazine published in Inverness, Ca., and author of *Sexual Solutions* (New York: Simon and Schuster, Inc., 1981).

Carol Downer is a Director of the Feminist Women's Health Center in Los Angeles, Ca., and founder and board member of the National Abortion Federation. She is general editor and main author of *A New View of a Woman's Body* and *How to Stay Out of the Gynecologist's Office*.

Linda S. Fidell, Ph.D., is currently professor of psychology at California State University, Northridge. Her publications include *A Practical Guide to Multivaraite Statistics* (with B. Tavachnick) (New York: Harper and Row, 1982) as well as "Sex Role Stereotypes and the American Physician" (*Psychology of Women, Quarterly*); "Sex Differences in Psychotropic Drug Use" (*Professional Psychology*); "Characteristics of Androgynous, Undifferentiated, Masculine and Feminine Middle Class Women" (*Sex Roles*); "Employment Status, Role Dissatisfaction, and the Housewife Syndrome," (*Psychology of Women Quarterly*), and numerous colloquia and papers at professional meetings.

Suza Francina is a free-lance writer who specializes in health and nutrition. She is a graduate of the Institute for Yoga Teacher Education in San Francisco. For the past ten years she has written a weekly health column for the *Ojai Valley News* and her articles have appeared in the *Yoga Journal, Well-Being, The Holistic Health Handbook,* and other publications. She is author of *Yoga for People Over 50* (Devin-Adair, London, 1977) and other health-related books.

Alyce Green is Psychophysiologic Therapist and Consultant for the Clinical Biofeedback and Psychophysiology Center at the Menninger Foundation in Topeka, Kansas. She is Co-Director of the Voluntary Controls Program, Research Department, at the Menninger Foundation. She was one of three Menninger psychophysiologists who studied yogic control of physiological processes in India (1974). She has lectured throughout the United States and in several foreign countries. Alyce Green has authored a number of papers. She has co-authored with Elmer Green: "Voluntary Control of Internal States, Psychological and Physiological," in *Biofeedback and Self-Control,* An Aldine Annual, Chicago, 1971; "Biofeedback: Rationale and Applications," in the *International Encyclopedia of Neurology, Psychiatry, Psycho-Analysis and Psychology,* Benjamin B. Woolman, ed. (New York: Van Nostrand Reinhold Company, 1977), and *Beyond Biofeedback* (New York: Delacorte Press, 1977).

Doris Haire, R.N., is President of the American Foundation for Maternal and Child Health, past Chairman of the National Women's Health Network, and the current Chairman of the Network Committee on Health Law and Regulation, as well as past President of the International Childbirth Education Association. Her publications include "How the Food and Drug Administration Determines the 'Safety' of Drugs—Just How Safe is 'Safe'?", "The Pregnant Patient's Bill of Rights," published by National Women's Health Network, New York, 1980; and "The Cultural Warping of Childbirth," *Journal of Environmental Child Health,* June, 1973. She brought about the first congressional hearing on "Obstetric Care in the U.S., 1978."

Jennifer Jacobs, M.D., is currently a homeopathist at the Herring Family Health Clinic, Berkeley, Calif. Her publications include "Attitudes of Women and Men Physicians," *American Journal of Public Health,* November 1979, and "Comparison of the Productivity of Women and Men Physicians," in *JAMA,* vol. 237, 1977. She presented a paper on "Science and Homeopathy" in 1980 at the International Foundation for the Promotion of Homeopathy and California State Homeopathic Medical Society annual meeting. Her current research interest is the application of computer technology to homeopathic case analysis and clinical research. She has also developed a training program for lay midwives.

Mara Klempner is a holistic health and nutrition consultant in San Francisco specializing in women's health care.

Mirka Knaster, M.S., is a medical antropologist currently living in India and studying the art and science of massage as it applies to healing.

Judith Lasater, Ph.D., is a physical therapist with a doctorate in East-West Psychology; a teacher of Hatha Yoga at the Institute for Yoga Teacher Education, San Francisco; founder and contributing editor of *Yoga Journal magazine;* and President of the California Yoga Teachers Association. She is author of several books including *Rediscovery of the Body* (New York: Dell Publishing Co., Inc., 1977); and *Yoga for People over Fifty,* Suza Norton, (aka Francina) ed. (London: Devan-Adair, 1977).

Angela Longo, Ph.D., biochemist and acupuncturist, has researched biochemical diagnosis of pre-disease states at the Linus Pauling Institute, Menlo Park, Calif. She is organizing a traditional Chinese medical society focused on applied clinical research. She was recently a professor of Chinese medical theory and holistic health studies at San Francisco State University and helped found the first holistic health department in a university.

Helen Marieskind, Dr. P.H., is Executive Director of Vision Services in Seattle. She is also editor of the *Journal of Women and Health* and author of *Women in the Health System: Patients, Providers and Programs* (St. Louis: The C. V. Mosby Company, 1980). Marieskind is author of the Department of Health, Education and Welfare report *Caesarian Sections in the U.S.* 1980. She formerly taught community health and research methodology at the State University of New York/College of Old Westbury.

Richard B. Miles is Assistant Dean of the Graduate School of Consciousness Studies and Director of the Graduate Program in Clinical Holistic Health Education at John F. Kennedy University in Orinda, Calif. He chaired the national conference "Hidden Health Hazards in Our Environment" at the University of California, Berkeley, in March 1982. He is co-author of *Freedom from Chronic Disease* (Los Angeles: J. P. Tarcher, Inc., 1979), and contributor of the lead articles for *The Holistic Health Handbook* (Berkeley, Calif.: And/Or Press, 1978), and *The New Healers* (Berkeley, Calif.: And/Or Press, 1980).

Regina Markell Morantz, Ph.D., is a teacher of women's history, and social history of medicine at the University of Kansas. For several years she has been working on a historical study of women physicians in America. She has served as the Academic Consultant and Principal Interviewer for the Oral History Project on Women in Medicine at the Medical College of Pennsylvania. Dr. Morantz is the author of "The Lady and her Physician," in L. Banner and M. Hartman, eds., *Clio's Consciousness Raised, New Perspectives on the History of Women,* New York: 1974; "The Connecting Link: The Case for the Woman Doctor in 19th Century America," in R. Numbers and J. Leavitt, eds., *Sickness and Health in America,* Madison, 1978; "Making Women Modern: Middle Class Women and Health Reform in 19th Century America," *Journal of Social History,* vol. 10 (June 1977); and "Professionalism, Feminism, and Gender Roles: A Comparative Study of Nineteenth Century Medical Therapeutics," in the *Journal of American History,* vol. 67 (December 1980).

Susanne Morgan, Ph.D., is a medical sociologist at the University of Southern California and

Professor of Women's Health at U.C.L.A. She is the author of *Coping with a Hysterectomy: Your Own Choice, Your Own Solutions* (New York: The Dial Press, 1982).

Freda Morris, Ph.D., psychologist, founded and directs the Hypnosis Clearing House, Inc., Oakland, Calif., an educational and training organization. She has been Assistant Professor of Medical Psychology at U.C.L.A. Medical School where she taught the uses of hypnosis in psychotherapy and medicine. She is author of *Self-Hypnosis in Two Days* (New York: E. P. Dutton & Co., Inc., 1975), and *Hypnosis with Friends and Lovers* (New York: Harper & Row, Publishers, Inc., 1979). She is co-authoring a textbook on hypnosis in business and industry.

Sandy Newhouse is a marriage, family, and child counselor and psychologist who has published on various cross-cultural topics in medicine and psychology.

Ann Patterson has done in-depth investigation into Western and Eastern massage and health practices. As a member of the Alternative Therapies Unit at San Francisco General Hospital, she instructs health professionals and patient groups in massage, acupressure, and relaxation through body awareness. Ann has written the *Acupressure Workbook* as a manual of instruction for her courses.

Linus Pauling, Ph.D., biochemist, has contributed greatly to the understanding of molecular structures, particularly with regard to chemical bonding. He is the only person who has received two unshared Nobel Prizes: one for Chemistry in 1954 and the Peace Prize in 1962. He was educated at the California Institute of Technology, Pasadena, and in Europe. He is the author of many articles and books. Some of those dealing with his theories on megadoses of Vitamin C and bonding are *Vitamin C, the Common Cold, and the Flu*, 1978. He co-authored *Orthomolecular Psychiatry: Treatment of Schizophrenia* with David Hawkins, 1972. His lifelong contributions are too numerous to list.

Jeanne Rose has studied medical herbology and botanical pharmacy for 25 years and has taught herbalism in California colleges. She is author of *Herbs & Things, The Herbal Body Book*, 1978 and *The Herbal Guide to Inner Health* (New York: Grosset & Dunlap, Inc., 1980), *Kitchen Cosmetics* (Panjandrum/Aris Books) and *The Herbal: A Guide to Living* (New York: Bantam Books, Inc., 1978). She has also authored chapters in many holistic health books. Ms. Rose has been mentioned in the *Contemporary Authors' Who's Who*, the *International Authors' Who's Who*, and most recently, the *World's Who's Who of Women*.

Linda Ruiz is a free-lance artist working in Palo Alto, CA. She is active in the women's peace movement. She contributed most of the illustrations in this book as well as the cover.

Angwyn St. Just, R.N., M.A., has been Rolfing since 1978. She studied nursing at Johns Hopkins Hospital in Baltimore and continued her graduate work in Art History and Renaissance Sculpture at the University of California at Berkeley. While engaged in her doctoral studies there, she learned of Ida Rolf's work and turned her attention to the possibility of "sculpting people." She writes and lectures in the San Francisco Bay area.

Barbara Seaman is the author of *Free and Female*, 1972, *Women and the Crisis in Sex Hormones*, and *The Doctors' Case against the Pill*, 1969, as well as a contributor to dozens of periodicals. She has been an editor and columnist at *Ladies Home Journal* and *Family Circle*. She is founder of the National Women's Health Network. She was cited by the Library of Congress for having raised sexism in health care as a worldwide issue and also cited by the Department of Health, Education and Welfare for introducing the concept of patient labeling on prescription drugs. Most recently, Ms. Seaman served on the National Task Force on DES and has been a consultant to the government's Contraceptive Research Branch. She has also testified at various Senate and congressional hearings.

David S. Sobel, M.D., is chief of preventive medicine at the Permanente Medical Group in San Jose, Calif., and a contributing editor of *Medical Self-Care* magazine, published in Inverness,

Calif. He has edited *Ways of Health: Holistic Approaches to Ancient and Contemporary Medicine*. (New York: Harcourt, Brace & Jovanovich, 1979).

Frances Tappan, Ph.D., is Professor Emeritus and Retired Associate Dean of the School of Allied Health Professions at the University of Connecticut. Dr. Tappan has a private practice in physical therapy and has authored the book *Healing Massage Techniques: A Study of Eastern and Western Methods*. (Reston, Va: Reston Publishing Company, 1978).

Joan Lamb Ullyot, M.D., is a well-known marathon runner, writer, and lecturer. During six years at the Institute of Health Research in San Francisco, she helped develop the unique "Health-Watch" program. In her athletic career, she has completed over 40 marathons, including the Boston Marathon, and has been on national and international championship teams. She is the author of two best-selling books: *Women's Running* (Mountain View, Calif.: World Publications, 1976) and *Running Free* (New York: G. P. Putnam's Sons, 1980), and is a regular columnist for *Running* and *Women's Sports* magazines.

Frances Vaughan, Ph.D. and clinical psychologist, is a Professor of Psychology at the California Institute of Transpersonal Psychology. She has taught classes on the psychology of meditation and does professional training in transpersonal psychotherapy. She is past President of the Association for Transpersonal Psychology and an editor for the *Journal of Transpersonal Psychology* and the *Journal of Humanistic Psychology*. She has published numerous articles on transpersonal therapy, is author of *Awakening Intuition* (New York: Doubleday/Anchor, 1979), and is co-editor with R. Walsh of *Beyond Ego: Transpersonal Dimensions in Psychology* (Los Angeles: J. P. Tarcher, 1980).

Andrew T. Weil, M.D., has served with the National Institute of Mental Health, Washington, D.C., and as a Fellow of the Institute of Current World Affairs in New York. He is presently Research Associate in Ethnopharmacology at the Harvard Botanical Museum, Adjunct Professor of Addiction Studies at the University of Arizona, and President of the Beneficial Plant Research Association in Carmel Valley, Calif. He is author of *The Natural Mind: A New Way of Looking at Drugs and the Higher Consciousness* (Boston: Houghton Mifflin Company, 1980) and the *Marriage of the Sun and Moon: A Quest for Unity in Consciousness* (Boston: Houghton Mifflin Company, 1980).

Kay Weiss, M.P.H. (Master of Public Health) has researched, lectured and published extensively on women's health. She has been affiliated with Stanford Research Institute, the University of California, Baylor College of Medicine; M.D. Anderson Research Hospital, and other institutions. She has promoted consumer health information through the media since 1971 when she was instrumental in organizing congressional hearings on the misuse of a prescription estrogen hormone drug (DES). Her work until recently has focused on analyzing the adverse effects of current medical treatments. In this book Ms. Weiss presents a sampling of newer forms of health care based on alternative, eastern and ancient perspectives which represent safer and more natural forms of self-treatment. She now resides in Albany, CA.

Louise Wensel, M.D., has studied and practiced acupuncture for 18 years, is a member of the National Acupuncture Research Society, and served on the AMA's Committee on Acupuncture in 1974. She has also served on the faculties of Johns Hopkins Medical School, the University of Florida, and the University of Arizona, where she acted as gynecologist as well as psychiatrist. Since 1973 she has been the director of the Washington Acupuncture Center, which has treated over 20,000 patients with acupuncture in Washington, D.C. and St. Petersburg, Florida. Her publications include: "Review of Acupuncture Therapy," *Johns Hopkins Magazine*, July 1973; *Introduction to Acupuncture* (Valkyrie Press, 1973 and 1977); *Acupuncture in Medical Practice* (Reston, Va.: Reston Publishing Co., 1980).

WOMEN'S HEALTH CARE
A GUIDE TO ALTERNATIVES

WOMEN'S HEALTH CARE
A GUIDE TO ALTERNATIVES

Part One

CURRENT CRISES AND CONTROVERSIES IN WOMEN'S HEALTH CARE

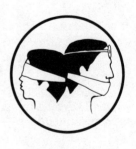

Kay Weiss

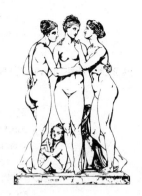

The United States is thought to have the best medical care system in the world, yet in every area of women's medical treatment there are controversies and crises caused by inappropriate and dangerous treatment. In the following eight chapters, some major areas of health care are discussed, and the problem inherent in current treatment practices are reviewed. These surveys of the quality of existing medical treatment of women provide an explanation of why many consumers of health care are turning away from orthodox medical care toward nontraditional alternatives.

INADEQUATE SCIENTIFIC TESTING, ESPECIALLY IN WOMEN'S HEALTH CARE

Roughly 90 percent of all medical care practices have not been subjected to reasonable scientific tests of efficacy and safety, according to the federal Office of Technology Assessment. Summaries of several studies show that only about 50 percent of professional health care now provided in the United States is effective; the other 50 percent is either ineffective or harmful. Technological advancement in medicine appears to be increasing the risks of medical care for routine procedures.

A committee of women doctors recommended in 1980 that the American Medical Association (AMA) address specific issues in health care for women: it urged the AMA to examine more aggressively the need for such controversial operations as hysterectomies and radical breast cancer surgery, to monitor more strongly the unnecessary prescription of tranquilizers and antidepressant drugs, and to improve medical attitudes toward the treatment of menopausal symptoms.

The committee also called on the AMA's scientific councils to pay increased attention to the diet, nutrition, and exercise needs of women, to work toward developing mutual respect between physician and female patient, and to encourage doctors to offer their patients, particularly women, more adequate explanations of diagnosis and treatment.

SCIENTIFIC MEDICINE'S VIEW OF WOMEN'S AILMENTS

The medical scientific view of female psychophysiology has undoubtedly contributed to many of the current problems in the medical treatment of women. Women have historically been regarded by medical science as neurotic. An examination of medical texts by sociologists reveals a typical pattern in the interaction of women patients and male physicians: (1) women's physical diseases are not taken seriously by physicians, (2) women are often referred to psychiatrists for symptoms of undiagnosed organic disease, and (3) women undergo far more unnecessary surgical removal of their sex organs and are prescribed far more sex hormones in the treatment of common ailments than men are. Dangerous side effects of drugs and techniques are minimized or not even mentioned to the female patient. And thousands of experimental drugs and techniques are applied to women, often without their informed consent (Adams and Cowan 1972).

This mistreatment of women has historically been rationalized, albeit subconsciously, by the theory of the inevitability of women's passivity and suffering. "The idea of suffering is an essential part of her life," states one gynecology text (Wilson *et al.* 1971). In the text, medical students are instructed in painful treatments for all of women's life stages: in sex, contraception, pregnancy, birth, and menopause. The text implies that painful menstrual cramps have no organic basis but are the result of "personality disorders," "guilt," or "neurotic predispositions." Medical students are taught that many ailments of pregnancy (such as nausea and headache) are the result of the fear of pregnancy, and that most women will need a labor-inducing drug to give birth. It is also suggested that menopausal symptoms are the result of psychological factors. Medical diagnosis even extends to a judgment of the patient's personality, as indicated by the following quotations from the same text:

> The very act of coming to the physician puts the patient in a parent-child relationship. . . . By the patient's dress, walk, makeup and attitude in answering questions, a judgment of her personality begins. . . . The physician notices whether the patient is reacting to the interview in a feminine way or whether she is domineering, demanding, masculine, aggressive. . . . The patient should be questioned about the sexual aspects of her life. . . . When the patient fails to respond and seems to be unduly emotional about the discussion, her transfer to a psychiatrist is indicated.

> The traits that compose the core of the female personality are feminine narcissism, masochism, and passivity.

The normal sexual act . . . entails a masochistic surrender to the man. . . . There is always an element of rape. The (normal) woman gives up her outwardly oriented active and aggressive strivings for the rewards involved in identification with her family . . . and sacrifices her own personality to build up that of her husband.

Scully and Bart (1973), in their analysis of obstetrics and gynecology textbooks of past decades, found that in some areas the texts revealed a greater concern with the patient's husband than with the patient herself, and they tended to foster sex-role stereotypes.

In the last decade, the women's movement has succeeded in changing many of the historical medical attitudes toward women that have resulted in inappropriate and poor treatment. The health consumer movement has also achieved many gains in improving the quality of health care. Yet the medical care offered women during their life stages is still characterized by a lack of effectiveness, safety, and consideration.

Chapters One through Eight call attention to these problems and present data regarding the inadequacy of even the most accepted, time-honored, scientifically based treatments in gynecological, obstetrical, and general care. Areas covered include contraception, pregnancy and childbirth, treatment of menstruation and menopause, unnecessary female surgery, and the inappropriate prescribing of drugs.

Part Four of this book then presents articles that make positive suggestions for improvements by describing alternatives to orthodox, traditional, technological medical care.

REFERENCES

Adams, A. and G. Cowan, "The Human Guinea Pig: How We Test New Drugs," *World*, December 15, 1972.

Scully, D., and P. Bart, an article in *American Journal of Sociology*, January 1973.

Willson, J.R., C. Buchanan and E. Carrington, *Obstetrics and Gynecology*, 4th ed., Chapters 4 and 8. St. Louis: The C. V. Mosby Company, 1971.

LISTING OF WOMEN'S HEALTH ORGANIZATIONS

The following list was compiled by Mara Klempner.

American Medical Women's Association
2302 East Speedway Boulevard
Tucson, AZ 85719
(602) 795-2677

Boston Women's Health Book
  Collective
465 Mt. Auburn
Watertown, MA 02172
(617) 924-1271

Center for Medical Consumers and
  Health Care Information, Inc.
237 Thompson Street
New York, NY 10012
(212) 674-7015

Coalition for the Medical Rights of
  Women
1638B Haight Street
San Francisco, CA 94117
(415) 621-8030

Coalition for the Reproduction Rights
  of Workers
1917 I Street, NW
Washington, DC 20006
(202) 822-0661

Concern for Health Options,
  Information, Care, and
  Education (CHOICE)
1501 Cherry Street
Philadelphia, PA 19102
(215) 567-2904 hotline

D.E.S. Action Project
Canton, MA 02021
(617) 828-7461

Feminist Action Alliance, Inc.
1300 Spring Street, NW
Atlanta, GA 30309
(408) 872-7544

Feminist Women's Health Center
6411 Hollywood Boulevard
Los Angeles, CA 90028

Gerontological Society of America
1835 K Street, NW
Washington, DC 20006
(202) 466-6750

Health Evaluation and Referral
  Service (HERS)
1954 W. Irving Park Road
Chicago, IL 60613
(312) 248-0166

Health Policy Advisory Center
  (Health PAC)
17 Murray Street
New York, NY 10007
(212) 267-8890

Health Writers, Inc.
306 N. Brooks Street
Madison, WI 53715
(608) 255-2255

Herpetics Engaged in Living
  Productively (H.E.L.P.)
260 Sheridan Avenue
Palo Alto, Ca 94306
(415) 321-5134

International Center for Research
  on Women
1010 16th Street, NW
Washington, DC 20036
(202) 293-3154

La Leche League International, Inc.
9616 Minneapolis Avenue
Franklin Park, IL 60131
(312) 455-7730

Margaret Sanger Center
380 2nd Avenue
New York, NY 10010
(212) 677-6474

Medical-Legal Consultation
c/o Kay Weiss
811 Evelyn Avenue
Albany, CA 94706

National Abortion Federation
110 E. 59th Street, Suite 1019
New York, NY 10022
(212) 688-8516

National Abortion Rights Action
  League
825 15th Street, NW
Washington, DC 20005
(202) 347-7774

National Association of Parents and
  Professionals for Safe
  Alternatives in Childbirth
(NAPSAC)
Route 1, Box 267
Marble Hills, MO 63764
(314) 238-2010

National Foundation for Women's Health
342 W. 22nd Street
New York, NY 10011
(212) 924-6863

National Organization for Women
3800 Harrison Street
Oakland, CA 94611
(415) 834-7897

National Self-Help Resource Center
1722 Connecticut Avenue, NW
Washington, DC 20006
(2)2) 387-1080

National Women's Health Network
2025 I Street, NW, Suite 105
Washington, DC 20006
(202) 233-6886

National Women's Health
    Organization
110 East 59th Street
New York, NY 10022
(212) 355-5420

Planned Parenthood Federation of
    America
810 7th Avenue
New York, NY 10019
(212) 541-7800

Reproductive Freedom Project
American Civil Liberties Union
132 W. 41st Street
New York, NY 10036
(212) 944-9800

Standing Committee on Women's
    Rights
American Public Health Association
Washington, DC 20036
(202) 789-5600

Women and Health Round Table
Federation of Organizations for
    Professional Women
2000 P Street, NW
Washington, DC 20036
(202) 466-3544

Women's Action Alliance, Inc.
370 Lexington Avenue
New York, NY 10017
(212) 532-8330

Women's Health Concerns
    Committee
1324 Locust Street
Philadelphia, PA 19107
(215) 546-3048

Women's Occupational Health
    Resource Center
School of Public Health,
    Columbia University
60 Haven Avenue
New York, NY 10017
(212) 781-5719

Chapter One

CONTRACEPTION 1984

Barbara Seaman

In 1960 much of the world was enjoying what the *New Scientist* has called "a high state of anticipation for the easy technological fix" (1981, p. 261). The Pill and the IUD were welcomed as great advances for women. Indeed, Clare Boothe Luce probably voiced a majority view when she told a reporter from the *Los Angeles Times* that, with the Pill:

> Modern woman is at last free, as a man is free, to dispose of her own body, to earn her living, to pursue the improvement of her mind, to try a successful career [Seaman 1969, p. 65].

For their first decade of widespread use, the Pill and IUD enjoyed a "diplomatic immunity"* originating in concern for world population. They were never intended for educated women in developed countries, who in fact became the principal adopters. In a 1951 letter to raise funds for Pill research, Margaret Sanger, champion of the diaphragm, opined:

> I consider that the world and almost our civilization for the next 25 years is going to depend upon a simple, cheap, safe contraceptive to be used in poverty-stricken slums and jungles, and among the most ignorant people. . . . I believe that now, immediately, there should be national sterilization for certain dysgenic types of our population who are being encouraged to breed and would die out were the government not feeding them [Vaughan 1970, p. 25].

Thirty years later, Dr. Min-Chuch Chang, a recipient of research monies channeled through Ms. Sanger, was to affirm:

*Term coined by Dr. David Clark, University of Kentucky, at the 1966 annual meeting of the American Academy of Neurology.

> The oral contraceptive was made merely for the population explosion. . . . We worked on the oral contraceptive for population control rather than to allow young people to have a good time [Associated Press 1981]

Consumer disenchantment with the IUD and Pill started in the 1970s. For example, 15.3 percent of Planned Parenthood clients requested the IUD at their initial 1970's visit; but by 1980, the figure was down to 4.5 percent (Planned Parenthood Federation 1981, p. 12; Campbell 1982). U.S. pharmacy purchases of oral contraceptives also dropped, from more than 10 million in 1974–1975 to a low of slightly over 6 million in 1981 (Information Program 1982). The decline in Pill prescriptions seemed directly related to patient package inserts—warnings that the Food and Drug Administration (FDA) ordered pharmacists to start dispensing with Pill prescriptions in 1975. The FDA has also ordered providers (doctors and clinics) to give IUD users a printed warning.

STERILIZATION—NOT AS SAFE AND SIMPLE AS IT SOUNDS

Sterilization figures are not available beyond 1976, but at that time, the popularity of both the female and male procedures was increasing sharply. In 1965, among U.S. married couples over 30 who used any method of fertility control, 17 percent had been sterilized (10 percent female and 7 percent male). By 1976, 41 percent of these couples were sterilized (21 percent female and 20 percent male) (Campbell 1982).

Although many women are delighted with the outcome of their sterilization procedures, others avow that these have been overpromoted as safe and simple. In addition to injuries that occur at the time of the surgery, including occasional deaths, up to 25 percent of sterilized women complain of severely increased menstrual disorders and other gynecological problems. The hysterectomy rate is also significantly higher in women who have been previously sterilized.

A backlash against female sterilization has occurred in feminist, civil rights, and health consumer organizations, and it is possible that there may have been some leveling off or decrease in female sterilization since 1976.

There may also have been a recent decrease in vasectomy, a safer and less expensive procedure as the male vas is located outside the main body (Seaman 1972). No deaths have been reported in the United States for at least a decade. Nonetheless, for some men the recovery period is uncomfortable, and others suffer psychological effects. There is also concern that vasectomy may entail some as yet undetected long-range effects on the autoimmune system, but the evidence thus far is reassuring (Petitti, in press).

As word has passed among women that no form of sterilization is quite as safe, simple, or reversible as it is often made to sound, surgeons have given substantial attention to developing "improved" techniques. So-called "band-aid" or "belly-button" sterilization was much touted during the 1970s, but it proved to have as many or more complications than the old-fashioned "tying off" of tubes. Enough women died or had severe intestinal injuries from the coagulation or electrical current instruments used in the new procedures that the CDC (Center for Disease Control) recently issued a bulletin pleading for information that would help clarify the risks (May/June 1982).

"Mini" or "laparoscopic" sterilization techniques have had another side effect that was quite rare with the older surgical procedures: pregnancy! *Subsequent pregnancies occur in 1 to 3 percent of all patients.* Very often, these pregnancies are life-threatening because the Fallopian tubes have somehow rejoined well enough to permit sperm to fertilize an egg but not well enough for the fertilized egg to pass on through to the uterus. Thus an "ectopic" pregnancy develops in the tubes producing a medical emergency.

Understandably, there is a new upsurge in research to develop nonsurgical sterilization techniques. For example, an experimental plug made of silicone rubber has been developed to plug the Fallopian tubes; and Methylycanoacrylate, a chemical that causes scarring, has also been used for tubal blockage. The procedures are performed vaginally without any cutting of the abdomen. However, in theory, some of the methods may prove to have a high reversibility rate—an important issue to many women in this age of delayed childbearing and multiple marriage. Even the silicone plug, which is considered the most promising of the new methods, is unlikely to prove carefree. Among the first 375 patients given the plug at Lankenau Hospital in Philadelphia, 6 pregnancies occurred. Of the first 1000 patients, 2 developed chronic pain, and 1 developed pain and fever (Broznan 1982).

As with other methods such as the Pill or IUD, consumers have pointed out that "when the side effect happens to you, it's 100 percent." One woman, at first pleased with her band-aid sterilization, experienced an increase in length and pain with each successive menstrual period. In addition to having to accept a less strenuous job, she soon became pregnant and had to have an emergency hysterectomy, after which she suffered from severe hot flashes. This is an exception, but not so much of an exception that women should remain unaware of the potential.

BACK TO THE BARRIERS?

In recent years the return to barrier methods has been steady and quite marked. Diaphragms, condoms, spermicidal foam, and foaming suppositories account for most of the increase, but some clinics and individual practitioners are also dispensing cervical caps and vaginal sponges. Indeed, among the health-conscious, "back to the barriers" seems to be the order of the day. Many women are asking, "If a method is so dangerous that it requires a doctor's supervision, why should I use it just for birth control?" (Seaman 1978).

In the July 1981 issue of *Fertility and Sterility*, Drs. Howard J. Tatum and Elizabeth Connell-Tatum published an article entitled "Barrier Contraception: A Comprehensive Overview." This was of particular interest since Dr. Tatum, formerly of the Population Council, was developer of the "Copper-T," an intrauterine device, while Dr. Connell-Tatum was a 1960s popularizer of the Pill. Their new article concluded with the following surprising statement:

> Barriers are regaining their rightful position in our contraceptive armamentarium as more and more questions are being raised about the real or potential adverse side effects of systemic and intrauterine contraceptives. . . . There is evidence throughout the world of the growing popularity and use of locally acting, mechanical and/or spermicidal contraceptive methods. . . .

Barrier methods were originally described 4000 years ago in our earliest known medical text, the *Petri Papyrus* from Egypt. But it was not until the nineteenth century that mechanical barriers such as the condom and diaphragm were first mass-produced. If they are properly fitted and used, these devices can be highly reliable—almost on a par with the Pill and certainly equal to the IUD. Barriers can interfere with the spontaneity of the sex act, and many persons find them unaesthetic. However, some couples or individuals who dislike, say, the diaphragm, find that they adapt well to the cervical cap, sponge, or certain types of condom. With determination, consumers can find a method (and a schedule for using it) that is not too obtrusive.

The Diaphragm

At Planned Parenthood clinics in the United States, diaphragm use among those adopting a specific method at their first visit climbed from 4.3 percent in 1973 to 12.9 percent in 1980. The private practice figure is probably higher because it is time-consuming to fit a beginner with a diaphragm and to train her in its correct use, so the public clinics who have neither the personnel nor funds to encourage diaphragm acceptance would have fewer clients adopting this device. In addition, family planning clinics normally make a profit on the Pills which they sell to clients, but do not make a profit on barriers. "Other" methods, presumably spermicides and condoms, have also jumped among first-time clients, from 6.1 percent in 1974 to 26.1 percent in 1980 (Planned Parenthood Federation 1981).

The diaphragm comes in 12 sizes, with a diameter range of 50 to 105 mm.; and all have spring-reinforced rims. There are several designs that behave quite differently; the conscientious diaphragm provider should allow clients, or patients, to try them all and to make a choice. The diaphragm should not be inserted more than 3 or 4 hours before intercourse as the spermicide that is used with it is deemed essential to the contraceptive effect. Evidently, in many women, the diaphragm gets displaced during sexual arousal, making the spermicide a necessity.

However, there has long been a small group of practitioners who claim that the "dry" diaphragm can be highly effective. In New York City, Dr. Edward Stim has reported that a small diaphragm (thin-rimmed arching size 60) is effective "dry," or without spermicide (1980). In London, Dr. Connie Smith at the Marie Stopes Clinic is attempting to replicate Stim's finding. Stim and Smith both maintain that we still have remarkably little understanding of the subtleties of diaphragm use. Ordinarily, a woman is given the largest size of diaphragm that fits her comfortably, so that it will wedge across her vagina tightly. In contrast, the theory behind the smaller "dry" diaphragm is simply that it sits like a saucer over the cervix and is *not* ridged between the vaginal walls. Hence, it is less subject to displacement when walls balloon. The dry diaphragm is removed, rinsed, and replaced every 24 hours in Connie Smith's regimen. (It is, however, always left in place for 8 hours after intercourse.) Whether the pregnancy rate is acceptable remains to be seen; but should it turn out to be, the "dry" diaphragm will undoubtedly become popular.

Diaphragm Prescriptions.   One factor hindering more widespread use of the diaphragm is the fact that in most states it is classified a "prescription only" item. Physicians in effect act as "middlemen" in the distribution of diaphragms; thereby raising the cost to the consumer. If diaphragms could be readily bought over-the-counter, the woman who knew her size and diaphragm model could walk into the drugstore and buy one without the necessity of first obtaining a prescription. She would also have the option of having it fitted by a nurse or paramedic, health care providers who charge less but are frequently more skilled than physicians in fitting the device.

Cervical Cap and Contraceptive Sponges

The cervical cap, an ancient device that was first mass-produced in the 1830s, outsold the diaphragm in many European countries but never developed a following in the United States. In recent years, women's health clinics and some individual practitioners have begun importing it from the Lamberts Company in England. The cap is a thimble-shaped rubber device that stays on the cervix by suction. It can be retained longer than the diaphragm and requires less spermicide. (Some long-term cap users who find that their caps have never been displaced often omit the spermicide altogether. Others substitute natural products such as aloe jelly or olive oil.)

In Europe, many women left their cap in place from menses to menses. However, most current providers advocate a regimen of no more than 24 to 72 hours. In the United States, the National Institute of Health is financing studies to determine the precise efficacy and safety of the cap, and to see whether the design might be improved. The range of present sizes is limited, and at least one-quarter of women who apply for the cap are informed by careful providers that they are not a close enough "fit." In addition, some women have difficulty with insertion, and especially removal.

With all of the drawbacks to the still-imperfect cap, at least two-thirds of the women who start on it say they are very pleased with it at one- and two-year follow-ups (Roshan, Lauersen, and Koch). This is probably a higher continuation rate than for the Pill and the IUD.

Experiments are also underway to develop a semi-permanent cap with a one-way valve so that fluids can be expelled. The one-way cap is perceived as being a bit like a denture and not surprisingly, its codeveloper *is* a dentist.

In author George Orwell's vision, *1984* was the target year during which all of our post-World War II technological dreams and nightmares would be realized. The irony is that today's big contraceptive "news" is the revival of the sponge—a barrier device at least as old as the Jewish Talmud.

Writings from the past show that the original sponge—the sea sponge found in nature—was used by many peoples and cultures throughout history. The ancients, 18th century French society women as well as prostitutes, and 19th century British feminists, all availed themselves of this contraceptive method. In the United States, as recently as the 1930s, slices of sea sponges with strings attached for easy removal were sold in drug stores, along with instructions cautioning the user to dip them in vinegar before insertion.

The new sponge, which went on sale on July 1, 1983 in California and in 11 other western states, is made of polyurethane. It is marketed under the name TODAY and is permeated with a spermicide, Nonoxynal-9. A non-prescription item, TODAY costs about a dollar, can be left in place for 24 hours, and is removed by pulling a loop. One size fits all.

Several consumer groups have filed objections to TODAY, and by mid-July 1983 a Congressional hearing was called. The debate centers over several issues, medical and political. These are:

1. Do plastic polymers cause cancer?
2. Does Nonoxynol-9 cause cancer or birth defects, specifically in the high, untested dosages TODAY delivers?
3. Is TODAY as reliable as the manufacturer claims? The World Health Organization (WHO) has set a standard for new contraceptives of less than 6 pregnancies per woman per year. Initial trials on *Today* failed to measure up to the standard, but the manufacturer argues that this was due to improper use, and has improved the instructions.

4. Might the sponge cause Toxic Shock Syndrome if women unwittingly leave it in during menstruation?

5. Is the product overpromoted and overpriced? Recognizing that the sponge is an age-old device, can the development and clinical tests which cost the U.S. taxpayer at least $1.7 million to develop a modern version be justified?

6. Considering the unanswered questions concerning safety and efficacy, the heavy promotion and the unexpectedly high price, consumer groups—and Congress—are raising the question of conflict of interest in FDA's approval. At least two physicians who have, or have formerly had, influential positions at FDA now serve as advisors to VLI, which manufactures TODAY. One of these physicians is Dr. Elizabeth Connell-Tatum whose new declaration of interest in barrier methods is cited above.

With testing of the "dry" diaphragm, and efforts to revive and improve the various cervical caps and sponges, it may well be that by the end of the 1980s, a far wider range of acceptable barrier methods will be available to women. Imperfect as the cap still is, for example, many users greatly prefer it to the diaphragm. Some say it is more comfortable, and others deem it more convenient, or less "messy." Others express appreciation that it can be put into place hours or days before sexual intercourse (Seaman and Seaman 1978).*

Spermicides

Ironically, just as the reliability and acceptability of chemical spermicides have been acknowledged, these methods have been linked to a possible increase in the risk of birth defects. Spermicides are sometimes classified as a barrier and sometimes as a chemical method. In Western science, Leeuwenhoek was the first to observe, in 1677, that rainwater immobilized dog spermatozoa (1941, p. 128). After Leeuwenhoek, other researchers noted that sperm are susceptible to organic and inorganic salts and to heavy metals such as copper and mercury (Quatrefages 1953).

But, by whatever method, and hard as it is for the Western mind to accept, effective formulas for vaginal spermicides appear in early writings as far back as the nineteenth century B.C. As early as the fourth century B.C., Aristotle suggested oil of cedar and frankincense and olive oil to block the cervix, while earlier yet, Cleopatra and other prosperous Egyptians used a vaginal paste mixed from honey, sodium carbonate, and dried crocodile dung (Himes 1970; Baker 1935; Seaman and Seaman 1978). Possibly through

*See references on Fischer, Scheinin, Ridgewald, Lione and Cancer Controversy for background for this section.

trial and error the ancients discovered that environments that were strongly acidic or strongly alkaline were hostile to sperm. Eighth-century Indian writers describe the use of rock salt, dipped in oil or honey. By the twelfth century, the Moslems had suppositories or tampons based on these ingredients.

Chemicals that are strong enough to kill off sperm may potentially have other side effects, either local or systemic. As Susan Jordan of the National Women's Health Network puts it, "The more the action, the more the reaction." In the 1950s, consumer concern regarding the toxicity of available spermicides led to the withdrawal of several popular brands.

The last of the popular products that still contained mercury even in the 1970s was Koromex, made by Holland-Rantos. By the mid-1970s, it had been clearly demonstrated that chemicals inserted in the vagina can be absorbed systemically. Specifically, it was also demonstrated—in Japan— that vaginally-absorbed mercury can cause birth defects to a developing mouse fetus (Bernstein 1974). Under pressure from consumer groups and the FDA, Holland-Rantos finally removed the mercury from Koromex but did not recall existing supplies (FDA 1974; 1975). Thus, for several years after the change of formula, many women continued to receive the mercury-based spermicide! When Holland-Rantos did switch, most of its products were not based on Nonoxynol-9, which is the basis of most spermicides that are on the market today. Instead, the company used a slightly different chemical called Oxytoxynol. This is important because the currently marketed brand of spermicide that has been tentatively associated with birth defects is, indeed, Koromex (Jick et al. 1981).

The testing was started in the mid-1970s, at a point where some of the subjects may have been receiving the older Koromex with mercury. Others received a product that contained Oxytoxynol, which may or may not be significantly different from the more widely used Nonoxynol-9. Research into the safety of current spermicides has had so little attention that it is difficult to draw any conclusions. For the time being, women who conceive while using a spermicide, especially a Koromex product, might wish to take the possibility of birth defects into account.

Whether spermicides might pose some subtle and still-unrecognized hazards to the germ cells, ovaries, or other organs has not been thoroughly investigated. No known deaths or hospitalizations have been associated with currently available products, and they seem to provide some protection against many sexually transmitted diseases including herpes (Singh, Cutler, and Utidjian 1977; Singh et al. 1972). They have lately come to be viewed as much more reliable than was previously thought. Nonetheless, long-range safety will not be firmly established until a good deal of further research is executed.

Some spermicidal products are not considered sufficiently reliable for "solo" use. These include creams and jellies, which are generally prescribed or suggested in conjunction with the diaphragm, condom, or cervical cap. Foams such as Emko and the newer foaming suppositories such as the

Encare Oval and Semicid are more effective by themselves since they disperse better. All spermicides are available over-the-counter without a prescription or the need for a "fitting."

Response to the aesthetics of spermicides is highly personal. Women who do not lubricate heavily often say that they like the foams, although sometimes their partners may develop a mild allergic reaction to a particular brand. A frequent complaint about the suppositories is that they cause burning or dripping.

Even within the same category of spermicide, and even when the same chemicals are used, there are some differences in "behavior," or consumer acceptability. For example, among satisfied users of the cervical cap, the most frequent "nuisance" complaint is that when left in for two days or longer, it may create an unpleasant odor upon removal. This odor can be removed by soaking in a baking soda or vinegar solution. The odor rarely occurs when spermicides are omitted. Nonetheless, Dr. James Koch and other cap providers have reported that, for unknown reasons, Ramses contraceptive jelly (based on Nonoxynol-9 like most of the others) is less odor-producing.

The Condom

Worldwide, the condom is the most widely used contraceptive today. Its popularity is increasing in the United States as males become more interested in sharing responsibility for birth control, and as both males and females grow increasingly wary of sexually transmitted diseases. Nonetheless, many consumers underrate the condom's reliability, which is better than 97 percent. Used in conjunction with a contraceptive cream or jelly, a 99 percent success rate can be obtained (Hatcher et al. 1979). Newer condoms are still more reliable: *Ramses-Extra*, for example, impregnated with Nonoxynol-9, is on a par with the Pill, according to a recent English study ("Birth Control News" 1983).

The quality of American condoms is consistently high, perhaps too high according to Dr. Philip Harvey, Director of Population Services at the University of North Carolina, Chapel Hill. If thinner condoms were permitted by the FDA, as are permitted in countries such as Japan, there might be a very slight loss in reliability (1 added pregnancy per 2.5 to 5 million acts of love), but this would be more than made up for by their greater sensitivity and the willingness of users (Harvey 1972). Condoms made from natural animal tissue (imported mostly from New Zealand and Australia) are said to transmit heat and provide a higher degree of sensitivity than latex products. Brand names of skin condoms include Schmid's Fourex and Crest's Skins.

Condoms are available dry or lubricated; the latter are generally preferred, for lubrication facilitates entry, decreases chances of breaking, and increases sensitivity. It is generally assumed by health professionals as well as by manufacturers that everyone knows how to use the condom. This is not necessarily so and the lack of instructions accompanying the packet sometimes results in the condom being used incorrectly. The most frequent instances of incorrect use are the following:

> failure to press out the air at the tip of the condom prior to application: approximately one-half inch at the end should be left to accommodate the ejaculate.
>
> failure to remove the penis from the vagina while it is still erect, so as to avoid spillage.
>
> failure to hold on to the rim of the condom while withdrawing the penis, to insure that the condom will not come off in the vagina.

According to some authorities, the wide availability of over-the-counter or machine-dispensed condoms along with their high degree of reliability, combined with good instructions and an aggressive advertising campaign, could do more to turn back the rising tide of teenage pregnancies than any other measure (ibid.; Seaman and Seaman 1978).

Many women cannot or will not trust their partners to take the initiative in contraception, but for those who do, it is clearly the male methods which are "best" for women's health. The new condoms which use spermicide as a lubricant are, apparently, as reliable as any contraceptive ever devised. Condoms also reduce the spread of sexually transmitted diseases, as do spermicides themselves. There may be some long-range still undetected health risks to women or unborn children from spermicide use, but in the case of condoms which incorporate spermicides, female exposure to the chemicals is minimal. The woman gets the benefit without the possible risk. Some men state that condoms are a nuisance, or reduce their sexual sensitivitiy. In blindfold tests, a majority of women cannot even tell whether their partners are wearing a condom.

In terms of more invasive methods, the "safest" choice for women is—male vasectomy.

METHODS OF NATURAL BIRTH CONTROL*

The Calendar Method

If all women had regular menstrual cycles, the calendar method would be glorious, for it would be simple enough to calculate the safe days before ovulation, the fertile days surrounding it, and the safe days after. Alas, cycles

*See references by Potter et al., Zuck, Ferin, and Ross and Piotrow for background for this section.

vary by an average of 7 to 13 days (over a year's time) during a woman's twenties and thirties, and by even greater amounts in her teens and later on as she approaches menopause. Thus the totally predictable 28-day cycle is rare.

Calendar rhythm, the grandmother of all "natural" contraceptives, was first advocated in the 1930s. To use this method, a woman records her menstrual history for 6 to 12 months to determine the intervals between her periods. Ovulation is assumed to occur 14 to 15 days before the onset of menstrual flow, and the woman who finds that her cycles are exceptionally regular needs to abstain from intercourse for only 6 days—3 before predicted ovulation and 3 days afterward. However, over the course of a year, no more than 5 to 15 percent of women remain entirely regular. To be at all safe, the majority must assume a 9-day fertile period—the 10th through 18th days of the cycles—during which they need to abstain. This calculation assumes 3 fertile days before ovulation, 1 to 2 afterward, and 4 more to allow for cycle variability. The point, of course, is to refrain from unprotected intercourse at least 72 hours in advance of ovulation, whenever that may occur. For women who have highly irregular cycles, the calendar rhythm method is no use at all.

The Temperature Method, or BBT (Basal Body Temperature)

In the 1930s the noting of temperature rise was recommended for women who had trouble conceiving, and in 1947 a Belgian doctor suggested that women practicing rhythm should record their daily temperatures. The temperature method is now proven to be more reliable (although much more troublesome) than the calendar method alone. A rise of about 0.5 to 1.0°F usually accompanies ovulation. By avoiding intercourse until 3 days after the temperature rise, and permitting it only in the remaining days before menstruation, a woman can prevent pregnancy with high reliability. A German study showed that strongly motivated women using BBT avoid pregnancy as successfully as women using the Pill.

It is the shift in temperature, not the number of degrees, that indicates ovulation. Thus, the readings must be taken daily in the morning, while still in bed, after at least 5 hours of uninterrupted sleep, and prior to eating, drinking, smoking, or conversation. Any activity can increase the BBT. Readings may be taken either orally or rectally, as long as the same method is always used. The rectal method is faster.

Temperatures do not rise during cycles where ovulation fails to occur. Thus when no increase is recorded, a woman cannot be sure whether she is having delayed ovulation or a cycle with none at all. The temperature method's greatest drawback is that it does not predict ovulation in advance, and hence requires a long period of abstinence. However, some experienced women can combine the calendar and ovulation methods. They record their menstrual cycles to estimate the preovulatory safe days, while using a thermometer to establish precisely when ovulation occurs. (Sometimes, a fever due to infection may lead a woman to think she's ovulated when she hasn't.)

As women proceed through their menstrual cycles, striking chemical changes occur. These can be charted with exquisite precision in lab tests of urine, blood plasma, cervical mucus, or vaginal and endometrial cells. Such tests have been developed for subfertile couples to help them conceive. Most are too complicated for a woman to try at home.

The Cervical Mucus (Billings) Method

Not surprisingly, the element in a woman's body that changes most noticeably during her monthly cycle is her cervical mucus—it is altered in quantity, structure, and water content as well as in chemical composition (Billings 1970 and 1973; Billings and Billings 1973).

This article does not allow sufficient space to properly describe the Billings Method and the variants on it. However, several good books are available for disciplined couples who wish to try it (see, for example, *No Pill, No Risk Birth Control* by Nona Aguilar [Rawson, Wade, 1980]), and counseling by organizations such as the "Couple to Couple League" is available as well.

Other Natural Birth Control Methods

In *Lunaception* by Louise Lacey, the author describes how she borrowed the findings of physicist Edmund Dewan, controlling the days she ovulates through the manipulation of light (1974). In Europe, Eugene Jonas and Kurt Rechnitz have developed a method called "cosmic birth control," which is based on the cycles of the sun and moon as well as on a woman's own ovulation timing (Rosenblum and Jackson 1974; Ostrander and Schroeder 1971).

In the self-help movement, some women practice natural birth control just through daily observation of their cervix. Techniques for self-examination of the cervix have been devised and promoted by two pairs of American health workers: Carol Downer and Lorraine Rothman who operate the Feminist Women's Health Center in Los Angeles, and the Connecticut mother-and-daughter team of Lolly and Jean Hirsch. When a woman is not on the Pill, her cervix goes through a monthly cycle of its own: tight and firm at the outset, to loose and droopy, to soft and moist, and then back again. There are color changes of the cervix as well: usually light pink at ovulation, dark pink as menstruation approaches, and purplish at pregnancy (*New Women's Survival Source Book* 1975).

Still other researchers such as Gerald Oster and Selmaree Oster at

New York's Mt. Sinai Hospital have been trying to develop simple saliva and urine tests that women could use (with a dipstick) to predict ovulation. In addition, the Osters have noted, women can be taught to observe their preovulation signs, including breast tenderness or discomfort in the abdomen, midsection, or back. Each woman has different "peculiarities," according to the Osters (1976; Oster et al. 1972).

In summary, although improved barrier methods are now being funded because manufacturers have reason to hope that they will earn back a profit, there is very little funding for techniques that would perfect natural birth control because the profit, if any, would be minimal.

ADVERSE EFFECTS OF ARTIFICIAL BIRTH CONTROL METHODS

The Pill and IUD

Defenders of the Pill and the IUD often observe, "Well, they're safer than pregnancy." However, it would only be legitimate to compare the Pill and IUD with pregnancy if women had no alternative but to use these risky methods or get pregnant. Even if this were the case, or even if a wealth of safer alternatives did not exist, the statement would no longer be substantially correct. In the May 28, 1982 issue of *JAMA*, researchers at the Center for Disease Control evaluated pregnancy versus contraceptive mortality risks in U.S. women from 1955–1975. The reproductive mortality rate had dropped dramatically: from 7.8 per 100,000 women, ages 15–44 in 1955, down to 2.1 in 1975. However, in 1955, 99 percent of reproductive deaths were pregnancy-related, whereas only 1 percent were linked to contraceptive use. In contrast, by 1975, only 53 percent of the deaths were pregnancy-related (due to miscarriages, abortions, ectopic pregnancies, and pregnancy-related complications), whereas 47 percent of the deaths were related to contraceptive use, chiefly use of the Pill.

Short of dying, significant numbers of women are left chronically impaired by the Pill, IUD, or sterilization.

Understandably, there is one side effect from the Pill and IUD that scientists and statisticians who are interested in population control are not likely to include in their calculations, that is, infertility. Here again, to the consumer this can be a devastating outcome, even though it may not directly threaten her physical health. Many users are temporarily sterile when they stop the Pill. It often takes months or years before normal ovulation and menstruation return. (In the women's self-help movement, it is widely believed, and taught, that nutritional programs that focus on replacing vitamins and minerals depleted by the Pill may help speed normal reproductive function.) Without any special intervention, pharmaceutical or nutritional, most women rendered infertile by the Pill do recover by the end of three or four years. However, there are certain "subgroups" who apparently do not, and these include very young women whose normal cycling is not yet established, as well as others whose cycles have been highly unpredictable (Seaman and Seaman 1978).

The IUD also affects subsequent fertility. Women who have used the IUD successfully and remove it in order to get pregnant do experience some delay, according to a major British report. Within two years after discontinuation, however, 92 percent give birth (Vessey et al. 1977). Incredibly, there has only been one large study of subsequent fertility in women who had their IUDs removed for *medical* as well as personal reasons. This study, performed in Taiwan, included past IUD wearers who had had trouble with their "loop," as well as women who had used it successfully and only took it out when they wanted to conceive. In Taiwan, the findings were even more ominous than for the Vessey study mentioned above. For women over age 30 it appears that the likelihood of conception, when desired, declines with duration of IUD use (Jain and Moots 1977).

There are several factors in post-IUD infertility. Users have an increased risk of ectopic pregnancy, which, in turn, often requires surgery that may render a woman sterile. Certain IUDs, such as the Majzlin Spring, an expulsion-resistant stainless steel device, have been removed from the market because, in after-the-fact testing, they tore up so many uteri. Apparently the main culprit in post-IUD sterility—and this can happen with any model, "old and reliable" or "new and better"—is PID, or Pelvic Inflammatory Disease.

IUD users have a four to ninefold risk of developing PID (an infection that invades the uterus, the tubes, and sometimes the ovaries) as compared to women who choose other methods. Many women with PID are lucky, especially if the condition is detected early. Vigorous treatment may prevent permanent harm. However, many PID victims wind up with severly scarred Fallopian tubes. Others require surgery which renders them infertile.

To add to the complexity of assessing risks, computations are normally based on current users. Little is known about effects that may be manifest as the ex-user proceeds through her life cycle. But, as a recent headline in *Newsweek* put it, "The Pill's Dangers Don't Go Away" (Seligman 1981, p. 54). In July 1981, the *New England Journal of Medicine* reported that women over 40 who had previously used the Pill for five to nine years run a 60 percent higher risk of heart attack than do controls; those who took the Pill for ten years or longer had a heart attack rate 2.5 times higher. The comforting note was that women who had used the Pill for five years or less did not demonstrate these increased risks. The Pill alters metabolism of fats and sugars, as well as blood pressure in many users. The longer the use, the greater the alteration; and in some consumers, values do not return to normal after discontinuation. This may explain why the risk of heart attack, and possibly stroke, continues.

By the fall of 1980 there were two developments that produced an effort to brush up the Pill's tarnished image. First, as noted, U.S. sales had dropped substantially since the appearance of a patient-package insert in 1975. This was understandably disturbing to manufacturers. Second, abortion rights appeared to be gravely threatened, while out-of-wedlock pregnancies continued to increase. The threat to abortion rights prompted some well-intentioned public health officials to start emphasizing the benefits of the Pill. Headlines stating "Birth Control Pills Are Called Safe" (UPI story 1980), or "Health Benefits of the Pill Found to Outweigh Its Drawbacks" (*New York Times* 1982) began to appear with some regularity. In its issue for September 21, 1982, the *National Examiner* ran a bold feature: "The Pill Can Prevent Cancer" (p. 5).

Walnut Creek Study Discredited

The first round of publicity had been sponsored by the G.D. Searle Co., a Pill manufacturer, and executed by Hill and Knowlton, a large public relations firm. Dr. Savatri Ramcharan, co-author of the Walnut Creek Report, a government-funded study of Pill safety had, toward the end, also accepted financing from 5 pill manufacturers (Searle, Mead Johnson, Ortho, Parke Davis, and Syntex), reinterpreted her earlier findings to make them seem more upbeat, and allowed Searle to send her on a nationwide publicity campaign. The Walnut Creek "findings" are considered inoperative for now. The data is being reanalyzed by Drs. Diana Pettiti and Shana Swan, two scientists who had previously withdrawn from the project.

Essentially, however, what Ramcharan tended to do was "blame the victim" instead of the Pill. For example, she did find more cervical and skin cancer in Pill users but she blamed these on their lifestyles, i.e., sexual "promiscuity" and "more sunbathing," respectively. Higher suicide rates in Pill users were attributed to their "emotional problems," and even the heart attacks and blood clots were attributed solely to smoking or sometimes to "physician bias." (The diagnosis of blood clots, Ramcharan suggested, is more likely to occur to a physician when he learns that the patient is on the Pill. [Oakie 1981; O'Malley 1981].) Reporters further discovered that, although this was omitted from her official bio, Ramcharan had also enjoyed an early association with G.D. Searle, when she worked at the Worcester Foundation with Drs. Pincus and Chang from 1957 to 1959, developing Enovid.

Biased Reports on Benefits of the Pill

Although the conclusions of the Walnut Creek study have been discredited, they are nonetheless frequently cited by defenders of the Pill. The health benefits of the Pill currently being suggested include *reduction in the incidence of benign breast disease*. (Center for Disease Control 1982; Ory 1981).

This has been confirmed in 11 studies and seems particularly true of brands that have a high ratio of progestin to estrogen. Certainly benign breast disease can be an uncomfortable condition; however, it is hardly as ominous as breast cancer.

Danger of Breast Cancer

The relationship between the Pill and breast cancer remains murky and will probably not be clarified for at least another decade. The breast is one of the sites where estrogens per se are often highly carcinogenic. Even workers, including males, who handle but do not ingest estrogen appear to be at increased risk of breast cancer. For example, in February 1982, Rutgers University in New Jersey closed Smith Hall, its largest classroom building, because the discovery of the hormone estrogen in several areas was deemed to be potentially responsible for the high rate of cancer among people working there. The link was first noted by the National Institute of Occupational Safety and Health, in conjunction with experiments at the Institute of Animal Behavior on Smith Hall's fourth floor (UPI story 1982; Michaels 1982).

Two popular estrogen products (Premarin for menopausal complaints and DES for problem pregnancies) started to come into widespread use in the United States in the 1940s, but it was not until the 1970s, three decades later, that their precise connection with cancers in various female organs was established. Thus it is unrealistic to expect that the cancer risks of the Pill, which did not come into widespread use until the 1960s, will be fully clarified before the 1990s.

So far, most broad studies have neither confirmed nor denied a connection between the Pill and breast cancer. However, at least two researchers (Paffenbarger and Black; see below) who have looked closely at certain "subgroups" reported that in these women, the Pill appears to increase the incidence of breast cancer. Late in 1979, Dr. Ralph Paffenbarger of Stanford University reported in the journal *Cancer* that women who have a history of benign breast disease and who take the Pill before the birth of their first child may substantially increase their odds of developing breast cancer. Six or more years of use in any woman with prior history of benign breast disease may also be an invitation to cancer—if Dr. Paffenbarger is correct (1979). Thus, ironically, although the Pill can subdue benign breast disease, it may, in some curious way, increase the patient's later odds of getting cancer!

Family history is an important factor in susceptibility to breast cancer, and in 1981, Dr. Maurice Black, Director of the Breast Diseases Institutes at New York Medical College in Valhalla, New York, told the American Association of Pathologists of a curious finding: According to his statistics, if a Pill user had a grandmother or aunt—but not, surprisingly, a mother or sister—who has had the disease, she is four times more likely than the population as a whole to develop breast cancer. For women who have such a family history, the risk of breast cancer remains double even after they have stopped taking the Pill (Black 1981). In this murky situation, it seems premature to advise women that the Pill is beneficial for the breast.

Other Health Benefits of the Pill Disputed

Other health benefits claimed for the Pill are that it *reduces ovarian cysts, ovarian cancer, endometrial cancer, iron-deficiency anemia, pelvic inflammatory disease (PID), ectopic pregnancy, and rheumatoid arthritis.*

The Pill may indeed reduce ovarian cysts because it supresses cyclical ovarian activity. On the other hand, microscopic studies of the ovarian tissue of long-term Pill users show many abnormal changes; according to Dr. W. P. Plate, a Dutch gynecologist, portions of the ovary resemble scar tissue (Seaman 1969, p. 160).

The possible reductions in ovarian and endometrial cancer that are now being claimed for the Pill could, if proven correct, be extremely important health benefits. The theory that may explain this reduction, if it exists, is that the progestins in the Pill have an "opposing" effect on the estrogen. There is, however, a central question that scientists attempting the pertinent studies have not been able to answer. That is, in concluding that Pill users may have less ovarian and endometrial cancer than nonusers, are they perhaps dealing with what one doctor has called a "survivor population"?

In contrast to the claimed benefits for ovarian and endrometrial cancer, the rate of early-stage cervical cancer is up to seven or eight times higher among Pill users than other women. This condition is sometimes treated with a limited procedure called "conization" of the cervix, but hysterectomy is more frequently performed. Another Pill-associated condition that leads to hysterectomy is the rapid growth of benign fibroids in the uterus. Even the Walnut Creek study acknowledged that there is a "significantly higher risk of uterine fibroma in users . . . [and a] higher rate of hysterectomy among them" ("Walnut Creek Drug Study" 1980, pp. 352–54).

In other words, women whose reproductive organs are sensitive to hormone stimulation apparently have an increased number of early hysterectomies (by the age of 39) if they take the Pill. Some of these hysterectomies are performed for malignancies of the cervix, and some for the rapid growth of fibroids. Thus, it may simply be that upon reaching the age where ovarian and endometrial cancer are likely to occur, the reproductive organs of hormone-sensitive women who used the Pill have already been removed. This is a thorny question that will take many years to resolve, but in the meantime it is surely premature to look on the Pill as a cancer preventative. Among other sites where some studies suggest that the Pill is associated with tumor growth are the liver, thyroid and pituitary, skin, and urinary tract.

It is true that Pill users have less chronic iron-deficiency anemia than nonusers since they do not actually menstruate; due to the manipulation of hormones, they undergo artificial withdrawal bleeding. On the other hand, because of the Pill's interference with normal metabolism, the *Journal of Reproductive Medicine* has stated:

> Biochemical and clinical findings point to an increased need for vitamin B_6. . . . The absorption of the major food form of "folic acid" is substantially impaired. . . . The Pill also appears to increase the requirement for vitamin C and perhaps for vitamin B_2 (riboflavin) and zinc. . . . [Theuer 1972].

It appears, as claimed, that users of combined Pill formulations may have few ectopic pregnancies; on the other hand, "mini" Pills (progestins) are associated with a higher than normal rate of ectopic pregnancies.

Pelvic inflammatory disease (PID) is also reported to be decreased in Pill users. This is clearly true compared to women with IUDs, but not compared to users of the barrier methods (Stadel 1982). For consumers who are concerned about preventing sexually transmitted diseases, the barrier methods probably remain the preferred form of birth control.

Claims that the Pill prevents some forms of rheumatoid arthritis are very thinly based. Some researchers, such as Dr. Giles Bole at the Rackham Arthritis Research Unit, University of Michigan, have reached quite the opposite conclusion. They find that in certain women, arthritis develops with use of the Pill or is worsened (Bole et al. 1969).

The Atlanta-based Arthritis Foundation has registered alarm at the suggestion that the Pill is good for arthritis victims. Dr. Frederick McDuffie, the foundation's senior vice president for medical affairs, points out that there is evidence that the Pill may trigger lupus erythematosus, a serious and sometimes fatal disease of the connective tissues that can resemble rheumatoid arthritis (McDuffie, 1983).

The current campaign to emphasize the health benefits of the Pill has made its impact on the FDA. Patient labeling is being prepared that is far more upbeat than the labeling that has been in use from the mid-1970s until the time of this writing. The present labeling, although weak on metabolic, nutritional, and nuisance side effects, is nonetheless fairly thorough, in contrast to the proposed revisions.

THE IUD—PROBLEMS AND MEDICAL COMPLICATIONS

IUDs have several problems as a contraceptive agent. In the first place, the pregnancy rate for women who retain IUDs is 1 to 6 per 100 users a year. The average with most devices is only 2 or 3 per 100. But this is only part of the story because many women cannot tolerate IUDs at all. Under the best circumstances, no more than 2 women in 3 are apt to retain IUDs for a year or longer. The number still using them after four years drops to 1 in 3. What has happened to all the others?

Some IUDs—7 to 20 out of 100 (this varies with the device in question, the skill of the inserter, and the age and number of pregnancies of the patient)—are spontaneously expelled. Most women notice when they've lost their IUDs, but 1 in 5 does not, and this person then assumes incorrectly that she is still protected. Another factor to be considered is that 3 to 35 IUDs in 100—a wide variance depending on model, clinic, and population group—are removed at the patient's request because of pain and bleeding. Also, the typical user of most devices has a two- to four-day increase in her period, and the amount of blood that she loses doubles or even triples. This may help explain why anemia is five times more common among women who choose this contraceptive method. Finally, in addition to removals for pain and bleeding, another 4 to 15 users out of each 100 must give up their IUDs for "other medical reasons," including infection.

Generally, older women and those who have had children can tolerate IUDs with least discomfort. The new copper and hormone devices perform best in young or childless women but pose special problems and dangers of their own (*Population Report* 1982, p. B–26), including an especially marked increase in ectopic pregnancies among Progestasert users.

However, the IUD is less deadly than the Pill. In nine years of use, from 1965 to 1974, the FDA received reports of "only" 39 IUD deaths in the United States out of an estimated 3 to 4 million users a year. But although the IUD is not as likely as the Pill to place a woman in the morgue, it is just as apt to place her in the hospital. According to FDA calculations,

> The hospitalization rates with intra-uterine devices are in the same order of magnitude as with oral contraceptives: 0.3 to 1.0 per hundred women years of use [Jennings 1974].

In short, both Pill and IUD users face a risk of associated hospitalization ranging from 1 to 300 to 1 to 100 per year, respectively. The IUD hospitalization figures would be higher yet if more doctors were conscientious about removing these devices whenever perforations occur.

The usual perforation rate for IUDs inserted by skilled specialists averages about 1 per 1000 insertions. In amateur hands, this rate is very much higher. Complicating the issue is the fact that some perforations are asymptomatic. Neither the woman nor her doctor can be sure whether a missing IUD simply fell out or migrated through her uterus. Most perforations occur or begin at the time of insertion, but this misfortune can happen at any time, even after five or six years. No IUD wearer should ever ignore a pain in her abdomen.

Infection rates second, after pain and bleeding, as the leading cause of IUD removal. Serious IUD infections are most apt to occur in association with insertion or venereal disease.

Women who adapt well to IUDs may more or less "forget them" and leave them in for years, or decades. This is inadvisable. After about the fifth or sixth year the rate at which severe infections erupt suddenly seems to climb back up.

Cellular changes in the lining of the uterus that are suspected by some pathologists to be precancerous also become more marked at this time ("Pathologic Changes Reported" 1968).

FDA has mandated that all IUD users receive a printed warning that includes information on risks and early signs that complications may be developing. Spot checks in several cities indicate that many providers are failing to give out the warning. Every IUD user is urged to request it.

Depo-Provera

Depo, an injectable contraceptive that is being sold abroad and used surrepticiously in many clinics in the United States, is under review for legal sale in this country. Nobody has any final statistics, but some health workers believe that Depo is almost equal to sterilization—and well ahead of the IUD—in the amount of infertility it causes.

As Judy Norsigian, chair of the Depo-Provera Committee of the National Women's Health Network, has stated: "Most women who are given Depo experience one or more of the following: chaotic menstrual patterns, weight gain, hair loss, fatigue, breast swelling or breast discomfort, limb pain, headache, depression, nausea and infertility, for as long as one to two years." (Norsigan, 1983). Depo also causes cancer in some test animals and significantly decreases high-density lipoproteins, which in turn is apt to increase the risk of heart attack, stroke, and other circulatory disorders. Depo may affect carbohydrate metabolism, raising blood sugar levels. It has also been linked to birth defects in animals and humans. So many women have suffered so many health problems from the Pill and IUD that the approval of Depo, which cannot be withdrawn from the bloodstream if complications ensue, is being vigorously contested by feminists and consumer groups (Ibid).

SUMMARY

For 20 years, the Pill, IUD, and sterilization have dominated contraceptive practice. These methods are continuing to gain adherents in developing countries and in some parts of Europe, but in the United States, England, and other European nations, a backlash—at least to the Pill and IUD—has developed. Consequently, there is a renewed interest in barrier methods and also in ovulation timing or "rhythm" birth control. There is much more funding than before for barrier research and reason to hope that these methods will soon be improved. There is also an awareness on the part of consumers that, when used with dedication, the barriers are highly reliable. The increase in sexually transmitted diseases is a further reason for the renewed popularity of barriers.

In the hands of committed users, rhythm methods can be quite reliable, although they require a great deal of discipline, and, at present, long periods of abstinence. The potential for making rhythm simpler clearly exists, but research monies for the pertinent biochemical studies are extremely meager.

Finally, due to a marked drop in the popularity of the Pill, consumers are now being subjected to a campaign to "resell" it. Some of the "positive" findings about the Pill that are being publicized may prove legitimate, although it is too soon to know for certain. Others are more dubious, and, in the meantime, new findings about negative effects are *not* being equally publicized.

One such negative effect that is of utmost gravity is that an increased risk of cardiovascular disease remains long after Pill use is discontinued. A second finding that has not been generally disseminated is the growing concern over the role of progestins. It was hoped that reducing the amount of estrogen in the Pill would eliminate most of the side effects, but by and large, this has not proven to be so. The progestins also contribute to adverse biochemical change. There are two basic progestin formulas used in most brands of the Pill, and it is presently suspected that Norethindrone, the most popular, is also the most intrusive (Stadel 1982). Funding for research into the specific effects of the different progestins, a matter that has been neglected for two decades of widespread Pill use, is just getting underway.

REFERENCES

Associated Press Interview, December 6, 1981.

Baker, J. R., *The Chemical Control of Contraception.* London: Chapman and Hall, 1935.

Bernstein, G. S., "Physiological Aspects of Vaginal Contraception: A Review," *Contraception*, 9 (1974), 333–45.

Billings, J. J., *The Ovulation Method*. Melbourne, Australia: Advocate Press, 1970.

———, *Natural Family Planning: The Ovulation Method*. Collegeville, Minn.: Liturgical Press, 1973.

Billings, J. J., and E. L. Billings, "Determination of Fertile and Infertile Days by the Mucus Pattern," in W. A. Urichio, ed., *Proceedings of a Research Conference on Natural Family Planning*. Washington, D.C.: Human Life Foundation, 1973.

"Birth Control News," *Vogue* Magazine, June 1983.

"Birth Control Pills Are Called Safe," UPI story, October 23, 1980.

Black, Maurice, an article in *Medical World News* (March 25, 1981), pp. 24–26.

Bole, G. G. et al., "Rhematic Symptoms and Serological Abnormalities Induced by Oral Contraceptives," *Lancet*, vol. I (1969).

Boston Women's Health Collective, 1976.

Broznan, Nadine, "Sterilization without Surgery Has Promise," *The New York Times*, September 6, 1982.

Campbell, Arthur A., Deputy Director, Center of Population Research, National Institute of Child Health and Human Development. Personal Interview, August 1982.

"Cancer Controversy for 'Sponge' Contraceptive," *New York Post*, July 14, 1983.

Center for Disease Control, "Oral Contraceptives and Cancer Risk," *Morbidity and Mortality Weekly Report*, vol. 31, no. 29 (1982).

——— "Oral Contraceptives in the 1980s," *Population Reports*, ser. 8, no. 6 (May/June 1982).

FDA, "Over-the-Counter Contraceptives and Other Vaginal Drug Products," *Federal Register*, 38 (May 16, 1974), 12840–42.

———, Advisory Committee, *Proceedings*, January 1975.

Ferin, J., "Determination de la Periode Sterile Premensdruelle par la Courbe Thermique" (Determination of the Premenstrual Sterile Period by Means of the Thermal Curve), *Bruxelles Medical*, 27 (1947), 2786–93.

Fischer, Mary A., "A California Scientist Remodels a Perpetual Problem's Ancient Solution: The Contraceptive Sponge," *People* Magazine, May 2, 1983.

Harvey, P. D., "Condoms—A New Look," *Family Planning Perspectives*, 4 (1972), 27–30.

Hatcher, R. A. et al., *Contraception Technology 1978–1979*, 9th rev. ed. New York: Irvington Press, 1979.

"Health Benefits of the Pill Found to Outweigh Its Drawbacks," *The New York Times*, July 18, 1982.

Himes, N. E., *Medical History of Contraception*. New York: Schocken Books, 1970.

Information Program, "Oral Contraceptives in the 1930s," *Population Report*, ser. 8, no. 6 (1982).

International Planned Parenthood Federation, International Medical Advisory Panel, "Statement on Intrauterine Devices," *IPPF Bulletin*, vol. 16, no. 6 (1981).

Jain, A. K., and B. Moots, "Fecundability Following the Discontinuation of IUD Use among Taiwanese Women," *Journal of Biosocial Science*, 9, no. 2 (1977), 137–51.

Jennings, J., "Report of the Safety and Efficacy of the Dalkon Shield and Other IUDs." Paper prepared by the ad hoc Obstetric-Gynecology Committee to the United States Food and Drug Administration, October 29–30, 1974.

Jick, H. et al., "Vaginal Spermicides and Congenital Disorders," *JAMA*, vol. 245 (1981).

Lacey, Louise, *Lunaception*. New York: Coward, McCann & Geoghegan, Inc., 1974.

Leeuwenhoek, A. V., "Observations di Anthoni Leeuwenhoek, de Natis e Semine Genitali Animalculis, 1677" (English trans.), *The Collected Letters of Anthoni Van Leeuwenhoek*, vol. 2, Amsterdam: C. Sweets, S. Zeitlinger, 1941.

Letter from Dr. Armand Lione, President of Associated Pharmacologists & Toxicologists, to Dr. Solomon Sobel, Food and Drug Administration, May 23, 1983.

McDuffie, Dr. Frederic, letter to Department of Health and Human Services, 1983.

Michaels, David, Department of Social Medicine, Montefiore Hospital, New York. Personal communication, 1982.

Miller, V., P. A. Klavano, and E. Csonka, "Absorption, Distribution, and Excretion of Phenylmercuric Acetate," *Toxicology and Applied Pharmacology*, 2 (1960), 344–52.

Murakami, U., Y. Kameyama, and T. Kato, "Effects of a Vaginally Applied Contraceptive with Phenylmercuric Acetate upon Developing Embryos and Their Mother Animals," in *Annual Report of the Research Institute of Environmental Medicine*, pp. 88–89. Japan: Nagoya University, 1955.

Nelson, N. et al., "Hazards of Mercury: Special Report to the Secretary's Pesticide Advisory Committee, U.S. Department of Health, Education and Welfare, November 1970," *Environmental Research*, 4 (1971), 1–69.

New Women's Survival Sourcebook. New York: Alfred A. Knopf, Inc., 1975.

"Non-Contraceptive Health Benefits from Oral Contraceptive Use," *Family Planning Perspectives*, vol. 4 (July/August 1982).

Norsigian, Judy, Testimony at FDA hearings on Depo, 1983.

Oakie, Susan, "The 12-Year Study of the Pill: More Questions Than Answers," 2-part article, *The Washington Post*, February 15–16, 1981.

O'Malley, Becky, "Who Says Oral Contraceptives Are Safe?" *The Nation* (February 14, 1981).

Ory, H., A. Rosenfeld, and Lyn Landman, "The Pill at Twenty," *Family Planning Perspectives*, vol. 2, no. 8 (1981).

Oster, G., and S. Oster, "Self-Test for Ovulation and Its Implications in Family Planning." Paper presented at the Centre Medical, Port-au-Prince, Haiti, January 25, 1976.

Oster, G. et al., "Cyclic Variation of Sialic Acid Content in Saliva," *American Journal of Obstetrics and Gynecology*, 144 (1972), 190–93.

Ostrander, S., and L. Schroeder, *Psychic Discoveries behind the Iron Curtain*. Englewood Cliffs, N.J.: Prentice-Hall, Inc., 1971.

Paffenbarger, R. S., *Cancer*, vol. 39 (1979).

"Pathologic Changes Reported in Study of Women Using IUDs," *Medicinal Tribune* (October 14, 1968).

"Pathologist Links IUDs Worn for Years with Infertility Risks," *Medical World News* (April 14, 1980).

Petitti, Diane, Kaiser Permanente. In press.

"The Pill Can Prevent Cancer," *National Examiner*, September 21, 1982.

Planned Parenthood Federation of America, 1981 Service Report. New York, 1981.

Population Report: Intrauterine Devices, ser. B, no. 4 (1982). A Johns Hopkins University publication with support of U.S. Agency for International Development.

Potter, R. G. et al., "Long Cycles, Late Ovulation, and Calendar Rhythm," *International Journal of Fertility*, 12 (1967), 127–40.

Quatrefages A. A., *Ann Sci Nat 3* series 13:111, 188 and *Ann Sci Nat 3* series 19:341, 1953. In Mann, T., *The Biochemistry of Semen and of the Male Reproductive Tract* (New York, John Wiley & Sons, 1964), p. 339.

Ridgewald, Dr. Gary, verbal communication, July 25, 1983.

Rosenblum, A., and L. Jackson, *The Natural Birth Control Book*. Boston: Tao Publications, 1974.

Roshan, Sarah, Nils Lauersen, and James Koch. Personal communication.

Ross, C., and P. T. Piotrow, "Birth Control without Contraceptives," *Population Report: Periodic Abstinence*, ser. 1, no. 1 (1974), pp. 1–5.

Scheinin, Rich, "New Puff Will Be Easy to Buy, Use," *USA Today*, May 25, 1983.

Seaman, Barbara, *The Doctors' Case against the Pill*. New York: Peter H. Wyden, Inc., 1969.

——, "A Skeptical Guide to VD and Contraception," *Free and Female*, chap. 7. New York: Fawcett Crest, 1972.

—— "Testimony of Barbara Seaman to Select Committee on Population, Fertility, and Contraception in America," *Contraceptive Technology and Development*, 3, no. 4 (March 7–9, 1978), 457–63. Also cited in report prepared by Select Committee on Population, U.S. House of Representatives, 95th Congress, *Fertility and Contraception in the United States*, December 1977.

Seaman, Barbara, and Gideon Seaman, *Women and the Crisis in Sex Hormones*, New York: Bantam Books, Inc., 1978.

Seligman, Jean, "The Pill's Dangers Don't Go Away," *Newsweek* (August 31, 1981).

Singh, B., J. C. Cutler, and H. M. D. Utidjian, "Studies on the Development of Vaginal Preparation Providing Both Prophylaxis against Venereal Disease and Other Genital Infections and Contraception. II: Effect in Vitro of Vaginal Contraceptive and Noncontraceptive Preparations of *Treponema Pallidum* and *Neisseria Gonorrhoae*," *British Journal of Veneral Diseases*, 48 (1977), 57–64.

Singh, B. et al., "Studies of the Development of Vaginal Preparation Providing Both Prophylaxis against Venereal Disease and Other Genital Infections and Contraception. III: In Vitro Effect of Vaginal Contraceptive and Selected Vaginal Preparations on *Candida Albicans* and *Trichomona Vaginalis*," *Contraception*, 5 (1972), 401–11.

Stadel, Bruce, doctor and consultant with Contraceptive Evaluation Branch, Center for Population Research, National Institute of Child Health and Human Development. Interview, September 1, 1982.

Stim, E. M., "The Nonspermicide Fit-Free Diaphragm: A New Contraceptive Method," *Adv. Planned Parenthood Physicians*, vol. 15 (1980).

Stryker, J. M., S. B. Sparber, and A. M. Goldberg, "Subtle Consequences of Methylmercury Exposure: Behavior Deviations in Offspring of Treated Mothers," *Science*, 177 (1972), 621–23.

Tatum, Howard J., and Elizabeth Connell Tatum, "Barrier Contraception: A Comprehensive Overview," *Fertility and Sterility*, vol. 6, no. 1 (1981).

Theuer, Richard, "Effects of Contraceptive Agents on Vitamin and Mineral Needs: A Review," *Journal of Reproductive Medicine* (January 1972).

UPI Story, February 16, 1982.

Vaughan, P., *The Pill on Trial*. New York: Coward, McCann & Geoghegan, Inc., 1970.

Vessey, M. P. et al., "Fertility after Stopping Different Methods of Contraception," *British Medical Journal*, 1, no. 6108 (1977), 265–67.

"The Walnut Creek Drug Study," *The Journal of Reproductive Medicine*, 25, no. 6, supplement (1980), 352–54.

White, M. K. et al., "Current Practice Concerning Time of IUD Insertion," *IPPF Medical Bulletin*, 11, no. 6 (1977), 1–3.

Zuck, T. T., "The Relation of Basal Body Temperature to Fertility and Sterility in Women," *American Journal of Obstetrics and Gynecology*, 36 (1938), 998–1005.

Chapter Two

PREGNANCY AND BIRTH: CURRENT TREATMENT

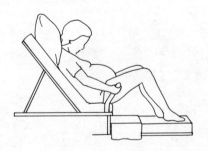

Doris Haire

> *There is no doubt in my mind that a significant proportion of the 4 million children and youths in the United States who are afflicted with mental and neurologic dysfunction are the victims of obstetric medications administered with the very best of intentions to the mother during labor and birth.*
>
> *[Doris Haire, President of the American Foundation for Maternal and Child Health]*

Few American infants are born today in optimal condition as nature intended them to be. The need to use resuscitative procedures to assist the newborn infant in taking its first breath has become so commonplace that such a neurologically depressed newborn infant is no longer considered a cause for alarm. The newborn infant's hands and feet, which normally should turn pink within the first five minutes after birth, more often than not remain pale and blue for hours, reflecting the inability of the narcotized newborn to pump oxygenated blood into its hands and feet. Does the poor oxygenation of the infant's hands and feet reflect a depletion of normal oxygen within the infant brain? A review of the medical literature indicates that no one has bothered to look.

The experience of birth has become so distorted by obstetric intervention in the United States that the average American obstretrician has probably never seen a truly normal birth and has no standards of normalcy against which to measure the condition of the infants he or she delivers.

EXAMPLES OF QUESTIONABLE DRUG USE AND OBSTETRICAL INTERVENTIONS

For example, until fairly recently it was considered ethical to administer a potent hormone (progesterone or Provera) to women in order to test for pregnancy. If the woman was not pregnant, the hormone would bring on her period. If the woman was pregnant, the drug exposed the fetus to the possibly dangerous effects of the powerful hormone at one of the most vulnerable periods of fetal development.

As another example, millions of pregnant women who complained of nausea and vomiting were offered an antinausea drug, Bendectin, now

35

suspected of possibly causing birth defects, even though the Food and Drug Administration (FDA) officers admitted during the September 15, 1980, FDA hearing on Bendectin that the drug had not been adequately tested for safety and effectiveness (Haire 1981).

Amniocentesis is also increasingly being used to test for fetal abnormalities. Yet there is no evidence to indicate that doctors are routinely informing women that there are inherent risks, such as spontaneous abortion following amniocentesis ("Hazards of Amniocentesis" 1978; Delaney 1981).

In addition, health care providers insist that the location of the fetus must be established by sonography before doing an amniocentesis. Sonograms (fetal imagery by means of high-frequency sound) are ordered during pregnancy on the faintest pretense of concern, although the FDA has cautioned that:

> increasing concern has arisen regarding the fetal safety of widely used diagnostic ultrasound in obstetrics. Animal studies have been reported to reveal delayed neuromuscular development, altered emotional behavior, EEG changes, anomalies and decreased survival. Genetic alterations have also been demonstrated in the invitro system. [Finkel 1979]

Yet the health care provider seldom advises the mother that an extensive study has shown that sonography does not, in fact, improve the safety of amniocentesis for the mother or her unborn infant (Nolan et al. 1981).

Estrogen drugs were administered to 6 million pregnant women in the United states between 1945 and 1971. These drugs are still being administered today to pregnant women on the assumption that they will forestall threatened abortion, even though the hormone is now known to be ineffective in preventing spontaneous abortion or miscarriage. Furthermore, it increases the possibility of the offspring developing precancerous and cancerous lesions (Herbst et al. 1971; American Academy of Pediatrics 1973) and reproductive failure (Herbst et al. 1981).

Although the FDA does not approve of the practice of using oxytocin to electively induce or stimulate labor, the practice is commonplace in certain parts of the United States. It is ironic that those obstetricians who fear a malpractice suit if they electively induce or stimulate labor with oxytocin and something goes wrong are likely to resort to amniotomy (the artificial rupture of the mother's membrane) for the same purpose. Amniotomy is a potentially dangerous practice that can lead to brain trauma because it increases the likelihood of umbilical cord prolapse, cord compression (Gabbe et al. 1976), and exaggerated disalignment of the fetal skull bones (Caldeyro-Barcia et al. 1974).

The excessive use of oxytocin in the United States to augment labor contractions in 25-50 percent of births, depending on the area of the country, reflects the fact that other drugs administered to the mother to reduce or eliminate her discomfort or pain during labor also reduce or eliminate the effectiveness of her contractions (Ralston and Shnider 1978).

Furthermore, administering pain-relieving drugs to the mother during labor virtually mandates that the mother must be confined to bed during labor in order to avoid the possibility of her falling or injuring herself. And Hoult (1977), Flynn (1978), Caldeyro-Barcia (1979), and others have shown that confining the mother to bed during labor and putting her in a lithotomy (lying down) position for the second (expulsive) stage of labor are practices that carry a potential for harm to both the mother and infant. The combined efforts of these three researchers have shown that confining a mother to bed tends to significantly:

(a) Prolong labor (by 2½ hours).
(b) Increase the mother's need for pain-relieving drugs and uterine stimulants.
(c) Increase the need for forceps extraction of the infant.
(d) Increase the incidence of abnormal fetal heart rates and poor Apgar scores in the newborn.

In addition, because the pain-relieving drugs administered to the mother frequently inhibit or obliterate the urge or the ability to push her baby out spontaneously, it is frequently necessary for the physician to do a large episiotomy in order to apply the forceps. And according to Dr. David Banta, Assistant Director of the U.S. Congress Office of Technology Assessment, contrary to what most women have been told, an episiotomy (the surgical incision made to enlarge the birth outlet) has *not* been shown to protect the pelvic musculature from damage but actually increases the likelihood of a serious third or fourth degree tear (1981; Thacker and Banta—in press).

Nor do women realize that the drugs administered to them during labor and birth may necessitate the questionable practice of early clamping of the umbilical cord so that the narcotized, neurologically depressed infant may be resuscitated.

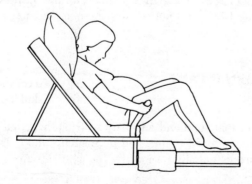

New delivery table adapted for physiological position for birth.

RESEARCH FINDINGS AND GOVERNMENT INACTION

Research by Brackbill, presented at the July 30, 1981 hearing held by the investigative arm of the U. S. House Science and Technology Committee, demonstrated that few women are sufficiently informed about the inherent risks to themselves and to their offspring of the drugs they are prescribed or offered during pregnancy, labor, and birth. Although these women give their consent to obstetric drugs, in most cases the mother's consent is of no legal relevance since it is not informed consent (1981).

For more than a decade, the author of this chapter has questioned the wisdom of the FDA's procedures and policies in regard to how that agency evaluates and regulates the safety of drugs, especially those drugs used in pregnancy and obstetrics. The author's research findings have been reported in a paper entitled, "How the FDA Determines the 'Safety' of Drugs—Just How Safe Is 'Safe'"? (Haire 1980a).

The report was intended as much for the Commissioner of the FDA as for the National Women's Health Network. This author became convinced of the need for such a report by the resistance encountered from various officials in the Bureau of Drugs when questioned regarding the FDA's evaluation of drugs, and, in particular, obstetric drugs. It became obvious that the FDA's inadequacies in this regard would not be brought to the Commissioner's attention by those responsible for the inadequacies. In keeping with this intent, a copy of each successive draft of the report was sent to Dr. Jere Goyan, then Commissioner of the FDA. Dr. Goyan and other FDA officers were repeatedly told that any inaccuracies in the report that the FDA could document as errors would be corrected. No such documentation has ever been offered.

During the preparation of the above report, the author learned that most of the drugs administered to women during labor and birth have never been approved by the FDA as safe for such use, and that none of these drugs has been subjected to a properly controlled scientific evaluation and found to be safe in regard to the drug's effects on the offspring's neurologic development. The FDA does not require the manufacturer to demonstrate such safety.

IMPACT OF DRUGS ON UNBORN INFANT

During the hours that surround an infant's birth, the brain is particularly vulnerable to drug-induced trauma and permanent injury. The other major organ systems are essentially formed by the first three or four months of pregnancy. It is the nerve circuitry of the brain and the rest of the central nervous system of the unborn child that are rapidly developing as labor begins, making these awesomely complex structures vulnerable to permanent damage from the drugs and procedures administered to the mother during that time.

Drugs administered to the mother during labor and birth rapidly filter through the placental membrane and enter the blood and brain of the fetus in a matter of seconds or minutes. While the fetus is connected to the mother's circulatory system, her system helps to eliminate the drug from both of their systems. However, if a drug is frequently or continuously administered to the mother during labor, there is a tendency for the drug to accumulate in the maternal and fetal blood and brain due to overload (Ralston and Schneider 1978).

Once the infant is born and the cord is clamped, those drugs that are present in the newborn infant's blood and brain are essentially trapped in the infant's circulatory system. Because the newborn's metabolic and endocrine systems are immature, the infant cannot readily break down and excrete the drugs. Thus the trapped drugs, or their potent metabolities, may continue to circulate in the newborn infant for several days or longer (ibid.).

What does this prolonged exposure to maternally administered drugs mean to the later neurologic development and behavior of the offspring? Drug-induced biochemical alterations within the brain of the about-to-be-born or newly born infant have the potential for permanently disrupting the normal linkup of the baby's brain cells by altering the biochemical markers that guide the cells into their proper places (Silver 1981). It is somewhat analogous to the unintentional spilling of a chemical over telephone wires that are being connected according to the color code at the end of each wire. The chemical removes the color from the wire ends. The technician must then continue to connect the wires, not knowing exactly which wires to connect with which. Thus the circuitry may be completed but it functions imperfectly.

Although the process of cell migration is not yet fully understood, present knowledge of neurobiology suggests that the normal biochemical message left along the pathway of the neuron by the preceding cell (as it travels to its proper place within the central nervous system) leaves a biochemical message that directs the next brain cell into place. Drug-induced changes in the biochemical message can disrupt this vital process ("The Brain" 1979).

Lesions, resulting from the death of cells due to drug-induced, prolonged reduction or deprivation of oxygen, can also disrupt the brain's circuitry by requiring the cells to find other routes by which to form the circuitry (ibid.).

The FDA's own guidelines for the evaluation of drugs used in pregnant women and in children (1977) acknowledge that drugs circulating in the bloodstream of the newborn infant penetrate the infant's brain and that once in the brain the drugs can adversely affect the rapidly developing nerve circuitry of the brain and central nervous system by altering the following brain processes:

(a) Neuronal maturation: the rate at which the nerve cells in the brain mature.
(b) Cell differentiation: the process by which the brain cells develop individual characteristics and capacity to carry out specific functions.
(c) Cell migration: the process by which the brain cells are guided into their proper place within the brain and central nervous system.
(d) Dendritic arborization: the interconnections of the branchlike nerve fibers as the circuitry of the brain is formed.

The FDA guidelines also point out that drugs in the newborn infant can disrupt the myelinization process of the infant's brain and central nervous system (ibid.). This is a physiologic process in which the nerve fibers are "insulated" with a fatlike substance called *myelin*. This insulation helps to assure that the nerve impulses—the messages to and from the brain—will travel their normal routes at the normal speed.

Any alteration or disruption in the development of the intricately complex nerve circuitry of the human brain has the potential for permanently altering the way in which the nerve signals travel to and from the brain and the way in which the brain processes information.

Dr. Donald Tower, Director of the National Institute of Neurological and Communicative Disorders and Stroke, made the following statement regarding the importance of the brain circuitry for the future development of the child:

> It is the biochemical circuitry—the biochemical messengers and relevant nerve cells in the brain—that forms the basis for mankind's behavior. [1978].

Dr. Roberto Caldeyro-Barcia, a renowned scientist in perinatal medicine and immediate past president of the International Federation of Gynecologists and Obstetricians, has issued his own warning:

> In the past forty years many artificial practices have been introduced which have changed childbirth from a physiological event to a very complicated medical procedure in which all kinds of drugs are used and procedures carried out, sometimes unnecessarily, and many of them potentially damaging for the baby and even for the mother. [1974]

CONTINUED USE OF DRUGS AND OTHER OBSTETRICAL INTERVENTIONS DESPITE POTENTIAL DANGERS

Despite the growing awareness that drugs administered to the mother can adversely affect the fetus, physicians continue to administer sedatives, tranquilizers, analgesics, regional anesthesia, uterine stimulants, and general anesthesia to women during childbirth, without advising them that none of these drugs has been subjected to a properly controlled scientific evaluation and shown to be safe for the offspring. Furthermore, none of the methods currently accepted by the FDA and the medical community is an adequate test to evaluate the safety of obstetric-related drugs in regard to their effects on the long-term development of the exposed offspring. Recent research by Colletti (1979) and Nelson and Ellenberg (1979) demonstrates that the FDA can no longer accept an Apgar score of 7 or higher as an indication of infant well-being.

Epidural anesthesia during labor and birth is often referred to by anesthesiologists as the "Cadillac" of anesthesia, yet research now indicates that the effects of regional anesthesia on the exposed offspring are not as innocuous as anesthesiologists would have us believe.

A six-week follow-up evaluation by Rosenblatt and colleagues of infants born to mothers who had bupivacaine epidurals demonstrated significant and consistent effects of bupivacaine throughout the six-week assessment period (1981). The initial effects of bupivacaine were cyanosis (a decreased oxygenation of the infant) and unresponsiveness. The infants' visual skills, alertness, motor organization, ability to control states of consciousness, and physiological response to stress were adversely affected throughout the six-week testing period. The intensity of the effects tended to correlate with the concentration of the drug in the cord blood at birth.

Research by Brazelton has demonstrated that epidural anesthesia puts the infant at the same factor of risk for neurologic damage as if the child had been born to a mother who had been subjected to semistarvation during the first seven months of her pregnancy (1979). Data from England show that an infant born to a mother who has had an epidural block is 20 times more likely than other infants to require rotational forceps delivery (Studd 1980). If the epidural block prolongs or disrupts labor, to the point where a Cesarean section is required, the fetal brain is further jeopardized by the greater levels of maternal drugs necessary in such major surgery.

Many of the drugs administered to the mother during labor and birth depress her central nervous system and can affect the fetus by lowering the mother's rate of respiration and her blood pressure. This combination of effects can interfere with the transfer of oxygen from the mother's circulatory system to the blood and brain of her unborn infant. Persistent fetal hypoxia (lowered oxygen saturation of the fetal blood) is considered by many scientists to be a greater threat to the fetal brain than is exposure to relatively short intervals of anoxia (complete cessation of oxygen).

Research by Ucko in England found that children with normal I.Q.'s who had been subjected to fetal hypoxia during labor tended to respond abnormally to stress (1965).

The mother, too, can be harmed or injured by the drugs administered to her during childbirth. The package insert of the regional anesthetic Marcaine cautions the reader as follows:

> *Reactions following epidural or caudal anesthesia also may include: high or total spinal block; urinary retention; fecal incontinence; loss of perineal sensation and sexual function; persistent analgesia, paresthesia, and paralysis of the lower extremities; headache and backache; and slowing of labor and increased incidence of forceps delivery.*

The fact that the FDA has permitted the manufacturer to place this important warning in the section of the package insert entitled "Allergic Reactions," long after its inappropriate placement has been brought to the agency's attention, demonstrates the FDA's willingness to permit manufacturers to bury the most important information regarding drug risks in the least notice-able sections of the package inserts.

Although the FDA has never approved the use of oxytocin and prostag-landins for the elective stimulation of labor, these uterine stimulants are frequently administered to women during labor in order to augment their contractions and speed up their labor. Such augmentation can adversely affect the fetal brain by increasing intracranial pressure and by inhibiting the normal transfer of oxygen from the mother's circulatory system to the fetal brain.

During a normal contraction, the maternal blood vessels that carry oxygenated blood through the uterine wall are constricted. During this period of diminished blood flow, the fetal brain is provided with a relatively constant supply of oxygen from oxygenated blood that has built up in the placenta's intervillous space during the resting intervals between contrac-tions. Therefore, any uterine stimulants that foreshorten these oxygen-replenished intervals, by making the contractions too long, too strong, or too close together, can increase the likelihood that brain cells will die. The situation is somewhat analogous to holding an infant under the surface of the water and allowing it to come to the surface to gasp for air but not to breathe.

Intracranial hemorrhage following amniotomy, forceps extractions, or vacuum extraction, conditions frequently associated with the use of obstretric drugs, is not likely to become evident until the child reaches an age (around 8 or 9 years) when he or she will be called upon to use the more analytic skills, such as those involved in mathematics. (Caldeyro-Barcia et al. 1974 b)

Many anesthesiologists have even convinced themselves that obstetric drugs can actually protect the fetal brain by reducing the mother's discomfort or pain, but in fact pain and discomfort do not cause damage to the infant brain through lack of oxygen or any other mechanism. Obstetrical drugs, however, can cause problems such as jaundice which can adversely affect the newborn infant's brain by altering the normal biochemistry of its blood.

The manufacturers of several potent pain-relieving drugs warn the practitioner that the drugs can elevate the infant's cerebrospinal fluid pressure beyond the normal level. If there is brain swelling induced by intra-uterine trauma, birth injury, or pathophysiology, the use of such drugs increases the possibility of brain damage (Brann and Myers 1975).

Drug-induced hypothermia, a condition whereby the infant cannot maintain its normal internal temperature, also can cause brain injury in the newborn because the infant must use the oxygen needed to maintain the integrity of the brain to instead turn its body "brown fat " into energy in order to maintain its normal internal temperature. Measures can be taken to reverse these drug-induced adverse effects, but there is no guarantee that such measures will be effective quickly enough to prevent permanent damage to the fetal brain.

PREVALENCE OF BRAIN DAMAGE AMONG THE GENERAL POPULATION

Behavioral scientists have found subtle brain damage to be far more prevalent among the general population than was once assumed (Silver et al. 1976). There are 4 million children and youths (1 out of every 10) in the United States today so severely neurologically or emotionally handicapped that they require special education and training. The fact that the majority of these impaired children, including those with cerebral palsy, were born within the normal range of gestational age and birth weight suggests that we should be more concerned about the neurological effects of obstetric drugs.

There is no doubt in this author's mind that a significant proportion of the 4 million children and youths in the United States who are afflicted with mental and neurological dysfunction are the victims of obstetric medications administered with the very best of intentions to the mother during labor and birth. It is impossible to ignore the fact that the drugs administered to the mother during labor and birth, and the procedures made necessary by such drug use, have the potential for adversely affecting the neurologic development of the exposed offspring, which may result in memory impairment, learning disabilities, and for some, in criminal behavior.

IMPROPER COMMERCIAL LABELING OF DRUGS

Despite the FDA guidelines for the evaluation of drugs used in pregnant women, which clearly acknowledge the potential adverse effects of drugs trapped in the infant's brain at birth, the FDA has permitted manufacturers to imply that the major risk to the fetus occurs when the drug is taken by the mother during the first three or four months of her pregnancy. This type of restricted caution is repeated in almost every package insert for obstretric drugs. None of the package inserts, however, cautions the reader that no properly controlled follow-up has been carried out on individuals exposed to the drug in utero and that, therefore, the drug may well have delayed long-term effects on the exposed offspring.

Although a substantial majority of package inserts have a section entitled "Usage in Pregnancy," very few have any information on the use of these drugs in obstetrics. Most of the drug inserts merely indicate that safe use in pregnant women has not been established. However, a significant number of these inserts *imply* that although safe use in pregnancy has not been established, *safe use in labor has been demonstrated*. They do this by stating that "safe use in pregnant women *other than in labor* has not been established" (emphasis supplied), or that "this does not exclude use in obstetrics," or other such ambiguous language. Since the vast majority of drugs whose package inserts include such wording have not, in fact, been approved by the FDA as safe for use in labor and delivery, the inclusion of such statements or words is clearly deceptive and misleading and should be prohibited by the FDA.

This author appreciates the fact that after many years of pressure from the women's health movement, the FDA's drug regulations have been revised so that all drugs known to be used in labor and delivery, whether approved for that use or not, will eventually have a separate section in the package insert entitled "Usage in Labor and Delivery," which will describe what is known and particularly what is not known about the effects of the drug on the long-term development of the child born of that delivery. For the manufacturer to continue to include undocumented assurances of safety leaves the manufacturer vulnerable to future litigation if time proves the use of the product to have adverse effects on the mother's physiology and on the subsequent development of the exposed offspring.

Although FDA officials and the pharmaceutical industry may say that FDA approval should not be considered the primary documentation of a drug's safety, the fact remains that if the manufacturer could document the safety of his product's use so as to obtain the FDA's approval of that use, then such approval would clearly enhance the sales of the drug for that purpose.

This is not to suggest that physicians should not be free to use a drug for a non-FDA approved use. However, it is felt that the health care professional and, in turn, the patient should be informed as to whether the intended use of the drug has or has not been approved by the FDA.

The women's health movement is keeping a close watch on drug labeling, drug advertising, and the FDA regulation of drugs that affect the lives of women and the lives of their families. Neither the FDA, the pharmaceutical industry, nor organized medicine can afford to continue to withhold information from the obstretric patient, information that she is entitled to have and the physician is obligated to provide her in order for her to make an informed decision as to whether to accept or forego the drug(s) offered her. (American College of Obstetrics and Gynecology 1974; Haire 1973, 1974, 1980*b*).

REFERENCES

American Academy of Pediatrics, "Stilbestrol and Adenocarcinoma of the Vagina," *New England Journal of Medicine*, 51, no. 2(1973), 297–98.

American College of Obstetrics and Gynecology, "Standards for Obstetric-Gynecologic Services," pp. 66–67, section on Informed Consent, 1974.

Banta, D., "The Risks and Benefits of Episiotomy," presentation at the 1981 Conference of the American Foundation for Maternal and Child Health, New York., 1981.

Brackbill, Y., "Informed Consent and Obstetric Drugs: An Ethical Hiatus," presentation to the U.S. House Science and Technology Committee's Subcommittee on Investigations and Oversight, Washington, D.C., July 30, 1981.

"The Brain," *Scientific American*, 241 (1979), 44–246.

Brann, A., and R. Myers, "Central Nervous System Findings in the Newborn Monkey Following Severe in Utero Partial Asphyxia," *Neurology*, 25, no. 4 (1975), 327–38.

Brazelton, T., "A Comparative Study of the Behavior of Greek Neonates," *Pediatrics*, 63 (1979), 279–84.

Caldeyro-Barcia, R., "Obstetrical Intervention: Its Effect on Mother, Fetus, and Newborn," presentation at the American Foundation for Maternal Health Conference, New York, 1974*a*.

——, personal communication, 1974*b*.

——*Physiological and Psychological Bases for the Modern and Humanized Management of Normal Labor*, Scientific Publication No. 858. Montevideo, Uruguay: Latin American Center of Perinatology and Human Development, 1979.

Caldegro-Barcia, R., et al., "Adverse Perinatal Effects of Early Amniotomy During Labor," *Obstetrics and Gynecology in Modern Perinatal Medicine*. Gluck, L. ed. Yearbook Medical Publishers, Chicago, 1974.

Coletti, L., "Relationship between Pregnancy and Birth Complications and the Later Development of Learning Disability," *Journal of Learning Disabilities,* 12 (1979), 25–29.

Delaney, B., "Second-Trimester Amniocentesis," *Obstetrics and Gynecology,* vol. 57 (1981).

FDA, *General Considerations for the Clinical Evaluation of Drugs in Infants and Children.* HEW Publication No. 77-3041, 1977.

Finkel, M., "Drugs and Other Hazards to the Fetus and Newborn," presentation to the National Foundation/March of Dimes Symposium on Drug and Chemical Risks to the Fetus and the Newborn Infant, New York, May 21, 1979.

Flynn, A., et al., "Ambulation in Labour," *British Medical Journal,* August 26, 1978, pp. 591–96.

Gabbe, S., et al., "Umbilical Cord Compression Associated with Amniotomy: Laboratory Observations," *American Journal of Obstetrics and Gynecology,* 126 (1976), 353–55.

Haire, D., "Cultural Warping of Childbirth," *Environmental Child Health,* 19 (1973), 171–91. Reprint.

———, "Pregnant Patient's Bill of Rights," report for the American Foundation for Maternal and Child Health, New York, 1974.

———"How the FDA Determines the 'Safety' of Drugs—Just How Safe Is 'Safe'"? American Foundation for Maternal and Child Health, New York, 1980*a*.

———, "Proposals for Improved Protection of the Unborn Child, presentation to the FDA Anesthetic and Life Support Drug Advisory Committee, Washington, D.C., February 19, 1980*b*.

———. "Research in Drugs Used in Pregnancy and Obstetrics," presentation at the hearings held by the U.S. House Science and Technology Committee's Subcommittee on Investigations and Oversight, Washington, D.C., July 30, 1981.

"Hazards of Amniocentesis," *British Medical Journal,* no. 6153 (1978), pp. 1661–62.

Herbst, A., et al., "Adenocarcinoma of the Vagina: Association of Maternal Stilbestrol Therapy with Tumor Appearance in Young Women," *New England Journal of Medicine,* vol. 284 (1971).

———, "Reproductive and Gynecologic Surgical Experience in Diethylstilbestrol-Exposed Daughters," *American Journal of Obstetrics and Gynecology,* 141 (1981), 1019–26.

Hoult, I., et al., "Lumbar Epidural Analgesia in Labour: Relation to Fetal Maeposition and Instrumental Delivery," *British Medical Journal,* January 1, 1977, pp. 14–16.

Nelson, K., and J. Ellenberg, "Neonatal Signs as Predicators of Cerebral Palsy," *Pediatrics,* 64, no. 2 (1979), 225–32.

Nolan, G., et al., "The Effect of Ultrasonagraphy on Midtrimester Amniocentesis Complications," *American Journal of Obstetrics and Gynecology,* 140 (1981), 531–34.

Ralston, D., and S. Schneider, "The Fetal and Neonatal Effects of Regional Anesthesia in Obstetrics, *Anesthesiology,* 48 (1978), 34–64.

Rosenblatt, D., et al., "The Influence of Maternal Analgesia on Neonatal Behaviour: II. Epidural Bupivacaine," *British Journal of Obstetrics and Gynecology,* 88 (1981), 407–12.

Silver, A., et al., "A Search Battery for Scanning Kindergarten Children for Potential Learning Disability," *Journal of American Academy of Child Psychiatry*, 15, no. 2 (1976), 224–30.

Silver, Michael, Department of Anatomy, Columbia University, College of Physicians and Surgeons, personal communication, 1981.

Studd, J., "The Effect of Lumbar Epidural Analgesia on the Rate of Cervical Dilatation and the Outcome of Labour of Spontaneous Onset," *British Journal of Obstetrics and Gynecology*, 87 (1980), 1015–21.

Thacker, S., and D. Banta, "Benefits and Risks of Episiotomy: An Interpretive Review of the English-Language Literature, 1860–1980," *Obstetrics/Gynecology Survey*, in press.

Tower, Donald B., "Presentation to the National Committee for Research in Neurologic Disorders," Alexandria, Virginia, 1978.

Ucko, L., "A Comparative Study in Asphyxiated and Non-Asphyxiated Boys from Birth to Five Years," *Developments in Medicine of Child Neurology*, 7 (1965), 643–57.

SUGGESTED READINGS

Banta, D., and S. Thacker, "Assessing the Costs and Benefits of Electronic Fetal Monitoring," *Obstet. Gynecol. Survey*, 34 (1979), 627–42.

Davis, Elizabeth, *A Guide to Midwifery: Heart and Hands*. Sante Fe, N.M.: John Muir Publications, 1900.

General Accounting Office (GAO), "Evaluating Benefits and Risks of Obstetric Practices,'" Report to the Congress by the Comptroller General, HRD-79-85, 1979.

Haverkamp, A., et al., "A Controlled Trial of the Differential Effects of Intrapartum Fetal Monitoring," *Am. J. Obstet. Gynecol.*, 134 (1979), 399–408.

Moyer, Linda, "What Obstetrical Journal Advertising Tells about Doctors and Women," in *Birth and the Family Journal*, vol. 2 (1975).

Noble, Elizabeth, *Essential Exercises for the Childbearing Year: A Guide to Health and Comfort Before and After Your Baby is Born*. Boston: Houghton-Mifflin Company, 1976.

Sousa, Marion, *Childbirth at Home*. Englewood Cliffs, N.J.: Prentice-Hall, Inc., 1076.

Wertz, R. W., and D. C. Wertz, *Lying-In*. New York: Schocken Books, Inc., 1979.

LISTING OF ORGANIZATIONS FOR PREGNANCY AND BIRTH

American College of Nurse-Midwives
1000 Vermont Avenue, N.W.
Washington, DC 20005
(202) 628-4642

American Foundation for Maternal
and Child Health
30 Beekman Place
New York, NY 10022

American Society for
    Psychoprophylaxis in Obstetrics
1523 L Street, NW
Washington, DC 20005
(202) 783-7050

Association for Childbirth at Home
National Headquarters
Box 1219
Cerritos, CA 90701
(213) 865-5123

International Childbirth Education
    Association
P. O. Box 20852
Milwaukee, WI 53220
(414) 476-0130

La Leche League International, Inc.
9616 Minneapolis Avenue
Franklin Park, IL 60131
(312) 455-7730

Moonflower Birthing Supply
Dept. M, Box 10006
Denver, CO 80210

National Association of Parents and
    Professionals for Safe Alternatives
    in Childbirth
P. O. Box 1307
Chapel Hill, NC 27514
(919) 732-7302

Chapter Three

TREATMENT OF MENSTRUAL AND MENOPAUSAL PROBLEMS

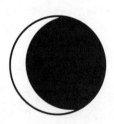

Kay Weiss

Medical treatment of menstrual and menopausal diseases is perhaps the facet of health care that women are most dissatisfied with and that is least scientifically based.

Although other aspects of women's health care—for example, obstetrical care and breast and uterine surgery—are controversial issues that make headlines, these affect far fewer women than do the menstrual and menopausal problems that afflict millions of women throughout their lives. Menstruation and menopause are the only physiological processes in which mild to severe discomfort is tolerated as a normal accompaniment to healthy functioning.

Menstrual "dis-ease" is reported by 50 to 75 percent of the 75 million adult women in the United States; and menopausal "dis-ease" is reported by 90 percent of menopausal women (Weidiger 1977). There is no safe and effective treatment known to alleviate these problems for all women. The symptoms of menstrual and menopausal diseases vary in severity, are recurrent, and often of lengthy duration. Many women spend up to 30 percent of their lives in misery for which there is no known medical relief.

Menstrual problems may include premenstrual syndrome (PMS), which is characterized by tension (physical and mental), depression, irritability, fatigue, and aching; as well as menstrual cramps, migraine headache, cycle irregularities, and profuse bleeding.

Menopausal symptoms are characterized by hot flashes, osteoporosis (thinning of bones), vaginal lining atrophy, and psychological symptoms (fatigue, headache, irritability, depression.)

A comprehensive review of current medical treatments as well as historical social attitudes toward menstruation and menopause can be found in Paula Weidiger's book *Menstruation and Menopause* (1977).

MENOPAUSE

Social Attitudes: Past and Present

Ancient societies treated menopausal women far better than our present society does, and some anthropologists attribute this fact to the absence of menopausal distress in pretechnological societies. In those early cultures, menopausal women, by virtue of their age and standing in the community, enjoyed positions of great respect. Rather than being held in low esteen because they had ceased to function economically and reproductively, they were the respected matriarchs of the extended family, looked up to as the conservators of wisdom and as resources for knowledge and skills.

In contrast, in our modern industrial society, menopausal women are considered relatively useless and are held in low esteem. This sense of being an outcast contributes to and exacerbates the hormonally based symptoms that usually accompany the decline in estrogen production.

The reaction of the medical profession toward menopausal problems differs markedly from that toward diseases far less prevalent and disturbing. Menopausal ailments, although considered serious enough to disqualify women from many jobs, do not appear to be serious enough to warrant investigation into their causes and cures. These ailments receive little research interest or funding in spite of the fact that women are a majority of the population and menopause is the midpoint in a woman's life, which today averages 77 years.

Symptoms and Current Medical Treatment

About 48 percent of menopausal women suffer hot flashes (vasomotor fluctuations), and half of those affected are acutely uncomfortable (McKinlay and Jeffreys 1974). The function and cause of hot flashes are still a mystery to medical science. They acompany the decline in estrogen production and reflect an instability of the autonomic nervous system.

Hot flashes are experienced by many women for up to two years and in some cases, for a much longer period of time. These symptoms may be treated effectively by replacement of estrogen (Estrogen Replacement or ER), albeit at a substantially increased risk of developing cancer of the uterine lining (endometrium), ovaries, and possibly breast (Judd et al. 1981). (See also Chapter Four on the use and abuse of sex hormones.) In addition, ER may be accompanied in some women by headache, nausea, and other symptoms.

Some investigators suggest that the increased risk of endometrial cancer is caused by the fact that only one of the ovarian hormones (estrogen) is being replaced without the progesterone that normally accompanies it. Progesterone counteracts the proliferative (overgrowth) effects of estrogen on the uterine lining, which can be an influencing precursor to the growth of endometrial cancer. Thus administration of estrogen with progesterone added for part of the cycle may simulate (mimic) a more normal hormonal profile. Other investigators claim that the addition of progesterone does not appreciably decrease the cancer risk and may even increase it (as in the sequential oral contraceptives), and, moreover, will reestablish monthly bleeding in the menopausal woman.

Psychological symptoms (irritability, fatigue, anxiety, insomnia, depression) and headaches are not improved by ER, and ER is classified by the Food and Drug Administration (FDA) as ineffective in the treatment of them. Estimates are that about 75 percent of prescriptions written for ER are unwarranted because they are unnecessary or ineffective for the purpose prescribed (Wolfe 1978).

Atrophy of the vaginal lining often follows menopause, making the vagina dry and intercourse difficult. Medical treatment is typically ER, although a safer and equally effective treatment would be topical applications of a lubricant such as coconut oil. Vaginal lubrication will also be increased if a women has an active sex life (Masters and Johnson 1977). Estrogen cream used vaginally carries the same risk as oral estrogen since the hormone is absorbed into the bloodstream.

Brittle bone disease (osteoporosis) can follow estrogen decline and may lead to fractures, which are a leading cause of death among older women. Some researchers believe that since the death rate from hip fracture is greater than that from endometrial cancer, it is wise to begin low dosage ER (0.3 or 0.625) mg.) at menopause to prevent osteoporosis and later fractures. However, it must be remembered that death from hip fractures generally occurs in women above age 90, whereas uterine cancer occurs in much younger women. Also, factors other than ER, such as exercise and diet, can decrease the likelihood of brittle bone disease and can help build bone density. Osteoporosis occurs more often in sendentary women than in active one. Sufficient dietary calcium, Vitamin D, and fluoride added to daily vitamins will help retard bone loss. Recent studies suggest that Calcitonin, an experimental hormonelike drug, or Stanozolol (Winstrol), an anabolic hormone, can benefit women with osteoporosis, although the side effects of these drugs are unknown and Winstrol tends to produce the masculinizing effects of male hormones.

Perhaps any treatment that stabilizes the autonomic nervous system may also help normalize hot flashes: tonifying the body could include methods like vigorous daily aerobic exercise, daily use of Ginsent (a thermoregulator), or sauna baths. The thermal-regulating effect of sauna on the body is a time-honored treatment in many cultures to tonify the body and prevent distress. It is known that both the regulation of estrogen production and the body's heating/cooling mechanisms are controlled by the same gland, the hypothalamus. Ancient Chinese medicine observed that heat receptors in the skin transmit information to the hypothalamus, which responds by heating or cooling the body (Farmilant 1981). Menopausal women are subject to hot flashes and sweats. Perhaps the regulation of the heating/cooling mechanism can also help regulate estrogen production.

See *Women and the Crisis in Sex Hormones* (Seaman 1978) for a discussion of natural treatments as alternatives to prescription drugs for the alleviation of menopausal symptoms.

MENSTRUATION

Some modern women who suffer debilitating symptoms during their periods envy their ancient sisters' ability to spend their menstrual periods in the retirement and seclusion of the "menstrual hut," freed of the obligation to work, cook, and serve their families.

Lack of Research and Little Effective Treatment

The troublesome symptoms and diseases of menstruation have received little research into their causes and little effective treatment. The medical profession in sophisticated societies has shunned menstruating women every bit as much as they were tabooed in primitive time. It is as if the medical profession has agreed that these problems are the result of women being inferior and cursed. Medical specialists have for too long ignored the study of menstrual and menopausal distress. The menstrual cycle has still not been sufficiently researched to provide answers to many basic questions: for example, What is the normal hormonal profile of the typical cycle in terms of estrogen and progesterone production? How does normal menstruation differ according to age and parity? What really constitutes "irregular" or "profuse" bleeding? Should hormones be used to "correct" these conditions, and if so, which ones (estrogen or progesterone) and in what dosages? What would the adverse effects of this treatment be?

The extent of menstrual and premenstrual distress is a health issue of grave concern that receives little attention from the medical profession. Fifty-two percent of female admissions to hospitals due to accidents occur during the paramenstrum; 46 percent of the acute admissions for psychiatric illness occur during this period; and 49 percent of the newly incarcerated female prisoners studied committed their crimes during this period. (Stadel and Weiss 1975). In England in 1981 in two separate cases, women were acquitted of murder because they had committed their crimes while under severe menstrual distress. Society seems to acknowledge the phenomenon of menstrual distress, while the medical profession tends to ignores it.

Premenstrual Syndrome (PMS)

Some 90 percent of women suffer from a complex of symptoms known as PMS, for which the chemical basis has not been found. The symptoms may differ among women, are variable and changeable, and last from one to ten days. These symptoms are experienced during most, but not all, months at a time prior to the menstrual period. The symptoms are classified by Budoff as follows (Budoff 1980).

Psychological: tension, irritability, anxiety, hostility, crying spells, lethargy, depression, and sleep disorders.

Neurological: tension headaches and neck aches, migraines, dizziness, fainting, and (rarely) seizures.

Glandular: tenderness and swelling of breasts.

Gastrointestinal: constipation, abdominal bloating, abdominal cramping, and craving for sweets or carbohydrate foods.

There is no agreed-upon treatment for PMS because little attention has been paid to the causes of the problem and because so many symptoms are found. Some scientists say that PMS is caused by hormone inbalance; others that it is the result of retention of water or salt, poor diet, calcium/magnesium deficiencies, or lack or aerobic exercise.

In a recent comprehensive review of the current medical treatments of PMS in the *British Journal of Psychiatry,* research studies that examined each treatment were reported on and criticized for their validity and reliability ("Treatment of Premenstrual Symptoms," 1979). In most studies the researchers administered a particular treatment to a small group of women patients without administering a placebo to a control group. The most valid studies were controlled studies that were double-blind (neither the physician nor the patient knows which treatment is being administered), enabling the effects of the treatments to be more objectively measured. The following treatments were reviewed:

Oral contraceptive: This treatment has not been proved in controlled double-blind studies to be effective in alleviating PMS, but the high-progestin pill is worth trying and can be helpful in some women.

Progesterone: The pure, nonsynthetic type of progesterone may be helpful and is being studied by Dr. Katherina Dalton, who theorizes that PMS is caused by a hormone imbalance in which there is too little progesterone in relation to estrogen (1964, 1977, 1978). Dalton reports that when pure progesterone is administered daily for the two weeks prior to the period, the remission of symptoms is complete in nearly 100 percent of cases. Pure progesterone is expensive and not absorbed orally; therefore it must be injected or taken by suppository. (Injection doses range from 50–100 mg. daily and must be tailored to individual needs.)

Progesterone taken premenstrually may delay the onset of the menses or cause irregular, scanty bleeding which in itself is not harmful but may be inconvenient.

Progestin (synthetic): Progestin is commonly available and orally absorbable, but some studies have found no benefit over the use of a placebo. One uncontrolled study (Taylor 1977) reported that 70 percent of women with PMS improved with dydrogesterone (Duphaston), but only symptoms of weight gain and bloating were relieved. Psychological symptoms and those of breast tenderness were not improved. A recent scrupulously conducted, double-blind controlled trial of progestin failed to establish its superiority over placebo (Sampson 1979).

Bromocriptine (a prolactin suppressent): This substance has been tried with some success on the theory that raised prolactin levels account for PMS.

Diuretics: A number of controlled studies have failed to demonstrate the superiority of diuretics over a placebo; leading researchers believe that fluid retention is not a cause of PMS. High dosages of prescription diuretics are more effective than over-the-counter brands but must be taken with potassium supplements.

Vitamin B^6 (Pyridoxine): Recent surveys indicate that when taken properly pyridoxine helps 80 percent of the women who take it for PMS. It does not affect hormone levels but rather changes the individual's response to them. To be effective it must be taken every day of the month in the amount of 1 gm. (500 mg. 2 times daily just before meals). Only U.S.P. breands (potency assured) should be used. (Personal communication, Paul Fitzgerald, M.D., Univ. of Calif. Medical School, 1982).

Psychoactive drugs: Tranquilizers and even Lithium have been prescribed in uncontrolled studies with mixed results. Marijuana may be helpful to some women. Alcohol is usually poorly tolerated and inadequately metabolized by the liver during the paramenstrum.

Inderal (Propranilol): Inderal decreases adverse sympathetic nervous system activity including vasodilation, migraine headaches, and high blood pressure in association with the menstrual period. (Fitzgerald 1982).

A complication of these research studies is that treatments have been applied to the whole collection of PMS symptoms—despite evidence that PMS is composed of a collection of distinct, though related, symptoms. If specific symptoms could be treated individually in a controlled manner, after first being rated and measured for severity, research would yield more definitive results.

Menstrual Cramps

Menstrual cramps are the most common cause of lost work and lost school hours in the United States today, accounting for 140 million lost working hours each year. Of the 75 million women in the United States who menstruate, nearly half have menstrual discomfort with some regularity. Of these, approximately 10 percent or 3.5 million are completely incapacitated for 1 to 2 days each month because of pain. It is hard to believe that a problem of such magnitude could go on for so long without prompting some interest among medical researchers.

Menstrual cramps in many women are severe and are compared with heart attack pain (angina) by one author (Budoff 1980). "Uterine angina" is a more descriptive term than "dysmenorrhea" for the severe pain of the uterine muscle contracting in the absence of sufficient oxygen. The uterus squeezes so hard that it compresses the blood vessels and cuts off the blood supply, which is very much like what occurs when the heart muscle has its blood supply cut off by a clot or blood vessel spasm during a heart attack.

For decades, women who suffered from painful menstrual cramps were told by physicians that their pain was purely psychosomatic. A 1971 gynecology textbook instructs the medical student in the diagnosis of menstrual cramps as follows:

> It is important to ascertain how crippling the symptom and how much emotional gain the patient is deriving from it. For example, does the whole household revolve around whether or not the mother is having menstrual cramps? Is the dysmenorrhea the locus for the expression of depression, anger, or a need to be dependent? The adult woman who presents this symptom very often is resentful of the feminine role. Each succeeding period reminds her of the unpleasant fact that she is a woman. . . . Menstruation symbolizes her role in

life. . . . To the immature girl menstrual blood comes from the same area as feces and urine; this causes her to transfer to menstruation the feelings she has toward these excretions. [Wilson, Beecham, and Carrington 1971.]

Traditionally women have been prescribed tranquilizers or narcotic pain relievers to treat menstrual cramps. But as early as 1973, a British physician identified the cause and treatment of dysmenorrhea. In 1967, it had been shown that women who had menstrual pain had five times the amount of prostaglandin in their menstrual fluid as did women who were without pain. Thus British researchers viewed dysmenorrhea as a physiologic problem, but American researchers continued to view it as a hysterical problem of complaining women. In addition, pharmaceutical companies declined to develop and market the drug because of a lack of interest on the part of American physicians. Eventually, Israeli researchers published in American journals in 1974 that prostaglandins play a role in the causation of dysmenorrhea (Schwartz et al.). These authors stated that excessive release of prostaglandins during menstrual breakdown of the lining of the uterus could lead to painful uterine contractions and could also account for the diarrhea and weakness that are commonly associated with dysmenorrhea. Many nonsteroidal antiinflammatory drugs such as Indocin and aspirin are weak inhibitors of antiprostaglandin.

Definitive controlled clinical trials were finally conducted by Dr. Penny Wise Budoff at State University of New York at Stony Brook to prove the effectiveness of prostaglandins in alleviating the age-old problem of menstrual cramps (1980). Today such brand name antiprostaglandins as Ponstel, Anaprox, Naprosyn, and others are available by prescription and can completely alleviate dysmenorrhea for many women. They carry no known adverse side effects.

CONCLUSION

The development of prostaglandins is an example of how menstrual and menopausal diseases can be conquered if there is interest in doing so and if they are assigned as a priority by federally funded research agencies.

In the last decade since the inception of the women's movement and the consumer health movement, physicians who treat menstruation and menopause have gradually begun to do so with greater attention and respect. New treatments are being tried, and although some are ineffective and dangerous, breakthroughs are being made.

GROUPS AND ORGANIZATIONS

Premenstrual Syndrome Action, Inc.
P.O. Box 9326
Madison, Wisc. 53715

REFERENCES

Budoff, Penny Wise. *No More Mentrual Cramps and Other Good News*, New York: Putnam, 1980.

Dalton, Katherina, *The Premenstrual Syndrome*. London: William Heinemann, Ltd., 1964.

———, *The Premenstrual Syndrome and Progesterone Therapy*. London: William Heinemann, Ltd., 1977.

——— "When Surgery Visits Come Like Clockwork: Is It PMS?" *Modern Medicine*, September 1978, pp. 37–40.

Farmilant, Eunice, "Working Up a Sweat," in *East-West Journal*, August 1981.

Hill, G. G., *British Medical Journal*, June 28, 1975.

Judd, H., et al. "Estrogen Replacement Therapy," *Obstetrics and Gynecology*, vol. 58 (1981).

Masters, W., and V. Johnson, *Human Sexual Response*. Boston: Little, Brown & Company, 1977.

McKinlay, J. M., and M. Jeffreys, "The Menopausal Syndrome," *British Journal of Preventive and Social Medicine*, 28, no. 2 (1974), 108–15.

Sampson, G. A., "PMS: A Double-Blind Controlled Trial of Progesterone and Placebo," *British Journal of Psychiatry*, 135 (1979), 209–15.

Schwartz, A., et al., "Primary Dysmenorrhea," *Journal of Obstetrics and Gynecology*, 44, no. 5 (1974), 709–12.

Seaman, Barbara, and Gideon Seaman, *Women and the Crisis in Sex Hormones*, New York: Bantam Books, Inc., 1978.

Smith, S. L., "Mood and the Menstrual Cycle," in *Topics in Psychoendocrinology*, ed. E. J. Sachar. New York: Grune & Stratton, Inc., 1975.

Stadel, B., and N. Weiss, "Characteristics of Menopausal Women: A Survey of King and Pierce Counties in Washington, 1973–74," *American Journal of Epidemiology*, 102 (1975), 209–16.

Stokes, J., and J. Mendels, "Pyridoxine and Premenstrual Tension," *Lancet*, 1 (1972), 1177–78.

Taylor, R. W., "The Treatment of Premenstrual Tension with Dydrogesterone," *Current Medical Research and Opinion*, Suppl. 4 (1977), pp. 16–22.

"The Treatment of Premenstrual Symptoms," *British Journal of Psychiatry*, 135 (1979), 576–79.

Weidiger, Paula, *Menstruation and Menopause*. New York: Delta Books, 1977.

Wilson, J. R., E. Beecham, and E. Carrington, *Obstetrics and Gynecology*, 4th ed. St. Louis: The C. V. Mosby Company, 1971.

Wolfe, Sidney, personal communication, Health Research Group, Washington, D.C. 1978.

Chapter Four

ESTROGEN HORMONE DRUGS: THEIR USE AND ABUSE

Kay Weiss

SEX HORMONE DRUGS—A MAJOR PUBLIC HEALTH PROBLEM

The use of prescription sex hormone drugs in the routine medication of women's life stages has become a major public health problem.

Estrogen, a female sex hormone, was first synthesized for medical use in 1938 and was employed in the treatment of women whose disorders were believed to be caused by low natural levels of estrogen. Thereafter, the uses for estrogen therapy multiplied. In the early 1940s, it was used to prevent complications of pregnancy such as threatened abortion and postpartum breast engorgement and to treat the estrogen decline of menopause and some forms of breast cancer. By the 1950s, almost any abnormality of the female reproduction system was being interpreted by physicians as due to a sex hormone imbalance and accordingly was treated with estrogens. Estrogen was prescribed for a wide variety of ailments such as diseases of the breast and uterus, menstrual and menopausal ailments, hormone "imbalances," acne, excessive growth at puberty, infertility, as a hormonal test for pregnancy, and even for nonsex-related diseases such as hypertension and migraine.

In the 1960s and 1970s, estrogen was promoted as an antifertility hormone, first as the oral contraceptive, then as a morning-after pill abortifacient. The hormone had come full circle from its early use to prevent abortion to its ultimate use as an abortifacient—an indication of the universal application of sex hormones in the treatment of women's ailments. By the 1980s, the use of estrogen hormones has become so ubiquitous that virtually every female in the United States who utilizes professional health care is offered estrogen by a physician at some time in her life.

Unlike many prescription drugs whose risks may be rationalized in the treatment of disease, the majority of estrogen drugs are taken by healthy

61

women for "elective" or nonmedical purposes. Furthermore, the effectiveness of many accepted uses of these drugs (with the exception of the oral contraceptive) has never been proven by scientific clinical trials, although professional belief in their efficacy persists based on clinical impressions of apparent benefits. The safety of these drugs has been the subject of much controversy and disagreement among scientists and federal health policy makers.

A wide range of serious adverse side effects has been associated with every use of these hormone drugs. Two unprecedented epidemics associated with estrogen use in young women have been recorded: (1) vaginal cancer, the first demonstration of human transplacental carcinogenesis, and (2) uterine cancer, the most dramatic increase in a cancer rate ever recorded by epidemiologists. Several current studies also point to the likelihood that widespread estrogen use will result in an increase in female breast cancer in the population. In spite of this, the use of estrogens in medical practice for elective uses has increased. Critics of this practice have therefore expressed concern that women consumers of estrogen drugs are not receiving accurate information about the risks of these drugs.

WIDESPREAD USE OF ESTROGEN DRUGS

Accurate data are unavailable on the extent of estrogen use in medical practice in the United States today. However, a survey of physicians indicates that about 90 million prescriptions are being written annually for a U.S. adult female population of 60 million (*National Disease and Therapeutic Index* 1975). Ten million take the oral contraceptive, and noncontraceptive estrogens are used by 15 to 30 percent of American women (Pettiti 1979). Another four million menopausal women take estrogen to replace declining levels of estrogen (*FDA Drug Bulletin* 1979). Other unknown millions of women have been given estrogen as a lactation inhibitor after childbirth, and millions more have taken estrogen as an experimental morning-after pill contraceptive (Weiss 1975). In addition, an unknown number of estrogen prescriptions are written every year for women for cosmetic uses like treatment of acne and thinning hair (National Cancer Institute 1977).

SAFETY AND EFFICACY OF ESTROGENS

In assessing the benefit-risk ratio in the taking of drugs, one must question whether the taking of any drug is necessary, safe, and effective. This chapter will deal in a later section with the question of whether many of the current uses of estrogen are really necessary. The following comments will be directed toward their safety and efficacy.

Questionable Effectiveness of Estrogen Drugs

Most uses of estrogens have never been subjected to proper clinical studies to prove their effectiveness. Instead, their use is rationalized on the basis of clinical impressions and isolated case reports of their effectiveness.

For most uses of estrogen, there are no reports in the medical literature about any well-controlled scientific studies conducted to prove the safe and effective use of estrogen in any dose or duration for the treatment of even generally recognized medical conditions, although there is much literature recommending its use (Holsten 1971). Moreover, some uses that have enjoyed scientific endorsement have been subsequently shown to be ineffective. Millions of prescriptions are still written for menopausal women for uses classified by the FDA as "not effective," "possibly effective," or "probably effective." As one example, the effectiveness of estrogen as a morning-after pill was originally reported as 100 percent (Kuchera 1971). Further study places its efficacy closer to 60 percent (Jones and McAllister 1977), which considerably lowers the benefit-risk ratio in view of its adverse effects. It was also recently recommended that by the FDA that doctors discontinue the use of estrogens to prevent postpartum breast engorgement, a time-honored practice in American obstetrics. This was after millions of women had received it, many without their knowledge, as a part of routine obstetrical care.

Adverse Effects

The adverse effects of estrogen preparations can range from unnoticed subclinical alterations of blood chemistry, to death from myocardial infarction or uterine cancer. A wide range of physiological systems are affected because the introduction of additional estrogen (an important and pivotal hormone in human biochemistry) acts on some 50 metabolic systems in all women who take estrogen, not just in those who experience and identify adverse effects.

Most adverse effects from estrogen drugs have been noted among women who take the oral contraceptive or estrogen replacement at menopause (ER), possibly because these are the most commonly used estrogens and the most thoroughly investigated. Since 50 million women in the world are taking the "pill," oral contraceptive users form the largest population in which to study the possible adverse effects of all estrogen drugs. Each year about 250 articles are published in the medical literature reporting on the wide range of adverse reactions that have been observed with varying incidences in women on the pill.

Noncancer Diseases.   Noncancer diseases that the pill has been shown to cause or exacerbate in susceptible women are: heart disease (myocardial infarction, coronary thrombosis, hypertension), visual disorders, cerebrovascular disease, liver tumors and jaundice, gallbladder disease, uterine fibroids, cervical erosion, cellular changes of varying severity in breast and cervix, anemia, gastrointestinal disease and nausea, vaginal infections, migraine and severe depression, skin diseases, loss of hair, chronic premenstrual syndrome, inability to conceive after discontinuing the pill, and distorted sex ratio (more females conceived after discontinuance) (McQueen 1978; Seaman and Seaman 1978). If a woman accidentally takes the pill during early pregnancy, she runs a double risk of having a child with congenital limb and heart malformations (Nora and Nora 1973).

Female Cancer.   Each year about 200,000 new cases of cancer of the estrogen target organs are diagnosed in American women (National Cancer Institute 1971). Of these, 90,000 are breast cancer, 37,000 are uterine cancer, 60,000 are cervical, 17,000 ovarian. It is not known what portion of these cancers estrogen drugs are responsible for promoting. The studies that would be required to prove such data would be difficult to conduct, partly because the latency period between exposure to a carcinogen and the development of cancer can be 20 years or longer. That is why it will not be known for sure whether the pill increases the occurrence of breast and uterine cancer until 20 years after its wide use began in the late 1960s.

Epidemiological studies can never prove that a factor like estrogen use is the cause of cancer. They can only demonstrate a statistical association between an increased taking of estrogen and an increased incidence of cancer in certain groups of women. Dr. Roy Hertz, former Chief of Endocrinology of the National Cancer Institute, talks about the unproven relationship between estrogen and cancer:

> Our inadequate knowledge concerning the relationship of estrogen to cancer in women is comparable with what was known about the association between lung cancer and cigarette smoking before extensive study delineated this overwhelmingly significant relationship. [1972]

He goes on to say that in addition to increasing the incidence of female cancer in the population, estrogen drugs can also promote or exacerbate existing latent cancer in women (ibid). About 225,000 American women are presently thought to have unexpressed breast cancer, which can exist for about six years before it can be detected.* One woman in 14 at some time

---

*Based on National Cancer Institute's projected annual rates of developing breast cancer.

in her life will develop it, so in using hormones like the oral contraceptive, we are exposing at least this portion of women to a substance known to stimulate preexisting cancer.

Epidemiological studies have pointed to an association between estrogen drugs and female cancer (Ziel and Finkle 1976; Smith et al. 1976). The cancer-causing potential of these drugs was documented in the 1970s, although this could have been predicted much earlier from a knowledge of basic physiology: under increased levels of estrogen, the cells of the estrogen target organs (breasts, uterus, vagina, liver, pituitary gland, bone marrow) are subjected to an increase in stimulation, raising the potential for cancer-promoting activity.

Although the carcinogenic potential of estrogens has been suspected for over 40 years and has already been demonstrated in animal studies, human clinical evidence of cancer was unavailable before 1971 when vaginal cancer in the daughters of women receiving estrogen during pregnancy was documented (Herbst et al 1971). Thereafter, studies of the association between other uses of estrogens and cancer in other sites of the female body were done. The use of ER (estrogen replacement) was shown to be associated with an unprecedented increase of uterine lining cancer in women (Weiss et al. 1976); sequential oral contraceptives were shown to increase the risk of uterine lining cancer; ER and estrogens taken during pregnancy (DES mothers) increased ovarian and breast cancer ("DES and Breast Cancer" 1978; Bibbo 1977); and the combination oral contraceptive increased the incidence of liver cancer (Mallory 1978; Mays et al. 1976) and brain cancer (pituitary adenomas) (Sherman 1978).

The rate of female cancer is rising in the population in association with rising rates of estrogen use (Greenwald et al. 1977). Between the second National Cancer Survey in 1947 and the third in 1969–1971, we see an increase in cancer of almost every estrogen-dependent site; ovarian,

TABLE 4–1. Estrogen preparations that are epidemiologically associated with increases in cancer of specific sites.

Cancer in Female Organs	Associated Estrogen Drugs
Breast (small increase)	ER (estrogen replacement) Oral contraceptive
Cervical invasive	
Ovarian	ER DES mothers
Endometrial	ER Sequential oral contraceptive
Vaginal	DES in utero
Liver	Oral contraceptive
Pituitary adenoma	Oral contraceptive

Arrows indicate the types of female cancer that increase with the use of estrogen drugs.

endometrial, vaginal, liver, pituitary, and a slight increase in breast cancer (Cutler et al. 1976). Only cervical cancer shows a decrease over the decades, probably owing to earlier detection with the Pap smear.

EARLY EVIDENCE OF THE CARCINOGENICITY OF ESTROGENS

Estrogen drugs have been developed, marketed, and FDA-approved in spite of the existence of studies proving them unsafe and ineffective. Evidence of the potential of exogenous estrogens to cause female cancer was available as early as the 1930s (Dutton, in press). As early as the 1930s, the American Medical Association advised caution in the use of DES and other estrogens in gynecological practice. In the years that followed, numerous articles appeared in the medical and scientific literature discussing the hormone-cancer relationship: by 1947 there were over 300 articles and by 1960, 500 articles discussing an estrogen-cancer relationship. In spite of this and studies early in the 1950s that showed DES ineffective in preventing miscarriage, the FDA and the medical community allowed millions of pregnant women to be given the drug. In 1969, still a peak period of DES use in pregnancy, even the *Physicians' Desk Reference* contained a warning against its use because of possible adverse reactions on the fetus. Yet the drug enjoyed great popularity with obstetricians in spite of its uselessness and carcinogenicity. Even four years after the vaginal cancer-DES link was discovered and the nation's physicians received FDA warnings against use of hormones in pregnancy, data show that in 1975, physicians wrote 533,000 prescriptions for the use of hormones during pregnancy, only about 10 percent fewer than were written in 1972 when such cases were approved (Maugh 1976).

MENOPAUSAL USES OF ESTROGEN

There are 32 million women over age 50 in the United States today, and about 4 million menopausal women take estrogen on a daily basis (*FDA Drug Bulletin* 1979). The average age of menopause is 49. However, many younger women report being encouraged by their doctors to begin taking estrogen. The consumer appears convinced that estrogen is effective in relieving the discomforts of menopause. These include vasomotor fluctuations (hot flashes), hormonal fluctuations (mood changes), vaginal dryness (making intercourse difficult), ageing skin, and the gradual development of osteoporosis (loss of bone density).

Prescribing physicians regard menopause and its declining levels of endogenous (produced inside the body) estrogen as a disease rather than as a normal ageing process, and they seek to alter a woman's normal physiology with ER. This involves risk because: (1) breast cancer in the general population is known to be increased among women whose age of menopause is late, implying that prolonged endogenous estrogen production influences cells of the breast; (2) exogenous estrogens in ER are implicated in an unprecedented risk of the incidence of uterine cancer; and (3) the type of estrogen use in ER (estrone) may be particularly carcinogenic (Cole and McMahon 1969; Sitreri and Schwartz 1974).

Critics of liberal prescribing of estrogen have pointed out that three-fourths of the prescriptions for ER are not warranted, either because they are unnecessary, or not effective, or because they offer benefits that are trivial in comparison to the risk of uterine cancer and the 20 percent incidence of nausea that accompanies their use (Wolfe 1978). Other side effects of ER include hypertension, gallbladder disease, and angina pectoris (Judd et al. 1981).

ER has been found to be effective for treatment of hot flashes, which 75 percent of women experience at the menopause. Short-term treatment is recommended for the shortest possible duration, but a survey found that the average amount of time spent on ER by most women is ten years (Stadel and Weiss 1975). ER is classified by the FDA as "probably effective" for the prevention of osteoporosis, a condition that requires long-term therapy, so this treatment is not recommended for all women. Osteoporosis affects 10 to 25 percent of postmenopausal women and can lead to bone fractures, especially in sedentary women. Although no research has been done into more natural ways to protect against normal bone loss, such as increased calcium in the diet, it is known that exercise can retard the loss of bone density. The FDA also classified estrogen as "not effective" for the treatment of nervous symptoms, anxiety, and depression. Yet of 8 million prescriptions examined in the survey, 598,000 were written for "symptoms of senility," 246,000 for "mental disorders," and 1 million for "special conditions without sickness" (ibid.).

The incidence of endometrial (uterine lining) cancer has increased rapidly during recent years, paralleling the increased postmenopausal use of estrogens. Data suggest that this rise in cancer followed the rise in estrogen use (Greenwald et al. 1977). In the 1970s, several studies were published to the effect that women who take ER are increasing their risk of developing uterine cancer by about 8 times, and for those who use it for more than seven years (as most users do), the increased risk is nearly 14-fold (Ziel Finkle et al. 1976).

If 4 million U.S. women are using ER and the increased rate of uterine cancer is 8 times more than the normally found 1 per thousand incidence in the general population, then ER may be causing an annual increase of 32,000 cancers in American women. New York State Cancer Registry data show an increase in endometrial cancer of 68 percent during the period 1960–1974 (Greenwald et al. 1977).

A thorough reevaluation of the medical indications for ER is urgently needed, along with research into alternative treatments. If a woman elects to take ER, she should ask her physician to prescribe the lowest dosage for the shortest period of time, preferably in a tapering dosage. She should avoid it if she has a family history of cancer or heart disease. Because of ER's recent association with uterine cancer, the manufacturer of Premarin (Ayerst) now advises physicians to prescribe it cyclically with progesterone. The addition of progesterone is thought to reduce the incidence of endometrial cancer, but progesterone does not prevent all of the adverse effects of estrogen, and addition of progesterone to ER results in the resumption of periodic vaginal bleeding. Critics claim there is insufficient evidence that sequential use of estrogen and progesterone will decrease the risk of cancer. Rather, the use of progesterone and estrogen in the sequential oral contraceptives was associated with an *increased* risk of uterine cancer.

A PROPOSAL TO MAKE ESTROGEN REPLACEMENT THERAPY (ERT) SAFER

Replacement therapy with synthetic hormones at menopause might be safer if the dosage were made to mimic the body's natural production of estrogen and progesterone. Since ovarian output of hormones varies every day in the month, replacement hormones should be taken in a different dosage every day to stimulate the normal premenopausal cycle. By taking ERT in this way, the chances of promoting cancer would be lessened. This is because the cells of the estrogen target organs (uterus, breast, and others) would be allowed the natural periodic rest from estrogen stimulation that endogenous hormone production allows and to which they are accustomed.

One factor in the growth of cancer in the estrogen target organs is continuous stimulation by estrogen, which encourages the proliferation of cells, including any existent mutagenic cells. If natural fluctuations of the hormone during the monthly cycle were copied, this would reduce the insult of continual estrogen stimulation to the target tissues.

Presently ERT is given in a continuous flat (and high) dosage, most often not even with progesterone added to counter endometrial proliferation.

TYPES OF ESTROGEN

Until recently, DES, a synthetic nonsteroidal estrogen, was the type used as menopausal ER, as well as for the morning-after pill contraceptive and for other uses. Recently there has been a switch to other types of estrogen (estradiol and others) because DES was shown to be carcinogenic. Premarin, a natural estrogen derived from pregnant mares' urine, is primarily used now for menopausal ER. However, endocrinologists warn that all estrogens, whether synthetic or natural, have the same effect on biochemical systems and carcinogenesis (Hertz 1972). The addition of any exogenous (from outside the body) estrogen over that produced by the body disturbs a natural balance, which even under ideal conditions is precarious, as demonstrated by the fact that many women with high endogenous estrogen profiles develop breast cancer.

Estrogen hormones probably do not *cause* cancer but rather act as growth hormones for existing latent cancer. Cancer is caused by mutations in the cell produced by viruses or carcinogens. The mutant cell multiplies during mitosis and responds to surges of hormonal stimulation. Estrogen can act to accelerate existing cancer or to transform hyperplasia into cancer.

"THE PILL"

In addition to the many noncancer diseases caused by or associated with the pill in susceptible women (many without high-risk profiles or family history of disease), the pill is associated with cancer.

The pill has apparently increased breast cancer in two population subgroups: (1) women with benign breast disease, and (2) women who took the pill before having their first child (Fasal and Paffenbarger 1975). Cervical cancer is also three times more common in women who have used the pill for at least four years as in women who never used it (Peritz et al. 1977). Uterine cancer in very young women has been associated with the sequential oral contraceptives (which employ estrogen for part of the cycle, then progesterone). Fatal liver tumors (both benign and malignant) are increased by eight times in pill users. Pituitary adenomas have been observed in women after they discontinue the combination pill. Malignant melanoma is also suspected to be increased in pill users.

Although these cancer diseases have been observed in small groups of pill takers, they are not yet statistically proven to be a result of the pill. As mentioned earlier, because of the latency period for cancer expression, epidemiologists cannot be certain whether the pill will result in a large-scale increase in female cancer until 20 years after widespread use of the pill began in the late 1960s.

However, according to Dr. Hertz, once a woman has taken the pill, she has permanently altered the cellular structure of her uterine lining:

> [Cancer of the endometrium] arises in a tissue which is delicately controlled by the hormonal balance in women. That the oral contraceptives disturb this balance is readily observable on microscopic examination of samples of this tissue. . . . It is important to appreciate that the renewed uterine lining is

generated from the persistent remnants of the same lining which has previously undergone these profound changes (of estrogen stimulation). Hence, the impact of these earlier cellular changes is transmitted to the subsequently developed tissues for the remainder of the patient's life. . . . [1972]

DES: A CASE STUDY IN HORMONE ABUSE

DES is a synthetic nonsteroidal estrogen whose use was favored over other estrogens because it was orally active and inexpensive to manufacture. It became popular for the treatment of pregnancy complications in the 1940s after two articles appeared in the medical literature claiming it to be effective (Karnaky 1942; Smith 1948). These studies were criticized as being inadequate, and in 1952, two major medical centers in Boston and Chicago used DES in controlled clinical experimentation on women attending their obstetrical clinics to prove or disprove its therapeutic value in pregnancy. In 1953 and 1958, several well-designed scientific studies were published in medical journals showing that DES was of no value in reducing the incidence of spontaneous abortion, prematurity, postmaturity, perinatal mortality, or toxemias in pregnancy (Dieckman et al. 1953; Goldzieher and Benigno 1958).

In addition to the findings regarding its uselessness, data on its carcinogenicity continued to accrue. Yet the safety and efficacy of prenatal DES seem to have been immune from questioning by obstetricians. DES continued to be widely prescribed to pregnant women who had any indication of a tendency toward miscarriage, in some cases simply as prophylactic "prenatal care." Between 1960 and 1970, an estimated 20,000 to 100,000 pregnant women per year were prescribed DES (Heinonen 1973). In sum, data suggest that after 1941, DES and other synthetic estrogens were prescribed to an estimated 6 million women in the United States before the practice was largely discontinued in 1971 (Weiss 1975).

Vaginal Cancer

In 1971, seven cases of an extremely rare type of cancer (clear-cell adenocarcinoma of the vagina or cervix) appeared in young women in one Boston hospital (Herbst, Ulfelder, and Poskanzer 1971). Following a suggestion of one of their mothers, an investigation was made and it was found that all of the mothers had been given DES during their gestation. In the following nine years, nearly 400 cases of this cancer in females ages 7 to 29 were reported around the country (Herbst 1979). Most of these women have been able to document that they were exposed in utero to DES some time between the 8th and 17th week of gestation, when the fetal vagina was forming. It is expected that more cases will develop as additional cohorts of DES daughters reach adolescence, when the cancer develops in response to increased stimulation of the vaginal tissues from rising levels of estrogen at adolescence. Peak incidence is at age 19, and it levels off after age 24. The risk of adenocarcinoma is estimated to be between .14 and 1.4 per 1000 exposed, meaning that reported cases will increase (Herbst et al. 1978). Over 80 deaths have occurred to date.

Vaginal Adenosis

It is believed that virtually all of the estimated 3 million DES daughters sustained damage to their genital tract during its development. Studies have shown that more than 90 percent of DES daughters have vaginal adenosis or cervical ectropion (Stafl et al. 1974). These are conditions wherein the exposed lining of the vagina or cervix is made up of glandular cells not covered by the normal protective layer of squamous epithelium. Like vaginal adenocarcinoma, adenosis was also an infrequently seen condition before prenatal DES use. Adenosis is not the precursor of adenocarcinoma, although it always accompanies it (Welch 1978). It is expected that this glandular layer of active cellular change will convert to normal squamous epithelium in most cases.

Squamous Cell Cancer of the Cervix or Vagina and Other Abnormalities

DES daughters may prove to be at increased risk of squamous cell cancer of the cervix and vagina. This more common type of cancer typically develops, in non-DES-exposed women, in the small area of exposed glandular cells (ectropion) on the cervix. However, in DES daughters, this area of active cellular change often covers the entire cervix and vagina and constitutes an area that is highly vulnerable to insult from physical, bacterial, and chemical agents. So far, 2 to 6 percent of adenosis patients studied have squamous cell dysplasia (precancer) or carcinoma in situ of the cervix (or more infrequently, of the vagina) (Robboy et al. 1978). This raises the question of whether adenosis (active squamous cell metaplasia) is on a continuum with squamous cell cancer. Pap smears are negative in 50 percent of cases during the dysplastic phase (Veridiano et al.). However, as more DES daughters with adenosis mature to the age when the incidence of squamous cell cancer of the cervix normally rises (after age 40), we may see an increased incidence of this type of cancer in them.

In addition to these developmental abnormalities of the cells of the genital tract lining, about two-thirds of DES daughters have congenital structural abnormalities of the uterus and cervix, which *may* make childbearing difficult. These are cervicovaginal ridges, small uteruses, and distortions of the cervical canal. A few DES daughters with malformation of the cervix have developed cervical incompetency during the second trimester of pregnancy (Goldstein 1978). DES daughters have ectopic (tubal) pregnancies 19 times more frequently than normal women. However, the majority of DES daughters who have tried have been able to have normal children. An as yet undetermined percentage of DES daughters also suffer from severe menstrual cycle imbalances.

Abnormalities in Males Linked to Prenatal Use of DES

There is a suspected but unproven association of DES exposure to testicular cancer in males at present. More commonly, nonmalignant abnormalities, epididymal cysts, small genitals, and abnormalities of the urethra have been reported (Bibbo, Gill, and Azizi 1977, Cosgrove et al. 1977). In one recent study it was found that about 25 percent of 163 DES-exposed males had nonmalignant abnormalities compared to only 6 percent of 168 controls (Bibbo, Gill, and Azizi 1977). In the same study, semen analysis of a smaller group of 38 exposed and 25 control subjects revealed decreased ejaculate volume and low-normal values for sperm density and motility. Severely pathologic semen were assessed in 28 percent of the 38 DES-exposed males compared to 0 in the controls. In a study in which male mice were exposed prenatally to DES, 60 percent were sterile and 15 of 24 animals had anatomic or microscopic anomalies of the testis (McLachlen, Newbold, and Bullock 1975).

These findings should be interpreted with caution, as the numbers of DES sons studied have been small. The implications of these findings for reproductive capacity in DES sons will not be known until further follow-up is done.

Effects in DES Mothers

Data from the University of Chicago obstetrics clinic where the original experiments were conducted with prenatal DES indicate that the women who took DES to prevent miscarriage may be at an increased risk of breast cancer, and to a lesser extent, of cervical and ovarian cancer.

DES: Banned for Cattle, Approved for Women

For over a decade, scientists had been lobbying to secure an FDA ban on DES as an additive to cattle feed because small residues of DES were remaining in beef marketed for human consumption. But not until vaginal cancer in women exposed to DES in utero was reported in 1971 did we have clinical evidence that DES could cause cancer in humans. Consequently, in 1972 the FDA banned DES as a cattle feed, even though residues of only 0.3 microgram were remaining in marketed beef. In contrast to this decision on cattle feed, in 1973 the FDA approved a new 250 mg. dosage of DES for use as a morning-after pill even though this amount represents 833,000 times the amount of DES banned for human consumption (Weiss 1975). And although approval of the morning-after pill was to be for "emergency uses only, such as rape and incest," there are no legal limitations on a physician's judgment of what constitutes an "emergency."

The Morning-After Pill

In spite of the carcinogenicity of lower doses of DES and its experimental status as a morning-after pill, some 2 million women continued to receive it through university health services and private physicians in the early 1970s. When this situation was called to the attention of a congressional investigating committee, the FDA quickly moved to approve the morning-after pill. This was done without first requiring the manufacturer to apply for an investigational new drug application (INDA) and in the absence of the three studies that are required by law (1962 Harris-Kefauver Amendment to the Food, Drug, and Cosmetic Act) to show safety and efficacy of a drug before approval. Instead, FDA approval was granted on the basis of one study at the University of Michigan student health service, which resulted in the claim that DES was 100 percent effective in preventing pregnancy in 1000 women exposed to unprotected intercourse (Kuchera 1971). Subsequent investigations of that study by an NIH committee revealed that there had been inadequate follow-up to determine if the pill had been effective, and further, that some pregnancies had occurred in the series but had been excluded from the official study. Also, not all of the 1000 women were at midcycle and therefore at risk of pregnancy. Two years and millions of prescriptions later, FDA approval for manufacture of the 25 mg. tablet of DES (ten tablets to be taken in a series) was revoked. At this time, manufacturers began producing 5-mg. tablets that physicians could legally prescribe in greater quantity as a morning-after pill.

In 1973, congressional subcommittee hearings on human experimentation examined the problem of widespread prescription of the morning-after pill and concluded that new legislation governing unapproved uses of drugs and informed consent of patients is sorely needed. The hearings concluded that FDA and HEW reliance on institutional peer review committees to monitor experimentation is inadequate. Evidence was presented that experimentation on humans is not limited to clinical trials but is sometimes part of the routine practice of medicine (Senate Committee on Labor and Public Welfare 1973).

A survey of women conducted at the university where the pilot study of the morning-after pill's effectiveness took place not only showed inadequate follow-up to determine the pill's effectiveness but also noted that its adverse effects had been overlooked, and that there had been inadequate testing of recipients for possible contraindications. Furthermore, none of the women in the study were asked if they were DES daughters (ibid.).

In spite of these facts and the revoked approval of DES as a postcoital contraceptive, in 1973 the Center for Population Research of the NIH awarded contracts to university health services and family planning agencies to test the effectiveness of other estrogens as morning-after pills in spite of the testimony of National Cancer Institute endocrinologists that all estrogens are as carcinogenic as DES (Hertz 1972).

The prescribing of the morning-after pill to young women places the present generation of DES daughters at particular risk. Further stimulation of target organs with the massive doses of estrogen could increase their risk of developing adenocarcinoma. Many may already have occult adenocarcinoma, the growth of which would be exacerbated by estrogen. Yet the specialized testing to determine if adenosis or adenocarcinoma is present (iodine stain test and colposcopy) is seldom if ever performed on a patient before a morning-after pill is prescribed.

Furthermore, in most cases, the morning-after pill is prescribed to alleviate only the fear of pregnancy, although the chances of actually becoming pregnant from one unprotected intercourse are only 4 to 10 percent (Tietze 1960). The morning-after pill itself is only about 60 percent effective (Jones and McAllister 1977), and if it fails to abort an incipient pregnancy, that embryo will be exposed to the effects of DES. Thus the development and regulation of the morning-after pill constitutes a typical example of scientific ambivalence in regard to the protection of the public from a dangerous, unnecessary, and ineffective drug.

SOCIAL, POLITICAL, AND ECONOMIC FACTORS IN ESTROGEN PROMOTION

There are social, political, and economic influences on scientific judgments made by physicians, medical researchers, and government regulatory agencies. Physicians may receive some form of financial benefit from representatives of the drug industry for prescribing certain drugs; medical researchers may be supported by funds from the drug industry when researching the safety and efficacy of drugs; and government regulatory agencies may share the interests of the drug industry rather than those of the general public.

Both industrial pressures and population control interests appear to have influenced FDA approval of the oral contraceptive, the antimiscarriage drug, and the morning-after pill prior to the accomplishment of sufficient testing to prove their safety. The antimiscarriage drug was developed during a period of social and economic pressure for population growth (1945–1955). Spontaneous abortion, a concomitant of many early pregnancies, was not viewed as a natural population fertility regulator but as a disease to be conquered. Conversely, in present times of overpopulation, the same drug is used to achieve the opposite effect: estrogen becomes an abortifacient (morning-after pill). With the development of both uses of estrogen as a fertility regulator, social and economic interests appear to take precedence over concern for the safety of women.

The profit motives of pharmaceutical companies is also a factor in the promotion of estrogen drugs. Since the synthesis of estrogens 50 years ago, drug firms have devised numerous uses for them and have advertised them to physicians in medical journals. In this way, the scientific direction of medical care is in part determined by the economic motives of a profit-making industry.

The pharmaceutical industry is a $5 billion industry that averages an 8 percent higher profit margin than other major industries (Kefauver Subcommittee 1960). Numerous congressional hearings have been held on questionable practices of the drug industry that result in products being promoted that are a known hazard to the public (Hertz, 1972, et al.). When so much profit is involved in the manufacture of estrogen drugs, it makes an objective assessment of their risks extremely difficult for industrial scientists. For example, the pharmaceutical industry earns $199 million annually from the manufacture of oral contraceptives (*Health Industries Handbook* 1977). Menopausal Premarin earns the industry another $40 million annually (ibid.). In 1962, the wholesale value of domestic shipments of estrogen (excluding contraceptives) was $15,422,000, and this increased by 437 percent to $82,777,000 in 1975 (Kefauver Subcommittee 1960). Sales of DES by its major manufacturer, Eli Lily Co., actually increased by 4 percent in the nine months following the news of the vaginal cancer link because of promotion of their new DES drug, the morning-after pill (Smith et al. 1976).

Under this private enterprise system, what is seen as best for the consumer's welfare (such as DES in cattle feed, the antimiscarriage drug, or the morning-after pill) is determined in part by an industry that profits from the manufacture and sale of the drug. FDA Chief Counsel explains that "industry is likely to challenge in the courts any FDA action where the net adverse economic impact exceeds the legal fees involved (National Academy of Sciences 1974).

Conflict of Interest and Laxity of FDA

Congressional subcommittees have examined potential conflicts of interest between the medical-research industry and governmental regulatory agencies, agencies that permit the profusion of new, often inadequately tested, prescription drugs on the market. Major drug companies spend approximately $3000 per physician annually to influence the nation's 200,000 physicians in their choice of drugs for their patients (Kefauver Subcommittee 1960). About half of the revenues of the AMA comes from advertisements that drug companies place in its journal. Medical researchers also may be supported by the drug industry when researching the safety and efficacy of new drugs. Approval of these drugs hinges on their scientific evaluation of research data. However, when conflicting results are obtained, the assessment in the final analysis becomes a subjective one—sensitive to benefits to the assessor. At present, scientific data evaluating new drugs are considered a trade secret of the industry.

The FDA oversees drug companies' activities by approving of new drugs to be marketed by the industry, ensuring their safety and efficacy. But critics of FDA performance have called attention to scores of instances over past years where regulatory judgments were influenced by the interests of the pharmaceutical industry. Many new drugs and combination drugs have obtained FDA approval for manufacture and sale on the basis of faulty or inadequate studies. FDA tolerance of the profusion of new, often inadequately tested prescription drugs on the market is unquestionably a major contributing cause of the vaginal and uterine cancer epidemics (Senate Committee on Labor and Public Welfare 1973).

Many pharmaceutical preparations have been used as time-honored medicines for major diseases when they are actually ineffective in treating those diseases and/or cause direct or latent injury. According to a Senate subcommittee on competition in the drug industry:

> There exists little convincing scientific evidence to support many of the cited indications for the use of drugs that are currently in good standing in medical practice. (Holsten 1971, p. 1202)

In 1970, the American Public Health Association sued the FDA to compel it to enforce the 1962 drug effectiveness amendments to the Food, Drug, and Cosmetic Act. The FDA was to remove more than 7000 drugs from the market. In 1979, although 482 of these drugs still remained, the agency said it regarded the program as substantially completed. The public spends an estimated $1 billion a year for these drugs ("Suit Forces FDA Agreement" 1980).

Federal regulatory agencies are reluctant to ban drugs and infringe on the rights of private corporate interests with whom they seem to share a symbiotic relationship. This reluctance of the FDA to ban a drug before absolute proof of damage has occurred in a significant number of people has been investigated by several congressional committees. For example:

> Despite urgent recommendation (in March 1971) and although DES had not been shown to be effective in preventing spontaneous abortion, FDA took no

action to inform physicians of the danger of DES use during pregnancy until November 10, 1971. . . . FDA's failure to act promptly in this instance delayed public health protection for 5 months and this delay might well have been substantially longer in the absence of the subcommittee's investigation of this matter. [Committee on Government Operations 1972]

And a spokesman for the California FDA has said this:

I cannot find reported in the medical literature any well controlled, scientific studies conducted to prove the safe and effective use of DES in any dose or duration for treatment of even the generally recognized medical conditions, although there is ample literature of endorsement. [Holsten 1971, p. 1202]

In 1974, Senate hearings examined claims by FDA employees that the drug industry dominates FDA decisions about approval of new drugs. FDA approval is supposed to hinge on a determination of their benefit versus risk to the consumer. However, congressional investigations have enumerated instances where definitions of benefit-risk ratio were made using drug industry rather than consumer criteria, i.e., where the risks to the consumer were not properly weighed against the benefits to the drug industry. Former FDA Commissioner James Goddard has stated:

The Drug Establishment is a close-knit, self-perpetuating power structure consisting of drug manufacturers, government agencies and select members of the medical profession. [Senate Committee on Labor and Public Relations 1973]

CONCLUSION

The period of DES use in pregnancy coincided with perhaps the strongest antifeminist period in recent history. No doctor would have allowed a mere woman, especially a pregnant woman, to express a medical opinion. A DES mother would have had little influence over her treatment when the doctor (and probably her husband) patronized her as an emotional, childlike creature, incapable of logical decision making. And the patient was so strongly conditioned to disbelieve in her own mental powers and abilities that even had she been aware of the risks, she would have been reassured by being told that she could not possibly know a medical fact that a doctor had missed (Molton 1982).

Little information is available today on whether women are giving informed consent to the prescribing of estrogens. These drugs are important causes of cancer among women, and to date no research has been done to determine if women are being informed by their physicians that the estrogen being prescribed has possible side effects of cancer and heart disease.

Clearly, informed consent in medical care is the strongest protective measure against malpractice. Women are increasingly protecting themselves by caring for their own health, by questioning their doctors on the details of treatment, and by avoiding unnecessary contact with the medical industry by using natural remedies and self-treatment wherever possible.

Many gynecology textbooks such as those discussed in Part I illustrate how misunderstandings of female psychophysiology have historically lead to inappropriate therapy of women and explain why sex hormones are still used today to routinely alter women's normal physiology. Since the synthesis of estrogen 50 years ago, numerous uses for these drugs have been created by drug companies, and diseases have been defined into existence to be treated by them. Thus, fertility is seen as a disease and the oral contraceptive created to cure it; lactation after childbirth is seen as a disease and estrogen given to stop it; and menopause is seen as a deficiency disease and treated with sex hormones.

REFERENCES

Antunes, C., "Endometrial Cancer and Estrogen Use. Report of a Large Case-Control Study," *New England Journal of Medicine,* 300, no. 1 (1979), 9–13.

Bibbo, M., "Ovarian Cancer Associated with Use of DES," *Progress Report, NICHHD* (National Institute of Child Health and Human Development), August 1977.

Bibbo, M., W. Gill, and F. Azizi, 'Follow-up Study of Male and Female Offspring of DES-Exposed Mothers," *Obstetrics and Gynecology,* vol. 49 (1977):

Cole, P., and B. McMahon, "Oestrogen Fractions during Early Reproductive Life in the Aetiology of Breast Cancer," *Lancet,* 1 (1969), 604–6.

Committee on Government Operations, *FDA Regulations of Oral Contraceptives.* House of Representatives, 91st Congress, 2nd Session. Washington, D.C.: U.S. Govt. Printing Office, 1970.

———, *Regulation of Diethylstilbestrol and Other Drugs Used in Food Producing Animals.* House of Representatives, 93rd Congress, House Report 93–708. Washington, D.C.: U.S. Govt. Printing Office, 1973.

Cosgrove, M., B. Benton, and B. Henderson, "Male Genitourinary Abnormalities and Maternal Diethylstilbestrol," *Journal of Urology,* vol. 117 (1977).

Cutler, S., S. Devesa, and T. Barclay, "The Magnitude of the Breast Cancer Problem," *Recent Results in Cancer Research,* vol. 57 (1976).

"DES and Breast Cancer," *FDA Drug Bulletin,* vol. 8, no. 2 (March–April 1978).

Dieckman, W., et al., "Does the Administration of Diethylstilbestrol During Pregnancy Have Therapeutic Value?" *American Journal of Obstetrics and Gynecology:* vol. 56 (1948).

Dutton, D., *Innovation in Medicine: Policy Making and the Public.* Stanford University, Health Services Research, in press.

Fasal, E., and R. Paffenbarger, "Oral Contraceptives as Related to Cancer and Benign Lesions of the Breast, *Journal of the National Cancer Institute,* 55 (1975), 767–73.

FDA Drug Bulletin, February–March 1979.

Goldstein, D., "Incompetent Cervix in Offspring Exposed to Diethylstilbestrol in Utero," *Obstetrics and Gynecology*, 52 (1978), 73S-75S (Suppl. 1).

Goldzieher, J., and B. Benigno, "The Treatment of Threatened and Recurrent Abortion: A Critical Review," *American Journal of Obstetrics and Gynecology*, 75 (1958), 1202–14.

Greenwald, P., T. Caputo, and M. Wolfgang, "Endometrial Cancer after Menopausal Use of Estrogens," *Obstetrics and Gynecology*, 50 (1977), 239–43.

Health Industries Handbook, Menlo Park, Calif.: SRI International, 1977.

Heinomen, O., "Diethylstilbestrol in Pregnancy," *Cancer*, 31 (1973), 573–77.

Herbst, A. "Epidemiology of Vaginal Adenocarcinoma—Current Case Factors," *American Journal of Obstetrics and Gynecology*, vol. 1 (1979).

Herbst, A., et al., "Complications of Estrogen Use: Clinical Studies," *Pediatrics*, 62, no. 2 (1978), 1151–59.

Herbst, A., H. Ulfelder, and D. Poskanzer, "Adenocarcinoma of the Vagina: Association of Maternal Stilbestrol Therapy with Tumor Appearance in Young Women," *New England Journal of Medicine*, 284 (1971), 878–81.

Hertz, R., *Testimony in Regulation of Diethylstilbestrol: Its Use as a Drug in Humans and Animal Feeds*. Committee on Government Operations, House of Representatives, 92nd Congress, Part 1, November 11, 1971. Washington, D.C.: U.S. Govt. Printing Office, 1972.

Holsten, W., "Protecting Patients from Drugs," *New England Journal of Medicine* vol. 285 (1971).

Jones, V., and A. McAllister, *The Effectiveness of Diethylstilbestrol as a Postcoital Contraceptive for Rape Victims*. Atlanta, Ga.: Center for Disease Control, 1977. Mimeographed.

Judd, H. et al., "Estrogen Replacement Therapy," *Obstetrics and Gynecology*, vol. 58 (1981).

Karnaky, H., "The Use of Stilbestrol for the Treatment of Threatened and Habitual Abortion and Premature Labor: A Preliminary Report," vol. 35 (1942).

Kefauver Subcommittee on Antitrust and Monopoly, Parts 22/23. U. S. Senate Committee on the Judiciary. Washington, D.C.: U.S. Govt. Printing Office, 1960.

Kuchera, L. "Postcoital Contraception with Diethylstilbestrol," *JAMA*, 218 (1971), 562–63.

Lipsett, M., "Estrogen Use and Cancer Risk," *JAMA*, 237, no. 11 (1977), 1112–15.

Mallory, A., "Hepatic Tumors and Oral Contraceptives," *Gastroenterology*, 75, no. 3 (1978), 517–18.

Maugh, T., "Irrational Drug Prescribing and Birth Defects," *Science*, vol. 194 (1976).

Mays, E. et al., "Hepatic Changes in Young Women Ingesting Contraceptive Steroids: Hepatic Hemorrhage and Primary Hepatic Tumors," *JAMA*, 235, no. 7 (1976), 730–32.

McLachlan, J., R. Newbold, and B. Bullock, "Reproductive Tract Lesions in Male Mice Exposed Prenatally to Diethylstilbestrol," *Science*, vol. 190 (1975).

McQueen, E., "Human Steroid Contraceptives: A Further Review of Adverse Reactions," *Drugs*, vol. 16, no. 4 (1978).

Molton, Lawrence, EVIST Project. Stanford University, Health Services Research, 1982.

National Academy of Sciences, *How Safe is 'Safe'? The Design of Policy on Drugs and Food Additives*. Washington, D.C.: U.S. Govt. Printing Office, 1974.

National Cancer Institute, *Third National Cancer Survey, 1969–71*.

———, *Diethylstilbestrol*, Monograph. Menlo Park, Calif.: SRI International, 1977.

National Disease and Therapeutic Index. Ambler, Pa.: IMS America, Ltd., 1975.

Nora, J., and A. Nora, "Proceedings of the Teratology Society" (St. Jovitte, Quebec), *Lancet*, vol. 1 (1973).

Peritz, E., S. Ramacharan, and J. Frank, "Walnut Creek Contraceptive Drug Study," *American Journal of Epidemiology*, vol. 106 (1977).

Pettiti, D., *JAMA*, 242 (1979), 1150–54.

Robboy, S., "Squamous Cell Dysplasia and Carcinoma in Situ of the Cervix and Vagina after Prenatal Exposure to DES," *Obstetrics and Gynecology*, 51, no. 5 (1978), 528–35.

Seaman, B., and G. Seaman, *Women and the Crisis of Sex Hormones*. New York: Bantam Books, Inc., 1978.

Select Committee on Small Business, *Task Force on Prescription Drugs*. U.S. Senate, 90th Congress, 2nd Session. Washington, D.C.: U.S. Govt. Printing Office, 1968.

———, *Competitive Problems in the Drug Industry*. Hearings before a Subcommittee on Monopoly. U.S. Senate, February–March 1973. Washington, D.C.: U.S. Govt. Printing Office, 1973.

Senate Committee on Labor and Public Welfare, *Quality of Health Care—Human Experimentation*, Part 1, 93rd Congress, February 21–22. Washington, D.C.: U.S. Govt. Printing Office, 1973.

Sherman, B., "Pathogenesis of Prolactin-Secreting Pituitary Adenomas," *Lancet*, 2, no. 8098 (1978), 1019–21.

Sitieri, P., B. Schwartz, and P. MacDonald, "Estrogen Receptors and the Estrone Hypothesis in Relation to Endometrial and Breast Cancer," *Gynecol*, 2 (1974), 228–38.

Smith, D., "Diethylstilbestrol in the Prevention and Treatment of Complications of Pregnancy," *American Journal of Obstetrics and Gynecology*, vol. 56 (1948).

Smith, D. et al., "Association of Exogenous Estrogens and Endometrial Carcinoma," *New England Journal of Medicine*, 293 (1976), 1167–70.

Stafl, D. et al., "Clinical Diagnosis of Vaginal Adenosis," *Obstetrics and Gynecology*, 43 (1974), 118–28.

"Suit Forces FDA Agreement to Remove 3,000 Medicines," *San Francisco Chronicle*, September 29, 1980.

Tietze, C., "Problems of Pregnancy Resulting from a Single Unprotected Coitus," *Fertility.and Sterility*, 11 (1960), 485–88.

Veridiano, N., L. Tancer, and E. Weiner, "Squamous Cell Carcinoma in Situ of the Vagina and Cervix after Intrauterine DES Exposure," *Obstetrics and Gynecology*, 52 (1978), 30S–33S (Suppl. 1).

Weiss, K., "Vaginal Cancer: An Iatrogenic Disease," *International Journal of Health Services*, vol. 5 (1975).

Weiss., N., D. Szekely, and D. Austin, "Increasing Incidence of Endometrial Cancer in the U.S.," *New England Journal of Medicine*, 294 (1976), 1259–62.

Welch, R., *Pathology Annual*, vol. 13 (1978).

Wolfe, S., Health Research Group, Washington, D.C., personal communication, 1978.

Ziel, H., and W. Finkle, "Increased Risk of Endometrial Carcinoma among Users of Conjugated Estrogens," *New England Journal of Medicine,* 293 (1976), 1164–67.

SUGGESTED READINGS

Fenichel, Stephen, and Lawrence Charfoos, *Daughters at Risk: A Personal DES History.* New York: Doubleday & Co., Inc., 1981.

Orenberg, Cynthia Laitman, *DES: The Complete Story.* New York: St. Martin's Press, 1981.

Chapter Five

WOMEN, DRUGS, AND PHYSICIANS

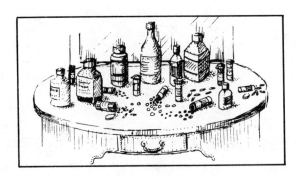

Linda S. Fidell

MISPRESCRIBING OF DRUGS: SPECIAL INPACT ON WOMEN

The misprescribing of drugs has special impact on women for several reasons. First, because women go to physicians more often than men do, they receive and fill 50 percent more prescriptions for drugs than men. Thus women are more involved with problems of effectiveness and safety of drugs. Second, because women tend to live longer, and because there are special problems associated with drug ingestion by the elderly, more women than men are affected by the use of drugs. Last, for one category of drug—the psychotropics or mood-modifiers such as Valium—women receive many more prescriptions than men do and many more than their number of visits to physicians would warrant.

Misprescribing can occur for a number of reasons. It can be the wrong drug for the illness, the wrong drug for the patient, the wrong dosage, the wrong frequency or duration of a drug, or the wrong drug in combination with other drugs the person is taking. Two recent studies, one by the Institute of Medicine of the National Academy of Sciences and one by the Institute of Medicine, question the prescribing practices of physicians (Elliott 1979). In another study of prescribing patterns in a major metropolitan medical center, Maronde et al. (1971) discovered numerous examples of misprescribing. For example, these authors found that sedatives and tranquilizers are particularly likely to be prescribed in too large a quantity or in dangerous combinations.

FREQUENCY AND SERIOUSNESS OF ADVERSE DRUG REACTIONS

The frequency and seriousness of adverse drug reactions have been a source of controversy for some time. Jick (1974) reports that 75,000,000 American adults regularly take one or more drugs, and 300,000 hospital admissions a year are for adverse drug reactions (excluding those for drug addiction and attempted suicide). Drug reactions leading to hospitalization are, in decreasing order of frequency, neurologic-metabolic, cardiovascular, cutaneous, and hematologic.

In addition to those hospitalized specifically for drug reactions, an additional 10 to 18 percent of patients have adverse drug reactions (usually gastrointestinal) while hospitalized, of which 13 percent may prove fatal (Caranasos et al. 1974). Jick (1974) estimates that about 30 percent of hospitalized patients have adverse drug reactions involving 3,000,000 hospitalized Americans annually and resulting in a total of 29,000 deaths.

Talley and Laventurier (1974) estimate that between 60,000 and 140,000 deaths occur annually in the United States due to adverse drug reactions. However, Stetler estimates that the number of deaths is closer to 2000 or 3000 and notes that many persons who die of adverse drug reactions were seriously ill or quite elderly to begin with.

TYPES OF DRUGS IMPLICATED

The drugs most frequently implicated in inappropriate prescribing are the psychotropics (major and minor tranquilizers, sedatives and hypnotics, stimulants, and antidepressants). These drugs, especially the minor tranquilizers such as Valium and Librium, are extremely popular. The FDA (1980) reports that 68,000,000 prescriptions were filled for minor tranquilizers, half of them for Valium, in 1978. Although widely regarded as harmless, more recent evidence has linked these drugs to both psychological and physiological dependence, even at regularly prescribed levels of ingestion (30–40 mg./;day). According to the Federal Alert Warning Network, 54,000 people needed emergency room treatment in 1977 for Valium misuse and overuse.

Further, in combination with alcohol, Valium has become a leading method of suicide. In an excellent article, Waldron (1977) has summarized many economic and social factors that have influenced physicians in regard to this extremely high rate of prescribing. Some of the relevant factors in patient-physician interactions have also been summarized by the author of this chapter (Fidell 1980).

Although in a nationwide survey conducted in 1970–1971 a majority of Americans considered the psychotropic drugs effective (Mellinger et al. 1974), there is reason to believe that these drugs are not always effective in treating the specific conditions for which they are frequently prescribed. For instance, stimulants are ineffective in promoting weight loss and are no longer recommended for that purpose. The prescribing of sedatives and hypnotics in treating insomnia has also been questioned. Cooper (1977) reports that although it has been reasonably well established that the barbiturates and the nonbarbiturate hypnotics are ineffective against insomnia after 14 days of use, in 1976 Nembutal was prescribed for an average of 42 days per perscription, Seconal was prescribed for 33 days, and Tuinal for 40 days. In another careful study of the effectiveness of psychotropics in the treatment of migraine, Parnell and Cooperstock (1979) reported that 41 percent of people suffering migraine had received prescriptions for psychotropics but found them generally less effective than exercise or various forms of meditation.

On a somewhat humorous note, Dunea (1977) reports that in one hospital where residents were prescribing psychotropic or analgesic drugs to an average of 125 out of 200 patients daily, an order by the Chief of Medicine requiring no more than 10 tablets at a time without a countersignature by a second physician reduced the prescription rate to 12 per day. Approximately $150,000 was saved yearly, and neither patients nor physicians complained overly much about the restriction.

Currently, 91 million prescriptions for sex-hormone drugs are being written annually for a U.S. adult female population of approximately 60 million (Weiss 1982). Of estrogens prescribed to postmenopausal women, estimates are that 75 percent are not warranted because they are either unnecessary or ineffective for the purposes prescribed (Wolfe 1975). Although short-term treatment is recommended, most estrogen prescriptions are given for an average of ten years (Stadel and Weiss 1975). In 1975, physicians wrote 533,000 prescriptions for hormones during pregnancy, although they are contraindicated because of adverse effects on the fetus (Maugh 1976).

Dunea (1977) reports that Americans use 26,000 tons of antibiotics at a cost of $1–2 billion annually. He concludes that there is "too much prescribing of antibiotics for viral illnesses, by telephone, without prior cultures, or for questionable prophylaxis" (p. 241). Graedon (1976) reaches similar conclusions, as do Silverman and Lee (1974), who estimate that 90 percent or more of prescribing of antibiotics is inappropriate.

CONTINUED PRESCRIPTION DRUG ABUSE DESPITE ADVERSE PUBLICITY

Sometimes prescribing of a drug continues despite widespread publicity concerning its adverse effects. Silverman and Lee (1974) report such a case with the Parke-Davis antibiotic Chloromycetin, still promoted in Third World countries (Silverman 1977), which can produce severe blood disorders and death. Hiatt (1975) reported similar events with an orally administered antidiabetic drug that was capable of producing serious cardiovascular disease. Likewise, routinely prescribed antihypertensive drugs can cause serious adverse effects. In many of these cases, the drug companies have continued to promote and physicians to prescribe a drug with serious side effects for several years after the adverse effects were documented and published.

And then there is the strange case of the analgesics. As Moertel et al. (1974) report, aspirin has repeatedly been found to be more effective in double-blind studies than a placebo, most over-the-counter drugs, and commonly prescribed nonnarcotic prescription drugs. Darvon, on the other hand, with more than 30 million prescriptions a year, has repeatedly been found to be equivalent to a placebo.

SEGMENTS OF POPULATION MOST AFFECTED

Some segments of the population experience misprescribing more often than others, presumably because they take drugs more frequently. Caranasos, Stewart and Cluff (1974) found that patients for whom drugs are more frequently misprescribed are disproportionately over 61 years of age, Caucasian, and female. The political and economic considerations that influence prescribing by physicians, particularly to elderly patients, have been summarized by Kayne (1978). Summaries of disproportionate prescribing of psychotropic drugs to women are also available (Cooperstock 1978, 1979, 1980; see also the following extract from Fidell 1981). Most recent studies show that physicians write two-thirds of their prescriptions for psychotropics for women.

Frequent prescribing of psychotropic drugs in particular has been linked to feelings of anger or dislike toward the patient, and to the social class of the patient—where lower-class persons get more prescriptions (Shader, Binstock, and Scott 1968). Physicians who prescribe fewer drugs of all kinds have better medical educations, smaller work loads, more progressive attitudes, and a tendency to look on each patient as a whole entity, and to take the symptoms of the patient as indicative of a physiological, and not psychosomatic, disorder (Mechanic 1970; Maronde et al. 1971).

There are also differences between prescribing practices here and in several other countries (Lawson and Jick 1976). For example, when hospitalized, a North American receives an average of nine drugs compared to the Scot's four drugs. In hospitals, differences in prescribing remain—even when symptoms and diagnoses are held constant; American physicians prescribe more numerous drugs for each indication, and 26 percent of Americans have adverse drug reactions compared to 15 percent of Scots.

RECOMMENDATIONS FOR CONTINUING PHYSICIAN EDUCATION IN PHARMACOLOGY

Many who have surveyed the literature on drug therapy (Elliott 1979; Koch-Weser 1974; Silverman and Lee 1974) point to the bewildering array of new drugs or old drugs in new combinations offered up yearly by the pharmaceutical industry, as well as to the insufficient training in clinical pharmacology and drug interactions given in most medical schools. It seems especially important that physicians be offered an extensive and continuing education in pharmacology, both before and after formal medical education, by some agency other than the drug companies. While waiting for such educational programs to develop, the consuming public can protect itself by consulting books like this one, the excellent article by Weg (1978) on changing metabolic and nutritional effects of drugs with ageing, and the book by Graedon (1976), which lists side effects of drugs, the dangers of their reactions with other substances, and alternative remedies that may be safer and equally effective.

SEX DIFFERENCES IN PSYCHOTROPIC DRUG USE

Psychotropic drugs are mood-modifying drugs such as minor tranquilizers (Valium, Librium), major tranquilizers (Thorazine), sedatives and hypnotics (Seconal, Quaalude), antidepressants (Elavil), and stimulants (Preludin, Dexedrine).* Over-the-counter versions of minor tranquilizers, sedatives, and stimulants are available in drugstores. . . . Because women are more involved with drugs in these categories than are men, this article explores the relationship between sex differences and the extent, origin, and persistence of use.

Extent of Use

It is estimated that at least half of adult women have used psychotropic drugs at some time for medical purposes (Program for Women's Concerns 1977). In 1977, of 51,000,000 Americans who used tranquilizers, 63% were women. Of 17,000,000 who used stimulants, 71% were women (National Institute of Drug Abuse 1978b). Women receive 71% of the prescriptions for antidepressants (Hughes and Brewin 1979). In 1977, approximately 8,500,000 women were introduced by prescription to tranquilizers, 3,000,000 to sedatives, and 1,000,000 to stimulants (National Institute on Drug Abuse 1978b). Over

*This section is excerpted and reprinted from *Professional Psychology*, vol. 12, no. 1, February 1981).

two-thirds of the prescriptions for psychotropic drugs are written to women, fewer than one-third to men (*FDA Drug Bulletin* 1980).

Valium, a minor tranquilizer first introduced in 1963, is now our most heavily prescribed drug. Between May 1976 and April 1977, 57,000,000 prescriptions were written for Valium (National Institute on Drug Abuse 1978a). Although advertised as an antianxiety agency effective in treating depression, evidence suggests that different effects on women may be produced at different stages of the menstrual cycle, with antianxiety produced premenstrually but restlessness produced during the postmenstrual phase (Shader 1978). These figures on psychotropic drugs underestimate their actual use in at least two ways. First, drugs may not be categorized as psychotropic drugs. Estimates of nonmedical use (e.g., to "get high" from nonmedical sources or without medical indicators) suggest that at least 1,200,000 Americans, half of them women, are involved nationwide with amphetamines, barbiturates, and tranquilizers (New York State Division of Substance Abuse Series 1978).

Sex differences in use of psychotropic drugs occur primarily when the source is a physician. Nonmedical use and over-the-counter use (Balter and Levine 1971) are approximately equal for women and men. Interestingly, prescription use is longer term and more consistent than nonprescription use (Fidell 1977).

Consequences of Use

Although some (Mellinger et al. 1974) have argued that psychotropic drugs, particularly minor tranquilizers, are safe and, if anything, underutilized, their harmlessness has recently been questioned on at least three grounds. The first is that their use probably promotes symptom reduction rather than resolution of underlying problems. Treatment by a nonmedical therapist usually encouraged behavioral change aimed at resolution of difficulties rather than adaptation to them, as does treatment with drugs.

Second, the safety of all categories of psychotropic drugs regarding dependence and withdrawal has been questioned. Although the dangers of the barbiturates and the stimulants have been recognized for some time, those associated with minor tranquilizers are just now becoming understood. Prolonged (4 months or more) and heavy (30–40 mg./day) use of Valium, for instance, can produce dependence and symptoms of withdrawal that mimic the symptoms for which the drug was originally prescribed (*FDA Drug Bulletin* 1980). Distinguishing between withdrawal and recurrence of original symptoms is, therefore, extremely difficult. It is estimated that between one and two million women have prescribed drug-related dependencies, many involving several drugs or a combination of drugs and alcohol (National Institute on Drug Abuse 1978b). About 60% of drug-related visits to emergency rooms are by women, over two-thirds of whom have attempted suicide (National Institute on Drug Abuse 1978b).

Origins of Use

Although the etiology of sex differences in use of psychotropic drugs is complex, there appears to be an unusually good fit between various attributes of the sex stereotypes and roles and the conditions under which psychotropic drugs are prescribed and used. . . .

The Patient.   One of the more consistent findings in the mental health area has been that women report more mental health symptoms than do men (Markush and Favero 1974; Phillips and Segal 1969). Depressive symptoms are reported by twice as many women as men (Weissman 1976). . . .

. . . If differences in mental health are real and the psychotropic drugs alleviate symptoms for women, then use of the drugs appears justified. If, however, the drugs are prescribed and used because of a failure to expect and discount sex-related differences in reports of mental health symptoms, then use is less justified.

The Physician.   Physicians, like other humans, are influenced by cultural stereotypes regarding women and men (Fidell 1980). Indirect evidence suggests that the sex stereotypes encourage physicians to attribute symptoms of women to psychological or psychosomatic difficulties and attribute those of men to organic imbalances. In the former case, but not necessarily the latter, a prescription for a psychotropic drug would result. Subsequently, Armitage, Schneidermann, and Bass (1979) provided more direct evidence that similar symptoms lead to different medical evaluations, depending on the sex of the patient.

Although physician expectations regarding sex differences may some-times result in a prescription for a psychotropic drug, another possible, more subtle factor deserves mention. Accurate diagnosis and effective treatment are by no means guaranteed all who seek medical attention, even those with organic disturbances. If the tests are negative and the physician's bag of diagnostic tricks is empty, he or she is still under pressure to do something. The patient may, in fact, demand treatment of almost any kind as justification for his or her expenditures of time, inconvenience, and monies. At this point, turning to psychotropic drugs may be extremely tempting. The patient may demand it, and the physician may fear losing the patient if nothing is done. . . . But even greater may sometimes be the need of the physician to shift "blame" for the illness back to the patient: If the symptoms can be attributed to emotion—the kind of problem properly treated by psychotropic drugs—then failure of diagnosis and treatment is not the physician's fault. Prescription for a psychotropic drug in this case meets many needs simultane-ously.

If the above-mentioned speculation is justified, then the most probable time during the course of medical evaluation for a psychotropic prescription to be received is at the point where everyone despairs of achieving a diagnosis. Some confirmation is available from Borgman (1973), who found that all of his drug abusing, middle-aged female subjects ($N = 25$) had first been introduced to psychotropic drugs during the course of prolonged but inconclusive evaluation for medical symptoms.

Not only is the physician a member of a culture with widely held stereotypic beliefs about women and men, but also she or he is a member of a medical subculture in which the stereotypes may be reinforced during training, in textbooks, and in advertising for drugs. Seidenberg (1979) suggests collusion between pharmaceutical firms and physicians, both of whom benefit from increased sales of psychotropic medications.

It should be noted that physicians are trained to dispense medicine, not to solve complex social, emotional, economic, and political problems. A sympathetic physician may see few alternatives to psychotropic medication for the woman with such problems. Lack of information regarding appropriate referrals to private or community mental health facilities or to treatment facilities for patients who have psychotropic drug dependencies leaves both the patient and the physician with few alternatives to the use of psychotropic drugs. . . .

. . . Zola (1966) found that physicians are influenced both by *what* is reported and *how* it is reported. Symptoms stoically reported are taken more seriously than those emotionally reported. Mechanic (1972) concluded that sex stereotypes tend to produce stoicism in the medical behavior of males and emotionality in the medical behavior of females.

Persistence of Use

Sex stereotypes not only contribute to the origins of prescriptions for psychotropic drugs but may also contribute to persistence in use of them. Low self-esteem has been identified as the one reliable correlate of both drug and alcohol abuse. For the woman with truly dysfunctional patterns of psycho-tropic drug use . . . , reduced self-esteem has been reported (Borgman 1973; Maginniss 1979). People who feel that they are not worthwhile do not see the point in resisting the temptation of chemical relief, however temporary. Dependence on drugs, of course, increases feelings of worthlessness; and so it goes.

Growing acceptance of drugs also facilitates persistent use. In 1975 (Fidell 1977), 54% of women questioned thought it better to take drugs than to go through a day tense and nervous, and 48% thought it better to use drugs than to spend a sleepless night. Acceptance of use of drugs is increasing, and so are the indicators for their use in the medical literature (Lennard et al. 1970).

. . . Neither physicians nor mental health professionals are trained·to recognize the indicators of drug dependency. Drug-related problems are rarely covered in any detail in professional training for clinical psychologists, psychiatrists, or physicians.

REFERENCES

Armitage, K., L.J. Schneidermann, and R. A. Bass, "Response of Physicians to Medical Complaints in Men and Women," *JAMA* (1979), 2186–87.

Balter, M. B., and J. Levine, "Character and Extent of Psychotherapeutic Drug Use in the United States." Paper presented at the Fifth World Congress on Psychiatry, Mexico City, 1971.

Borgman, R. D., "Medication Abuse by Middle-Age Women," *Social Casework*, 54, no. 9 (1973), 526–32.

Caranasos, G. J., R. B. Stewart, and L. E. Cluff, "Drug-Induced Illness Leading to Hospitalization," *JAMA*, 228, no. 6 (1974), 713–17.

Cooper, J. R., ed., *Sedative-Hypnotic Drugs: Risks and Benefits*. HEW Publication No. (AD)78–592, 1977.

Cooperstock, R., "Sex Differences in Psychotropic Drug Use," *Social Science and Medicine*, 12b (1978), 179–86.

————, "A Review of Women's Psychotropic Drug Use," *Canadian Journal of Psychiatry*, 24 (1979), 29–33.

————, "Special Problems of Psychotropic Drug Use among Women," *Canada's Mental Health*, 28, no. 2 (1980), 3–5.

Dunea, G., "Shopping-Bag Syndrome," *British Medical Journal*, 2 (1977), 240–41.

Elliott, J., "Physician Prescribing Practices Criticized; Solutions in Question," *JAMA*, 241, no. 22 (1979), 2353–60.

FDA Drug Bulletin, February 1980, pp. 2–3.

Fidell, L. S., "Psychotropic Drug Use by Women: Health, Attitudinal, Personality, and Demographic Correlates." Paper presented at the 85th Annual Meeting of the American Psychological Association, San Francisco, August 1977.

————, "Sex Role Stereotypes and the American Physician," *Psychology of Women Quarterly*, 4, no. 3 (1980), 313–31.

————, "Sex Differences in Psychotropic Drug Use," *Professional Psychology*, 12, no. 1 (1981), 156–62.

Graedon, J., *The People's Pharmacy*, New York: Avon Books, 1976.

Hiatt, H. H., "Protecting the Medical Commons: Who Is Responsible?" *New England Journal of Medicine*, 293, no. 5 (1975), 235–41.

Hughes, R., and R. Brewin, *The Tranquilizing of America: Pill Popping and the American Way of Life*. New York: Harcourt Brace Javanovich, Inc., 1979.

Jick, H., "Drugs—Remarkably Nontoxic," *New England Journal of Medicine*, 291, no. 16 (1974), 824–28.

Kayne, R. C., ed., *Drugs and the Elderly*, revised. Los Angeles: University of Southern California Press, 1978.

Koch-Weser, J., "Fatal Reactions to Drug Therapy," *New England Journal of Medicine*, 291, no. 6 (1974), 302–3.

Lawson, D. H., and H. Jick, "Drug Prescribing in Hospitals: An International Comparison," *American Journal of Public Health*, 66, no. 7 (1976), 644–48.

Lennard, L. L., et al., "Hazards Implicit in Prescribing Psychoactive Drugs, "*Science*, 169 (1970), 438–41.

Maginniss, C., *Women's Dependency on Prescription Drugs*. Testimony given in the hearing before the Select Committee on Narcotics Abuse and Control, House of Representatives, September 13, 1979. U. S. Government Printing Office, Washington, D.C., 1979.

Markush, R. E., and R. V. Favero, "Epidemiologic Assessment of Stressful Life Events, Depressed Mood, and Psychophysiological Symptoms—A Preliminary Report," in B. S. Dohrenwent and B.P. Dohrenwent, eds., *Stressful Life Events: Their Nature and Effects*. New York: John Wiley & Sons, Inc., 1974.

Maronde, R. F., et al., "A Study of Prescribing Patterns," *Medical Care*, 9, no. 5 (1971), 383–95.

Maugh, T., "Irrational Drug Prescribing and Birth Defects," *Science*, vol. 194 (1976).

Mechanic, D., "Correlates of Frustration among British General Practitioners," *Journal of Health and Social Behavior*, 11, no. 2 (1970), 87–104.

——, "Reponse Factors in Illness: The Study of Illness Behavior," in E. G. Jaco, ed., *Patients, Physicians and Illness*. New York: The Free Press, 1972.

Mellinger, G. D. et al., "An Overview of Psychotherapeutic Drug Use in the United States," in E. Josephson and E. E. Carroll, eds., *Drug Use: Epidemiological and Sociological Approaches*. Washington, D.C.: Hemisphere Publishing Company, 1974.

Moertel, G., et al., "A Comparative Evaluation of Marketed Analagesic Drugs," *New England Journal of Medicine*, 286, no. 15 (1974), 813–15.

National Institute on Drug Abuse, "Top 26 Problem Drugs in the U.S.," *NIDA Capsules*, February 1978a.

——, "Women and Prescription Drugs," *NIDA Capsules*, April 1978b.

New York State Division of Substance Abuse Series, *Drug Use in New York State: A Report on the Nonmedical Use of Drugs among the New York State Household Population*, December 1978 (Box 8200, New York, N.Y. 10047).

Parnell, P., and R. Cooperstock, "Tranquilizers and Mood Elevators in the Treatment of Migraine: An Analysis of the Migraine Foundation Questionnaire," *Headache Journal*, 19, no. 2 (19798), 78–89.

Phillips, D. L., and B. E. Segal, "Sexual Status and Psychiatric Symptoms," *American Sociological Review*, 34 (1969), 58–72.

Program for Women's Concerns, National Institute on Drug Abuse, *Women and Drugs: Data from the National Survey*, November 1977.

Seidenberg, R., *Women's Dependency on Prescription Drugs*. Testimony given in the hearing before the Select Committee on Narcotics Abuse and Control, House of Representatives, September 13, 1979.

Shader, R., "Drug Treatment of Premenstrual Distress," in A. F. Fisher, ed., *Women's Worlds*. HEW Publication No. (ADM) 78-660, 1978.

Shader, R. I., W. A. Binstock, and D. Scott, "Subjective Determinants of Drug Prescription: A Study of Therapists' Attitudes," *Hospital and Community Psychiatry*, 19 (1968), 384–87.

Silverman, M., "The Epidemiology of Drug Promotion," *International Journal of Health Services*, 7, no. 2 (1977), 157–66.

Silverman, M., and P. R. Lee, *Pills, Profits and Politics*. Berkeley: University of California Press, 1974.

Stadel, B., and N. Weiss, "Characteristics of Menopausal Women: A Survey of King and Pierce Counties in Washington, 1973–74," *American Journal of Epidemiology*, vol. 102 (1975).

Stetler, C. J., "Letter to the Editor: Drug-Induced Illness," *JAMA*, 229, no. 8 (1974), 1043–44.

Talley, R. B., and M. F. Laventurier, "Letter to the Editor: Drug-Induced Illness," *JAMA*, vol. 229, no. 8 (1974).

Waldron, I., "Increased Prescribing of Valium, Librium, and Other Drugs—An Example of the Influence of Economic and Social Factors in the Practice of Medicine," *International Journal of Health Services*, 7, no. 1 (1977), 37–59.

Weg, R. B., "Drug Interaction with the Changing Physiology of the Ages: Practice and Potential," in R. C. Kayne, ed., *Drugs and the Elderly*, revised. Los Angeles: University of Southern California Press, 1978.

Weiss, K., "The Use and Abuse of Sex Hormones in Medical Practice," in A. Stromberg, ed., *Women, Health, and Medicine*. Palo Alto, Calif.: Mayfield, 1982.

Weissman, M. M., "Depressed Women: Traditional and Nontraditional Therapies," in J. L. Claghorn, ed., *Successful Psychotherapy*. New York: Bruner/Mazel, Inc., 1976.

Wolfe, S., Health Research Group, Washington, D.C., personal communication.

Zola, I., "Culture and Symptoms: An Analysis of Patients' Presenting Complaints," *American Sociological Review*, 31, no. 2 (1966), 615–30.

SUGGESTED READINGS

Editors of Consumer Reports, *The Medicine Show*. New York: Pantheon Books, Inc., 1974.

Graedon, Joe, *The People's Pharmacy*. New York: Avon Books, 1976.

Graedon, Joe, and Therese Graedon, *The People's Pharmacy 2*. New York: Avon Books, 1980.

Hughes, Richard, and Robert Brewin, *The Tranquilizing of America*. New York: Harcourt Brace Jovanovich, Inc. 1979.

Long, James, *The Essential Guide to Prescription Drugs*. New York: Harper & Row, Publishers, Inc., 1977.

Nellis, Muriel, *The Female Fix*. Boston: Houghton Mifflin Company, 1980.

Silverman, Howard, and Simon Gilbert, *The Pill Book*. New York: Bantam Books, Inc., 1979.

Silverman, Milton, and Philip Lee, *Pills, Profits and Politics*. Berkeley, Calif.: University of California Press, 1976.

Wolfe, Sidney, and Christopher Coley, *Pills That Don't Work*. New York: Farrar, Straus & Giroux, Inc., 1981.

Chapter Six

BREAST SURGERY: CURRENT TREATMENT

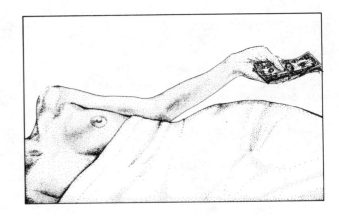

Kay Weiss

Breast cancer strikes 90,000 women in the United States every year and kills 37,000 of them. Now, many women believe that the American medical profession is doing as much harm to women's breasts as the disease is. Surgeons are performing mastectomies far more than is medically necessary; and technological medicine is causing breast cancer in many cases where none exists due to the use of prescription drugs (reserpine, estrogen, and some tranquilizers) and mammography (Kushner 1975; Budoff 1981; Corea 1977).

UNNECESSARY RADICAL SURGERY

It has long been known that the treatment for breast cancer that was developed 90 years ago, the Halsted radical mastectomy, which amputates the breast, underlying chest muscles, and underarm lymph nodes, is a mutilating procedure—one that is unnecessary for treating most women who have breast cancer; unnecessary because data from Europe and England where less disabling procedures have long been used have shown survival rates from breast cancer to be as favorable after minimal surgery as they are after the radical mastectomy.

Many surgeons have joined women's health advocates in speaking out against the unnecessary mutilation and disfigurement of thousands of American women every year with the radical mastectomy. But not until Rose Kushner (1975) a woman who had breast cancer, began to investigate this barbarous treatment and pressed her findings on governmental regulatory agencies did the medical profession adjust its approach to the treatment of breast cancer. In 1979, the National Institute of Health (NIH) finally advised physicians what the medical literature had for decades been supporting; that is, to replace the radical mastectomy with lesser treatment. (*JAMA* 1979, p. 14; *Obstetrics and Gynecology News* 1980, p. 41). This profound advancement in American medicine, achieved by an individual woman patient who gathered together scientific documentation to prove her case, took years and represents a small, although significant, improvement in breast cancer treatment.

Unfortunately, NIH stopped short of asking physicians to cease four other routine practices that unnecessarily mutilate or traumatize tens of thousands of women yearly: (1) the use of any mastectomy to treat early breast cancer, (2) the use of any mastectomy on women about to die from breast cancer, (3) cutting off of women's breasts before tests have been done to determine the stage (extent) of cancer and its cell type so that the most appropriate treatment can be chosen, and (4) the performing of mastectomies while women are still under general anesthesia from the biopsy and before they know whether they have cancer, a practice that is in decline but still exists in some areas.

For years, women consumer rights advocates have charged that Amer ican surgeons cut off womens breasts unnecessarily for financial motives. In 1979, the American College of Surgeons itself agreed that U.S. surgeons are doing radical mastectomies in favor of lesser procedures because insurance plans pay more for more extensive surgery.

Besides economic motives, the training of physicians has also contributed to the choice of radical surgery for breast cancer. American medicine is characterized by the mechanistic approach of removing the offending part without considering how the body system as a whole affects the part or is affected by it, to say nothing of the mental or emotional factors involved. In addition, physicians who treat cancer are trained heavily in surgery and are often unfamiliar with many of the new developments in radiation treatment. (Budoff 1980).

A radical mastectomy removes the breast along with the entire pectoral (chest) muscle and underarm lymph nodes. The result is a skeletonlike hollowness extending up to the collarbone on the affected side. Without the usual muscle and fat protection, the rib cage and inside of the body are mercilessly exposed to temperature variations, and there is shoulder weakness, swelling, stiffness, and susceptibility to infection of the affected arm. The lungs remain vulnerable throughout life. Women who have radical mastectomies often experience a major decline in their sex lives; about one-third stop having sex altogether.

The Halsted mastectomy was developed as the standard for routine use at at time when most women had not been diagnosed until they had extensive local spreading of the disease. Although there has been a sharp reduction in the number of radical mastectomies performed since 1979, mastectomies are still used too routinely—in 25 percent of all breast surgery in the United States. In a study reviewed by the American College of Surgeons (ACOS) 52 percent of 242 women had limited early (in situ) cancer, yet 44 percent had modified radicals or Halsted radicals with internal node biopsy. (Kushner, Rose, personal communication) In another study of 922 women, 57 percent underwent the debilitating mastectomies, although they already had distant metastases present, and simple palliative surgery could have been performed to reduce the tumor burden and make the patient more comfortable in the advanced stages of disease (Kushner Rose, personal communication).

ALTERNATIVE PROCEDURES AND SURVIVAL RATES

There is nothing that radical mastectomy can accomplish that cannot be achieved as well by lesser procedures (simple mastectomy, local excision or segmental resection, lumpectomy, partial mastectomy, or radiation). Radiation is as effective as mastectomy in treating early breast cancer when used alone or in combination with local excision (Rotman et al. 1979; *Breast Cancer Digest* 1979, p. 29).

The medical literature contains studies confirming that the difference in survival rates between various treatments for breast cancer is negligible or nonexistent after five years. In one study done in Italy, 710 women received treatment for breast cancer; half of these received Halsted radicals and half received lumpectomy and radiation. Total survival rates were 89 percent for the radical and 88 percent for the lumpectomy. Cancer-free survival rates were 83 percent for Halsted and 82.7 percent for lumpectomy (Bonadonna et. al. 1980, p. 3).

STAGE OF DISEASE SHOULD DETERMINE TREATMENT

The treatment given for breast cancer should be determined by the stage of disease, and tests should be conducted prior to surgery to determine whether the cancer is localized or has spread. These tests include blood tests, and bone, liver, and brain scans. Chest X-rays can indicate lung metastases, and current improvements in technology now enable occult micrometastases to be detected. New research promises that blood tests may soon be capable of detecting an antigen or tumor marker that will reveal cancer cells before a visible or palpable mass is present.

In Stage 1, cancer is confined to the breast, with no spread to the armpit lymph glands; in Stage 2, lymph nodes in the armpit are enlarged and firm and may contain cancerous cells that have spread from the breast;

in Stage 3, there are large tumors or there may be tumors that have spread to the armpit, above the clavicle, or have become fixed to the underlying chest muscle. In Stage 4, distant metastases are present. Fifty percent of breast cancer is detected in Stage I, and 35 percent in Stage 2 (Budoff 1981).

In patients with Stage 1 or Stage 2 disease, radiation plus lumpectomy is as effective as a mastectomy that removes the breast plus axillary lymph nodes but preserves the pectoral muscles. And interstitial radiation implant therapy in combination with external radiation yields survival rates that are comparable to surgical procedures. (Rotman et al. 1979; *Breast Cancer Digest*, 1979). Stage 3 and Stage 4 breast cancer are not good candidates for cure by mastectomy; simple palliative surgery should be performed to reduce the tumor burden and make the patient more comfortable.

MISDIAGNOSIS AND UNNECESSARY SURGERY

The one-stage biopsy/mastectomy approach in which the surgeon sends the biopsy specimen to the pathologist who reads it while the patient is still on the operating table has been the standard procedure until very recently. If cancer is found, the surgeon completes the mastectomy. This is convenient for the surgeon, yet it can result in an occasional irreversible error. In addition, it subjects women who have biopsies, most of whom will *not* have cancer, to unnecessary anxiety and fear that they may wake up without a breast.

Misdiagnosis of breast cancer resulting in unnecessary surgery has occurred too often in the past. In 1977, a federal advisory group of pathologists reviewed the early cancers (less than 1 cm. in size) detected in the National Cancer Institute breast cancer screening (mammography) demonstration program. They found that 66 of the lesions classified as malignant were, in fact, benign. Of the 66 women who apparently had no cancer, 53 were subjected to unnecessary mastectomies. News media coverage of this resulted in a demonstration of public outrage. Subsequently the advisory group announced there had been a mistake and that only 7 women had needlessly had their breasts amputated. (Corea 1977).

EARLY DETECTION

If breast cancer is found early, the type of surgery that is performed will be more limited, and the survival rate can be as high as 80 percent five years after treatment. About 90 percent of all breast cancer nodules are first found by the woman herself rather than by technological detection methods. Such methods include radiography, thermography, or ultrasound. Radiography or mammography should be reserved for high-risk women because it carries a small risk of actually inducing cancer by radiation. However, the newer-style mammography machines now produce less radiation, increasing the safety of this technique.

When performing breast self-examination, women should be alerted not to confuse benign cysts with cancer. Approximately 30 percent of women age 30-40 have benign cysts which usually disappear with the coming of menopause (Landon and Sommers 1978, p. 1231).

REVIEW OF TREATMENT OPTIONS

Consumers of breast cancer treatment care should be alerted that the following review of treatment options is ideal but may not be offered by physicians without a specific request from the patient:

1. The biopsy should be done by needle aspiration under local anesthesia if possible; more extensive and expensive surgical biopsies are often done unnecessarily. Eight out of ten biopsies have benign diagnoses. Needle biopsies prevent much emotional trauma, physical disfigurement, and expenditure of money.

2. Biopsy results should be made available to the patient before treatment is commenced so that she may join in the decision about the type of therapy. The myth that the cancer could "spread like wildfire" if the breast is not removed immediately has been disproved by many studies.

3. Extent and stage of disease should be determined before therapy is performed. Therapy should be chosen based on the stage and histologic type of disease.

4. Early breast cancer should not be treated by mastectomy but rather by lumpectomy and postoperative radiation. Advanced breast cancer patients with distant mesastases should not be subjected to mastectomies.

CONCLUSION

Prevention of breast cancer requires more research into promising investigational areas, including the role of prescription drugs such as estrogens and reserpine (drug therapy for hypertension) and mammography, as well as lifestyle factors such as caffein consumption (Mintou . . .), dietary fat, and reproductive history.

Few surgeons will be enthusiastic about reviewing all the possible procedures for patients, yet some states now have laws requiring surgeons to discuss with patients all options for treating breat cancer.

Ideally, surgery should not be the treatment of choice for any disease. The surgical removal of a breast that has been invaded by cancer is an admission that medical science does not yet understand cancer, what causes it, how to prevent it, or how to control it in a more sophisticated, specific way.

REFERENCES

Bonadonna, G., U. Veronesi, and P. Valagusta, *Clinical Cancer Letter*, vol. 3, no. 10 (1980).

The Breast Cancer Digest, Bethesda, Md.: Office of Cancer Communications, National Cancer Institute, 1979.

Budoff, Penny Wise, "No More Radical Mastectomies." in *No More Menstrual Cramps and Other Good News*. New York: Putnam, 1980.

Corea, Gena, *The Hidden Malpractice: How American Medicine Treats Women as Patients and Professionals*. New York: William Morrow & Co., Inc., 1977.

JAMA, July 6, 1979.

Kushner, Rose, *Breast Cancer: A Personal History and Investigative Report*.New York: Harcourt Brace Jovanovich, Inc., 1975.

Landon, Parsons, and Sheila Sommers, *Gynecology*, 2nd ed. Philadelphia: W.B. Saunders Company, 1978.

Minton, Foecking et al, "Caffein, Cyclic Nucleotides, and Breast Disease," in Budoff, Penny. op cit.

Obstetrics and Gynecology News, January 10, 1980.

Rotman, Marvin et al. "Radical Therapy for Breast Cancer," *Journal of Reproductive Medicine*, 23, no. 1 (July 1979), 13–20.

SUGGESTED READINGS

Check, William, "Benign Breast Lumps May Regress with Change in Diet." *JAMA*, vol. 241, no. 12 (March 1979).

Crile, George, Jr., *What Women Should Know about the Breast Cancer Controversy*. New York: Pocket Books, 1974.

Greenfield, Natalee S., *First, Do No Harm* . . . New York: Two Continents, 1976.

Kushner, Rose, *Breast Cancer: A Personal and Investigative Report*. New York: Harcourt Brace Jovanovich, Inc., 1975.

Millman, Marcia, *The Unkindest Cut: Life in the Backrooms of Medicine*. New York: Morrow Quill, 1977.

Rollin, Betty, *First, You Cry*. Philadelphia: J. B. Lippincott Co., 1976.

Winkler, Win Ann, *Post-Mastectomy*. New York: Hawthorn Books, Inc., 1976.

Chapter Seven

HYSTERECTOMY: CURRENT TREATMENT

Susanne Morgan

Hysterectomy is the most common major operation performed in the United States today. Approximately 700,000 hysterectomies are performed annually, half of which are performed on women of reproductive age. And according to the Center for Disease Control (1980), as many as 500,000 of the 3.5 million hysterectomies performed on reproductive-aged women in the United States between 1970 and 1978 were done for questionable reasons (Greenspan 1981). Experts estimate that between 40 and 62 percent of women in the United States will have a hysterectomy by age 65. (Bunker 1977; Richards 1978). In addition, D & C (dilation and curettage of the uterus) is also considered to be frequently performed unnecessarily by the medical profession (Bunker and Bourse 1974).

Although technically *hysterectomy* refers only to the removal of the uterus and cervix, a *complete hysterectomy* involves removal of the uterus, cervix, fallopian tubes, and ovaries. In cases of cancer, a *radical hysterectomy*, removing also the pelvic lymph nodes, is performed.

The most common indication for a hysterectomy is the presence of uterine fibroid tumors—benign growths that are very common in middle age (25 percent of women develop them), and which generally shrink during menopause without surgery. Other examples of questionable indications for surgery include a number of benign diseases of the uterus, cervix, ovaries, or fallopian tubes (such as dysfunctional uterine bleeding), and endometriosis, uterine or cervical polyps, and pelvic inflammatory disease. Only about 10 percent of hysterectomies are performed for life-threatening conditions. (Greenspan 1981; Lewis 1969). Even a positive pap test does not necessarily mean a woman's life is endangered, and new evidence suggests that many pap tests are read incorrectly (Corea 1977).

RATES OF UNNECESSARY HYSTERECTOMY

Hysterectomy rates increase dramatically with increasing age. Women ages 35–44 have rates 20 times higher than those under age 25 (Greenspan 1981). Rates vary widely in different parts of the country and even within different parts of a state. The South has more than twice as many hysterectomies as the Northeast (Lewis 1969).

Some studies indicate that insured women undergo twice as many hysterectomies as uninsured women and that salaried physicians perform one-fourth fewer hysterectomies than physicians paid on a fee-for-service basis (House of Representatives Subcommittee 1976). Poor women, in public facilities, are most likely to have hysterectomies (Koepsell 1980). Hysterectomy rates are directly correlated to the number of gynecological surgeons in practice, and in the United States the rate is more than twice that in the United Kingdom, paralleling the fact that the United States has twice as many gynecological surgeons (Bunker 1970). Most of the increase in hysterectomies noted by the Center for Disease Control is due to increasing rates among white women. The hysterectomy rate for black women has been consistently high: between 9 and 10 percent 1000 women (Center for Disease Control 1980).

The increase in hysterectomy rates may be partially due to improved detection of disease (so that women are obtaining necessary treatment that was unavailable in the past) or to the occurrence of new diseases for which hysterectomy is the only appropriate treatment (ibid). Although these factors can contribute to an increased rate, the weight of evidence continues to indicate that many hysterectomies performed in the United States are unnecessary.

To determine the number of unnecessary hysterectomies, researchers use several methods. One method is to review hospital records and categorize the surgeries as necessary or unnecessary, based on a list of preset criteria. As early as 1946, a study revealed that at least one-third of all the hysterectomies in the United States had been performed on women with normal uteri. In a 1977 Canadian study, between 17 and 59 percent of hysterectomies were unjustified according to the criteria for acceptable indications (Dyck 1977). A recent study by the Center for Disease Control estimated that 5 to 15 percent of the hysterectomies were done for reasons that did not appear to be justified (Greenspan 1981).

Another approach to determining the rate of avoidable surgery is to obtain a second opinion from a physician other than the one recommending surgery. One study evaluated a program within union health plans where second opinions were paid for by the insuror and found that the second opinion disagreed with the first recommendation for surgery at a high rate: 21 percent when the second opinion was mandatory, and 43 percent when it was voluntary (McCarthy and Widmer 1974). Critics of second opinion programs point out correctly that two doctors disagreeing does not mean the first was wrong (Emerson and Creedon 1977). However, second opinion programs do reduce the number of surgeries performed, and a high level of disagreement over the necessity of surgery suggests that many are unnecessary.

REASONS FOR AND AGAINST SURGERY

When medical professionals investigate unnecessary use of hysterectomy, what indications do they consider appropriate? The list of acceptable indications in the Canadian study (Dyck 1977) includes many abnormalities that are not life-threatening, such as endometriosis, benign ovarian growths, dysfunctional uterine bleeding, or pelvic congestion syndrome. Thus, the rates of "unnecessary" hysterectomies do not include marginally necessary hysterectomies but only those not medically justified at all: hysterectomies done in the absence of functional or organic pathology, elective hysterectomies, sterilizations, and those performed for prevention of possible future disease. Proponents of elective hysterectomy refer to the uterus after childbearing as a useless organ that ought to be removed (Wright 1969). James H. Sammons, the Executive Vice-President of the American Medical Association, recommends hysterectomy to women who request it for relief of anxiety about getting cancer or conceiving children (1977).

Hysterectomy is never a rational alternative to tubal ligation. It is 5 to 7 times more expensive, has a complication rate of 10 to 22 times higher, and a death rate far higher than tubal ligation (Hibbard 1972). Yet until active intervention was offered by consumer groups, hysterectomy was promoted as a form of sterilization, and despite federal guidelines, continues to be a common sterilization procedure (Swenson 1979).

Prevention is often a reason given for elective hysterectomy, and proponents point to the high rate of uterine cancer as the reason for removing the healthy uterus of a woman who wants no more children. However, the death rate in any year for uterine cancer is less than that for unnecessary hysterectomy; and for any one woman who has no reason to predict cancer, the decision is between a known immediate risk—surgery—and an unknown future one—cancer.

In a cost-benefit analysis of elective surgery, Cole estimated that if all women in this country were given a hysterectomy at age 35, the costs would be almost $3 billion (Cole and Berlin 1977). The calculated savings of $1.4 billion would include the costs of prevented cancer, gynecological care, pap tests, contraceptives, menstrual preparations, and care for Downs Syndrome children. Even in this "coolly rational" calculation, elective hysterectomy was not cost-justified. We might note also that we do not hear proposals for elective prostrate surgery, although the mortality rate for prostate cancer is similar to that for uterine cancer.

Estimates of unnecessary hysterectomy are always made at the policy level. For any individual woman, the choice is far more complex. She must weigh the severity of her difficulty against the probability of problems after hysterectomy. At an individual level, a woman may choose a procedure that statistically would be considered unnecessary.

MORBIDITY AND MORTALITY

Why is unnecessary hysterectomy an issue? To consumer activists the answer is obvious, and yet many physicians and their patients do not seem to be aware that any unnecessary surgery should be avoided. The dangers of a general anesthetic are great, and most surgical mortality is due to anesthesia. The death rate from hysterectomy is estimated at .3 to .5 percent, and the rate of complications is 30 to 48 percent, including both minor complications such as fever, bleeding, urinary tract infection, pneumonia, and blood clots, and major complications such as damage to the intestine, vagina, bladder, or ureter (Dicker 1981). Vaginal hysterectomies carry a 25 percent morbidity rate and abdominal hysterectomies a 40 percent morbidity rate (Greenspan 1981).

OTHER CONSIDERATIONS: MENTAL AND PHYSICAL

Depression after hysterectomy is found in several studies to be consistently higher than after other similar procedures (Barker 1968; et al.). Some women experience a day of weepiness in the hospital; others become severely depressed, some as late as in the second year after surgery. This depression may be related to hormonal or symbolic factors or a combination of these. Although most women will not become depressed after hysterectomy, there is a risk (Newton and Baron 1976; Sloah 1978).

The unique symbolic meaning of the uterus to women is also a factor that must not be ignored (Drellich and Bieber 1958). Unnecessary or prophylactic hysterectomies are justified by doctors' beliefs that the uterus has only one function and that is to produce babies (Paulshock 1976; Wright 1969). Even if childbearing was the only function of the uterus, many women (and men) have a major interest in that function, and unnecessary hysterectomy will seem castrating to them.

Women are virtually never told about the sexual changes that can result from hysterectomy. Masters and Johnson (1969), among other researchers, have documented the role that the uterus plays in sexual arousal and the fact that women may experience reduced intensity of sexual arousal and satisfaction after the uterus is removed (Morgan 1978). Six recent studies of posthysterectomy sexuality revealed that 32 to 46 percent of women reported decreased sexual response (Zussman 1981). In addition, such operative complications as uterine or urinary tract infection can cause sexual problems. Permanent sexual dysfunction can also be caused by surgical errors in performing a hysterectomy (Masters and Johnson 1970).

In the recent past, many surgeons carelessly removed the ovaries along with the hysterectomy, stopping a woman's estrogen and androgen production and rendering her instantly postmenopausal. Often justified as preventing ovarian cancer, the practice of ovariectomy in premenopausal women is challenged today by medical experts as well as by consumer advocates (Corea 1977). A premature and abrupt menopause brings unnecessary risks and changes that are difficult to cope with. A woman who experiences premature menopause will probably be prescribed estrogen replacement therapy, although estrogen drugs are documented to increase the risk of uterine, ovarian, and breast cancer (NIH 1980; Weinstein 1980; Huka 1980). A woman who has undergone premature surgical menopause must weigh the risks of long-term estrogen replacement therapy (ERT) against the potential risk of osteoporosis and other menopausal symptoms, including sexual changes.

ALTERNATIVES TO HYSTERECTOMY

Alternative medical procedures to hysterectomy are too often disregarded. A myomectomy is an operation that will remove just the fibroid tumor and not the entire uterus. Also hormones can often successfully treat endometriosis, obviating the need for surgery. And sometimes simply watching and waiting can be an effective option. A specialist in infertility can sometimes be helpful in exploring alternatives to hysterectomy (Harrison 1979).

While watching one's condition and waiting to see whether hysterectomy is truly necessary, some women embark on healing programs with holistic practitioners. For example, some women have reduced fibroids by dietary changes (see Chapter Twelve) or successfully treated a prolapsed uterus with yoga programs (see Chapter Nineteen). Meditation and visualization have been successful in the treatment of cancer (Simonton and Simonton 1980) and acupuncture can relieve endometriosis (see Chapter Ten).

SOCIOLOGICAL AND ECONOMIC FACTORS THAT CONTRIBUTE TO HYSTERECTOMY RATES

The hospital-oriented, fee-for-service system of payment dominates U.S. medical care. Comparative studies of fee-for-service medical practices (financed by insurance plans such as Blue Cross-Blue Shield and Medicaid) and prepaid medical plans suggest that the incentive of fee-for-service medicine not only fosters more hospital admissions but also is responsible for as many as 50 percent more hysterectomies than prepaid plans employing salaried physicians (Larned 1977).

Obstetricians and gynecologists, faced with decreasing birthrates, may be turning to hysterectomy for a stable service they can provide. A recent HEW report has shown that unnecessary Caesarean sections are on the increase because of the decreasing birthrate and the economic incentive to perform them (Marieskind 1979).

The training of obstetricians and gynecologists also contributes to the high rate. The teaching hospital system requires many hysterectomies to be performed in order that students may be taught. Thus women who request tubal ligations are often encouraged to have hysterectomies instead (Scully 1980). In general, OB-GYNs are trained to do surgery instead of less traumatic procedures.

Historically, when abortion services are less available, sterilization procedures are more available, and some women who have been sterilized without their full consent have had hysterectomies instead of the lower risk tubal ligation. For nonwhite women, "hysterilization" is a form of social control both as individuals and as members of a group. Explicit and implicit population-control policies have resulted in the sterilization of one-third of Puerto Rican women and one-fourth of native American women in the United States (CARASA 1979).

RECOMMENDATIONS

Emphasis should be placed on the dissemination of information about the risks of hysterectomy and the safer alternatives. Concerned physicians and researchers should conduct local studies of hysterectomy rates. Consumer groups should provide information and support services for women and should monitor the actions of governmental and regulatory agencies. HEW guidelines on medical indications for hysterectomy should be complied with. Recent state supreme court decisions on informed consent require physicians to make clear the risks and alternatives to surgery. Medicine must develop alternatives to the surgical mentality so prevalent today.

REFERENCES

Barker, M.G., "Psychiatric Illness after Hysterectomy," *British Medical Journal*, vol. 2 (1968).

Bragg, R. L., "Risk of Admission to Mental Hospital Following Hysterectomy or Cholescystectomy," *American Journal of Public Health*, vol. 55 (1965).

Bunker, J. P., "Surgical Manpower: A Comparison of Operations and Surgeons in the United States and in England and Wales," *New England Journal of Medicine*, vol. 282 (1970).

——, *Testimony: Hearings on Quality of Surgical Care*. House of Representatives Subcommittee on Investigations and Oversight, Serial No. 95–32: 135, 1977.

Bunker, J. P., and B. W. Bourse, Jr., "The Physician-Patient as an Informed Consumer of Surgical Services," *New England Journal of Medicine*, vol. 290 (1974).

CARASA, *Women under Attack: Abortion, Sterilization Abuse, and Reproductive Freedom*. New York: Committee for Abortion and against Sterilization Abuse, 1979.

Center for Disease Control, *Surgical Sterilization Surveillance, Hysterectomy in Women Aged 15–44*. U.S. Department of Health and Human Services, Atlanta, Ga., 1980.

Cole, P., and J. Berlin, "Elective Hysterectomy," *American Journal of Obstetrics and Gynecology*, vol. 129 (1977).

Corea, G., *The Hidden Malpractice: How American Medicine Treats Women as Patients and Professionals*. New York: William Morrow & Co., Inc., 1977.

Dicker, R. C., "Complications Associated with Elective Hysterectomy in Reproductive-Aged Women." Paper presented to the American Public Health Association, 109th Annual Meeting, Los Angeles, 1981.

Drellich, M. G., and I. Bieber, "The Psychological Importance of the Uterus and Its Functions," *Journal of Mental Diseases*, vol. 126 (1958).

Dyck, F. J., "Effect of Surveillance on the Number of Hysterectomies in the Province of Saskatchewan," *New England Journal of Medicine*, vol. 296 (1977).

Emerson, R. S., and J. J. Creedon, "Unjustified Surgery Dilemma," *N.Y. State Journal of Medicine*, vol. 77 (1977).

Greenspan, J. R., "Hysterectomy Trends for Reproductive-Aged Women in the U.S., 1970–1978." Paper presented to the American Public Health Association, 109th Annual Meeting, Los Angeles, 1981.

Harrison, M., *Infertility: A Couple's Guide to Its Causes*. Boston: Houghton-Mifflin Company, 1979.

Hibbard, L. T., "Sexual Sterilization by Elective Hysterectomy," *American Journal of Obstetrics and Gynecology*, vol. 112 (1972).

House of Representatives Subcommmittee on Oversight and Investigations, *Cost and Quality of Health Care: Unnecessary Surgery*. 94th Congress, 2nd Session, 1976.

Hulka, B., "Effect of Exogenuous Estrogen on Post Menopausal Women: The Epidemiologic Evidence," *Obstetrical and Gynecological Survey*, vol. 35 (1980).

Koepsell, T., "Prevalence of Prior Hysterectomy in the Seattle-Tacoma Area," *American Journal of Public Health*, vol. 70 (1980).

Larned, D., "The Epidemic in Unnecessary Hysterectomy," in C. Dreyfuss, ed., *Seizing Our Bodies: The Politics of Women's Health*. New York: Vintage Books, 1977.

Lewis, C. E., "Variations in the Incidence of Surgery," *New England Journal of Medicine*, vol. 281 (1969).

Marieskind, H. *An Evaluation of Caesarean Section in the U.S.* U.S. Department of Health, Education, and Welfare, 1979.

Masters, W. H., and V. E. Johnson, *Human Sexual Response*. Boston: Little, Brown & Company, 1969.

———, *Human Sexual Inadequacy*. Boston: Little, Brown & Company, 1970.

McCarthy, E. G., and G. W. Widmer, "Effects of Screening by Consultants on Recommended Elective Surgical Procedures," *New England Journal of Medicine*, vol. 29 (1974).

Melody, G. F., "Depressive Reactions Following Hysterectomy," *American Journal of Public Health*, vol. 55 (1965).

Morgan, S., "Sexuality after Hysterectomy and Castration," *Journal of Women and Health*, vol. 3 (1978).

National Institute of Health, "Estrogen Use and Postmenopausal Women," *Consensus Conference Summary*, vol. 2 (1980).

Newton, N., and E. Baron, "Reactions to Hysterectomy: Fact or Fiction," *Primary Care*, vol. 3 (1976).

Paulshock, B. Z., "What Every Woman Should Know about Hysterectomy," *Today's Health*, vol. 54 (1976).

Raphael, B., "The Crisis of Hysterectomy," *Australia-New Zealand Journal of Psychiatry*, vol. 6 (1972).

Richards, B. C., "From Women to Women," *American Journal of Ob*, vol. 131 (1978).

Richards, D. H., "Depression after Hysterectomy," *Lancet*, vol. 7826 (1973).

Sammons, J. S., *Testimony: Hearings on Quality of Surgical Care*. Vol. 1. House of Representatives Subcommittee on Investigations and Oversights, Serial No. 95-32:135, 1977.

Scully, D., *Men Who Control Women's Health*. Boston: Houghton Mifflin Company, 1980.

Simonton, C., and S. Simonton, *Getting Well Again*. New York: Bantam Books, Inc., 1980.

Sloan, D., "The Emotional and Psychological Aspects of Hysterectomy," *American Journal of Obstetrics and Gynecology*, vol. 131 (1978).

Swenson, N., personal communication, 1978.

Weinstein, M. C., "Estrogen Use and Post Menopausal Women: Cost, Risks and Benefits," *New England Journal of Medicine*, vol. 303 (1980).

Wright, R. C., "Hysterectomy: Past, Present and Future," *Obstetrics and Gynecology*, vol. 33 (1969).

Zussman, L. et al., "Sexual Response after Hysterectomy-Oophorectomy: Recent Studies and Reconsideration of Psychogenesis," *American Journal of Obstetrics and Gynecology*, vol. 140 (1981).

SUGGESTED READINGS

Center for Disease Control, *Surgical Sterilization Surveillance, Hysterectomy in Women Aged 15–44*.

Koepsell, T, "Prevalence of Prior Hysterectomy in the Seattle-Tacoma Area." *American Journal of Public Health*, vol. 70 (1980).

Morgan, S., *Coping with a Hysterectomy: Your Own Choice, Your Own Solution.* New York: The Dial Press, 1982.

Newton, N., and E. Baron, "Reactions to Hysterectomy: Fact or Fiction." *Primary Care*, vol. 3 (1976).

Zussman, L. et al., "Sexual Response after Hysterectomy-Oophorectomy: Recent Studies and Reconsideration of Psychogenesis." *American Journal of Obstetrics and Gynecology*, vol. 140 (1981).

Chapter Eight

CAESAREAN SURGERY: CURRENT TREATMENT

Helen Marieskind

Between 1968 and 1979, Caesarean section rates in the United States rose 222 percent, from 5 percent to 16 percent of all births. What was historically an emergency procedure in ancient times (Findley 1939), and used with great moderation in recent times (Douglas et al. 1963) has in the last decade become a routine procedure, performed on approximately one in every six women giving birth (National Center for Health Statistics 1968–1981).

TYPES OF CAESAREANS

Caesarean section is a surgical procedure that involves an abdominal and uterine incision to remove the fetus. There are several different types of incisions: *low cervical* procedures account for about 87 percent of all Caesareans performed, and *classical incisions* account for another 4 percent. Other procedures such as *extraperitoneal* or *vaginal* Caesareans account for the remainder (Lowe et al. 1976).

A low cervical Caesarean section employs a horizontal crescent incision into the lower uterine segment with a similar incision into the abdomen just above the pelvic bone. This procedure is preferred for both physiologic and cosmetic reasons as the wound heals more strongly and the abdominal scar will be obscured in the pubic hairline.

A classical Caesarean employs a vertical incision (usually 5 inches in length) in the center of the upper segment of the uterus with a corresponding vertical incision in the abdomen. This procedure is quick and minimizes abdominal blood loss. Sometimes a vertical abdominal incision and a low cervical uterine incision will be combined to gain the benefits of each.

113

MORBIDITY AND MORTALITY CONSIDERATIONS

Although the use of sterile techniques and the availability of blood supplies and antibiotics have dramatically increased the chances of survival from Caesarean section for both mother and infant, the surgery is still undertaken with considerable risk and costs.

Physiological complications have been summarized by Shearer (1977). These include pain, depression, and exhaustion, gas (Alfonzo and Stichler 1978), infection (Hagen 1975; Gibbs et al. 1978), repeat Caesareans (Craigin 1961; Muller et al. 1961), hemorrhage (Ross and Galliford, 1974), adhesions (Polishuk et al. 1975), fistula (Frankel and Buchsbaum 1971), sinuses (Jain 1974), wound dehiscence (Schrinsky and Benson 1978), subsequent uterine rupture (Beachman et al. 1970), injury to adjacent structures (Hibbard 1976), complications of blood transfusions (Lowe et al. 1976), thromboemboli and thrombophlebitis (Arthure 1968), aspiration pneumonia (Baggish and Hooper 1974), anesthesia accidents, cardiac arrest and cerebral vascular accidents, and death. Pain, depression, exhaustion, and gas are experienced by almost all Caesarean patients, and until recently the 1916 dictum "Once a Caesarean, always a Caesarean" prevailed for almost all women (Craigin 1961). Institutions report that at least one-third of their Caesarean patients have some postoperative infection (Gibbs et al. 1972). Other complications are less frequent.

Data on death related to Caesareans are at present unclear and must be evaluated cautiously to determine whether the death is a result of the Caesarean per se (or procedures related to it, for example, anesthesia or antibiotic use) or whether it is caused by preexisting conditions that led to the Caesarean procedure. Where studies exist, however, maternal mortality from Caesareans is substantially higher than from vaginal deliveries. The estimates range from 2 times higher in California (Petitti et al. 1979), to 10 times higher in Georgia (Rubin et al. 1981), to about 26 times higher in Rhode Island (Evrard and Gold 1977). All authors caution against drawing absolute inferences from their data as discussed above.

The 1974 Professional Activity Study (PAS) revealed a maternal mortality rate of 80 per 100,000 sections compared with 27 per 100,000 for deliveries of all types. This rate may be even higher because the 133 Caesarean patients in this study many of whom were complicated cases and were transferred to other hospitals, were not followed (Marieskind 1979). The Professional Standards Review Organizations *(PSRO) Hospital Discharge Data Set* indicated a national Caesarean mortality rate in 1977 of .84 per 1000 Caesarean discharges (1978–1979).

PSYCHOLOGICAL COSTS AND OTHER COMPLICATIONS

Many mothers report psychological costs from Caesarean section. They may feel inadequate and guilty at not having delivered vaginally, hostility toward the infant, and/or have a sense of failure and of helplessness, especially if they are unaware of the reasons for the surgery (Alfonzo and Stichler 1978).

They are also physiological costs to the infant from Caesarean surgery; but, as mentioned earlier, it is difficult to distinguish factors deriving from the Caesarean per se as opposed to those present in the infant that led to the Caesarean (Benson et al. 1969). Complications arise principally from the effects of anesthesia and analgesic drugs (Bowes et al. 1970). These drugs may depress the infant or make the infant so sleepy as to mask serious abnormalities; or the infant may be delivered while its lungs are still immature (Maisels et al. 1977). This condition is known as hyaline membrane disease (HMD) or respiratory distress syndrome (RDS) and can be fatal because an infant's lungs lack sufficient pulmonary surfactant to get enough oxygen to supply body tissues (Hack et al. 1976). Allowing the infant to initiate labor when ready rather than practicing elective delivery at the mother's or at the obstetrician's convenience can contribute substantially to lowering the estimated 40,000 cases of HMD in the United States annually (Goldenberg and Nelson 1975).

FINANCIAL COSTS

The financial costs of Caesarean section may be direct, in the form of increased physician fees for the surgical delivery and for the longer hospital stay for mother and infant ($2500–$3500 as compared with $1000–$1800 for a vaginal delivery); or indirect, when a women experiences loss of productivity with the longer convalescence needed after a Caesarean section. Also, because of physical debilitation, a woman may require a home-helper to assist her in caring for other family members or for the new infant, thereby adding yet another financial cost.

RATIONALE FOR CAESAREAN DELIVERY

With the risks and high costs of Caesarean section, it is reasonable to ask why more and more sections are being done and why the national rate has increased so rapidly. What does Caesarean surgery do for a mother and baby?

Caesarean sections are performed when the surgery is believed to offer a better outcome than would be achieved by a vaginal delivery. Justifications for Caesarean may be *absolute* (there is no other method by which a living child can be delivered) or *relative* (the practitioner decides that abdominal delivery offers better chances for survival for both mother and child). Relative indications are largely subjective and most open to medico-legal interpretation (DeLee 1913) and to evaluation as to their necessity.

Analysts of the rapid rise of Caesareans are beginning to question the necessity for the large increase in the face of considerable risks, especially in the absence of causal evidence of improved outcomes. Also questioned are the beliefs, practices, and decision-making processes that have contributed to the rise.

ECONOMIC INCENTIVES

A combination of economic factors can exert influence toward the more profitable, in this case surgical, approach, while at the same time providing no incentive to persist with a vaginal delivery. One source has noted a decline in the number of births per obstetrician from 260.7 in 1963 to 144.9 in 1976 (Marieskind 1979). Yet, despite declines in morbidity and mortality rates and improved prenatal care during this period, the rate for deliveries with so-called complications has steadily increased. Also during this period, obstetrician-gynecologists have become top earners. Caesarean section may very well be attractive to the physician because it involves a predictable expenditure of time. The added length of stay for C-sections is also attractive to hospitals, particularly in light of the declining birthrate and empty obstetrical beds. In addition, third-party payment may influence the decision to section because the surgery is usually 100 percent covered, whereas vaginal deliveries are not completely covered.

CONDITIONS BELIEVED TO WARRANT CAESAREAN SURGERY

Although factors such as the shift in age of the childbearing population (National Center for Health Statistics 1966–1978), the increase in women with severe medical conditions such as diabetes or Herpes II who are giving birth (Minkoff and Schwarz 1980), and other miscellaneous elements such as economic incentives all play a part in the dramatic rise of Caesarean sections (Marieskind 1979), four principal kinds of physiological conditions may be said to account for this increase. Repeat Caesareans (the first condition) comprise approximately one-third of all Caesareans performed. Another third are performed for cephalo-pelvic (feto-pelvic) disproportion, or dystocia. Another 10 percent are performed for malpresentation (particularly breech) and fetal distress (Lowe et al. 1976; et al.) Other combined indications make up the balance. The reported incidence of these situations has increased dramatically over the last decade, but their basic roles as reasons for the surgery have remained unchanged for centuries. More women are simply being defined as having these recognized conditions. However, because such indications are relative and depend on subjective judgment, they are the most liable to scrutiny in regard to their necessity. Based on findings from scientific study, Caesarean surgery needs to be evaluated as to whether it offers an outcome sufficiently superior to vaginal delivery to offset its increased risks (Chalmers and Richards 1977).

Repeat Caesarean Births

The practice of uniform repeat Caesarean surgery for any subsequent pregnancies, although a well-established practice in the United States since 1916, has not been shown to be valid today (if indeed it ever was) by properly controlled scientific studies (Chalmers and Richards 1977; Merrill and Gibbs 1978).

Today, particularly when the majority of Caesareans employ a low cervical incision, which reduces the risk of uterine rupture thought to be more prevalent with a classical incision (Lowe et al. 1976; Dewhurst 1969), there is no solid medical evidence as to why at least 50 percent of women with a previous Caesarean cannot safely deliver vaginally in a subsequent pregnancy. Although a policy of individual evaluation with the possibility of vaginal delivery has always been the practice in most other countries and has been reported in the U.S. medical literature (Chalmers and Richards 1977; Douglas et al. 1963), it has only recently received national attention and subsequent cautious approval here (National Institute of Child Health and Human Development 1980).

In the national 1974 (PAS) study cited earlier less than 1 percent of women delivered vaginally after a previous Caesarean (Marieskind 1979). Since that survey, Merrill and Gibbs have reported that of 526 patients who were allowed a trial of labor, 59 percent delivered vaginally, doing so with slightly less morbidity than 108 similar patients not given a trial of labor (1978). A consensus conference on Caesarean childbirth sponsored by the National Institute of Child Health and Human Development (NICHD), after surveying the evidence, recommended that vaginal delivery after Caesarean should be offered in selected cases (1980).

Consumer health group and childbirth educators have responded more to these recommendations than physicians have (International Childbirth Education Association 1979; Young and Mahan 1980). Mahan, commenting in the International Childbirth Education Association's position paper, "Vaginal Birth Following Caesarean Section" (1979) notes that few who have experienced a Caesarean are offered the choice of possible vaginal delivery because of habit—that is, obstetricians are not taught this in their training and are not familiar with the scientific literature on the subject and are thus unable to evaluate its safety and advantages. Furthermore, since repeat section is the standard accepted practice, obstetricians are concerned that in the event of an adverse outcome after allowing a vaginal delivery, they will be at high risk for a malpractice suit. The opinions of the NICHD are likely to positively influence a change in this regard. Mahan further notes that the staff time needed to closely monitor a woman attempting a vaginal birth after a Caesarean (VBAC) is an incentive against allowing the practice. Other reasons given state that since patients have not requested VBAC, they do not want it. None of these reasons is based on medical evidence, and Mahan observes that such reasons can be counteracted with education for both physicians and patients. He also notes that as insurance companies become aware of the safety of VBAC and its potential cost savings, unnecessary Caesareans performed simply for the reasons of a previous Caesarean are likely to decline (ibid). As experience with VBAC increases in the United States, physician training and willingness to allow it will change.

Feto-Pelvic Disproportion and Dystocia

Cephalo-pelvic (feto-pelvic) disproportion and dystocia have become "catch-all" diagnoses to refer to conditions in which the fetus is believed to be too large for the mother to deliver vaginally as in cephalopelvic disproportion or where labor is not proceeding at an optimum pace because of dystocia (failure of the cervix to dilate). Despite the widespread use of Caesarean section and a belief that it will produce a less traumatized baby where dystocia is suspected, there are no uniform criteria by which dystocia can be defined either in regard to fetal-maternal size or in terms of an optimum length of labor by which an assessment of "failure to progress" can be made (National Institute of Child Health and Human Development 1980). Minkoff and Schwarz note that a tendency toward Caesarean will prevail once a diagnosis of dystocia has been made. This, combined with a decline in the use of midforceps, the stress of the monitor, and its use without an internal pressure transducer, led to the largest number of new sections in their study (1980). This is confirmed by other authors, several of whom have noted the vagueness of the diagnosis and that the increase for this indication has no relationship to the size of the infant being delivered (Hibbard 1976; Haddad and Lundy 1978; Coady 1980).

Although textbooks maintain that labor should be terminated if the duration of the second stage exceeds two hours, thereby creating a legal concern if this standard is not followed, at least one study (Cohen 1977) showed no adverse outcomes on perinatal or neonatal mortality by allowing a longer second stage. However, this does not infer that a long second stage should be ignored; rather, it should be evaluated carefully before proceeding with "potentially traumatic operative procedures merely because [patients] have not delivered within two hours after the second stage has begun . . ." (Cohen 1977.)

Again, legal concerns, training, the belief that Caesarean section produces a superior outcome, and the influence of technology all have combined to increase Caesareans for the indication of dystocia (Minkoff and Schwarz 1980).

Malpresentation

The use of Caesarean section for malpresentation (anything other than head down), particularly breech, has increased to the point where many institutions report that 80 to 90 percent of such presentations are delivered by Caesarean. (Women who do have vaginal breech deliveries are frequently reported as having arrived at the hospital with the infant almost born.)

Although Caesarean section is unquestionably essential for safe delivery of some malpresentations, the evidence in favor of vaginal delivery of the breech presentation normal birthweight infant is compelling (Collea et al. 1978). Investigators have concluded that:

> although perinatal morbidity occurs with vaginal breech delivery, the significant maternal complications of elective Caesarean section make Caesarean section for term frank infants an unattractive policy. [Collea et al. 1978.]

The shift to Caesarean section for breech delivery has obscured any careful scientific evaluation of its advisability as a preferred technique. Furthermore, the pool of vaginally delivered breech infants from whom physicians may gain knowledge and experience has diminished rapidly (Minkoff and Schwarz 1980). A new "prevailing community standard" has also appeared, creating the possibility of a malpractice suit in the event of a poor outcome following a vaginal delivery of a malpresenting infant. In addition, acceptance of Caesarean section has almost eliminated the teaching of the external cephalic version, an ancient skill for externally manipulating the fetus in utero in turn to normal presentation—head down position (Ranney 1973).

Electronic Fetal Monitoring (EFM)

The influence of the fetal monitor and the fetal distress it measures on the Caesarean section rate have been extensively studied and debated (Paul et al. 1977). The controversy focuses on the accuracy of the interpretation of the recordings: whether they indicate fetal stress or distress; whether the added information is of sufficient value to offset complications and costs of monitor use; and/or whether monitor use actually causes an increase in Caesareans.

Despite debate over the use of electronic fetal monitoring (EFM) for all patients, it is in widespread use in the United States and has become a "prevailing community standard." Failure to use EFM in the event of an adverse outcome may place a physician at legal risk.

In contraposition to this, it should be noted that physician inexperience can lead to inaccurate monitor tracing interpretation and a subsequent Caesarean, as can failure to follow a distress reading with fetal scalp sampling prior to deciding on surgery (Paul et al. 1977). Use of the monitor itself may lead to maternal stress and the release of catecholamines, which produce vasoconstriction, and in turn can stress the fetus (Minkoff and Schwarz 1980). This causes a fetal distress reading that is responded to with Caesarean section.

Minkoff and Schwarz note that further education of obstetricians in accurately interpreting monitor tracings, education of the mother about the value of the monitor, and use of fetal scalp sampling may reduce the Caesarean rate for the indication of fetal distress (1980). Other authors have also noted the need for more appropriate monitor use (Neutra et al. 1978).

CONCLUSION

The physical conditions discussed above as well as the EFM factor do not stand alone as reasons for the rise in the rate of Caesarean section. Other factors such as economics, physicians' training and beliefs, malpractice fears, and technological innovations all affect decisions and practices. However, the present evidence does not demonstrate superiority of outcome from Caesarean section in many instances. It is this interweaving of factors that obscures thinking and affects medical practice, making it all the more important that scientific studies be pursued and their data rigorously analyzed. The costs of Caesarean section are too high for the practice to be utilized unnecessarily.

REFERENCES

Alfonzo, D., and J. Stichler, "Exploratory Study of Women's Reactions to Having Caesarean Birth," *Birth and the Family Journal*, 5 (1978), 88–94.

Arthure, H., "Maternal Deaths from Pulmonary Embolism," *Journal of Obstetrics and Gynecology of the British Commonwealth*, 75 (1968), 1309–12.

Baggish, M. S., and S. Hooper, "Aspiration as a Cause of Maternal Death," *Obstetrics and Gynecology*, 43 (1974), 327–36.

Banta, H. D., and S. B. Thacker, *Cost and Benefits of Electronic Fetal Monitoring: A Review of the Literature*. Washington, D.C.: National Center for Health Services Research, DHEW (PHS) 79–3245, 1979.

Beachman, W. D. et al., "Rupture of the Uterus at New Orleans Charity Hospital: A Report of 101 Cases and Comparison with the Previously Reported 96 Cases," *American Journal of Obstetrics and Gynecology*, 106 (1970), 1083–97.

Benson, R. C. et al., "Fetal Compromise during Elective Caesarean Section," *American Journal of Obstetrics and Gynecology*, 105 (1969), 579–88.

Bowes, W. A. et al., "The Effects of Obstetrical Medication on Fetus and Infant," *Monographs of the Society for Research in Child Development*, vol. 35, no. 4 (1970).

Chalmers, I., and M. Richards, "Intervention and Causal Interference in Obstetric Practice," in *Benefits and Hazards of the New Obstetrics*, T. Chard and M. Richards, eds. Philadelphia: J. B. Lippincott Company, 1977.

Coady, D. J., "Caesarean Section: Trends in Rates and Indications," *Journal of Women and Health*, 5 (1980), 9–22.

Cohen, W. R., "Influence of the Duration of Second Stage Labor on Perinatal Outcome and Puerperal Morbidity," *Obstetrics and Gynecology*, 49 (1977), 266–69.

Collea, J. V. et al., "The Randomized Management of Term Frank Breech Presentation. Vaginal Delivery vs Caesarean Section," *American Journal of Obstetrics and Gynecology*, 131 (1978), 186–95.

Craigin, E. B., "Conservatism in Obstetrics," *New York Journal of Medicine*, 104 (1916), 1–3.

Crawford, J. S., "The Anesthetist's Contribution to Maternal Mortality," *British Journal of Anesthesia*, 42 (1970), 70–73.

DeLee, J. B., *The Principles and Practice of Obstetrics*. Philadelphia: W. B. Sanders Company, 1913.

Dewhurst, C. J. "The Ruptured Caesarean Section Scar," *Journal of Obstetrics and Gynecology of the British Commonwealth*, 76 (1969), 137–43.

Douglas, R. G. et al., "Pregnancy and Labor Following Caesarean Section," *American Journal of Obstetrics and Gynecology*, 86 (1963), 961–71.

Evrard, J. R., and E. M. Gold, "Caesarean Section and Maternal Mortality in Rhode Island: Incidence and Risk Factors, 1965–1975," *Obstetrics and Gynecology*, 50 (1977), 594–97.

Findley, P., *Priests of Lucina: The Story of Obstetrics*. Boston: Little, Brown & Company, 1939.

Fortney, J. A., Section Head, Special Projects Department, International Fertility Research Program, Research Triangle Park, N.C., personal communication, 1978.

Frankel, T., and H. J. Buchsbaum, "Vesicocorporeal Fistula with Menourea," *Journal of Urology*, 106 (1971), 860–61.

Gibbs, R. S. et al., "Prophylactic Antibiotics in Caesarean Section: A Double-Blind Study," *American Journal of Obstetrics and Gynecology*, 114 (1972), 1048–53.

——, "Internal Fetal Monitoring and Maternal Infection Following Caesarean Section: A Prospective Study," *Obstetrics and Gynecology*, 52 (1978), 193–97.

Goldenberg, R. L., and K. Nelson, "Iatrogenic Respiratory Distress Syndrome," *American Journal of Obstetrics and Gynecology*, 123 (1975), 617–20.

Hack, M. et al., "Neonatal Respiratory Distress Following Elective Delivery: A Preventable Disease?" *American Journal of Obstetrics and Gynecology*, 126 (1976), 43–47.

Haddah, H., and L. E. Lundy, "Changing Indications for Cesarean Section: a 38-Year Experience at a Community Hospital," *Obstetrics and Gynecology*, 51 (1978), 133–37.

Hagen, D., "Maternal Febrile Morbidity Associated with Fetal Monitoring and Cesarean Section," *Obstetrics and Gynecology*, 46 (1975), 260–62.

Hall, J. E. et al., "Breech Presentation and Perinatal Mortality: A Study of 6,044 Cases," *American Journal of Obstetrics and Gynecology*, 91 (1965), 665–83.

Haverkamp, A. D. et al., "The Evaluation of Continuous Fetal Heart Rate Monitoring in High-Risk Pregnancy," *American Journal of Obstetrics and Gynecology*, 125 (1976), 310–20.

——, "A Controlled Trial of the Differential Effects of Intrapartum Monitoring," *American Journal of Obstetrics and Gynecology*, 134 (1979), 399–412.

Hibbard, L. T., "Changing Trends in Cesarean Section," *American Journal of Obstetrics and Gynecology*, 125 (1976), 798–804.

International Childbirth Education Association, Inc., "Vaginal Birth Following Cesarean Section," *ICEA Review*, 3 (1979), 1–8.

Jain, S. P., "Utero-Abdominal Sinus after Classical Cesarean Section," *Journal of Obstetrics and Gynecology of the British Commonwealth*, 81 (1974), 333–34.

Jones, O. H., "Cesarean Section in Present-Day Obstetrics," *American Journal of Obstetrics*, 126 (1976), 521–30.

Kelso, I. M. et al., "An Assessment of Continuous Fetal Heart Rate Monitoring in Labor—A Randomized Trial," *American Journal of Obstetrics and Gynecology*, vol. 131 (1978).

Lowe, J. A. et al., "Caesarean Sections in U.S. PAS Hospitals," *PAS Reporter*, vol. 14 (1976).,

Maisels, M. J. et al., "Effective Delivery of the Term Fetus: An Obstetrical Hazard," *JAMA*, 238 (1977), 2036–39.

Marieskind, H. I., *An Evaluation of Caesarean Section in the United States*. Washington, D.C.: U.S. Govt. Printing Office, 1979.

Merrill, B. S., and C. E. Gibbs, "Planned Vaginal Delivery Following Caesarean Section," *Obstetrics and Gynecology*, 52 (1978), 50–52.

Minkoff, H. L., and R. H. Schwarz, "The Rising Cesarean Section Rate: Can It Safely Be Reversed?" *Obstetrics and Gynecology*, 56 (1980), 135–43.

Minogue, M., "Vaginal Breech Delivery in Multiparas," *Irish Medical Journal*, 67 (1974), 117–19.

Morgan, E. S., and S. H. Kane, "An Analysis of 16,327 Breech Births," *Jama*, 187 (1964), 262–64.

Muller, P. F. et al., "Repeat Cesarean Section," *American Journal of Obstetrics and Gynecology*, 81 (1961), 867–76.

National Center for Health Statistics, *Final Natality Statistics*, 1966–1978.

———, *National Hospital Discharge Survey*, 1968–1979, and personal communications, March 1978, May 1979, February 1981.

National Institute of Child Health and Human Development, *Caesarean Section Consensus Report*. Washington, D.C.: U.S. Govt. Printing Office, 1980.

Neutra, R. R. et al., "Effect of Fetal Monitoring on Neonatal Death Rates," *New England Journal of Medicine*, 299 (1978), 324–26.

Paul, R. H. et al., "Clinical Fetal Monitoring: Its Effect on Cesarean Section Rate and Perinatal Morality: Five Year Trends," *Postgraduate Medicine*, 61 (1977), 160–66.

Petitti, D. et al., "Cesarean Section in California—1960 through 1975," *American Journal of Obstetrics and Gynecology*, 133 (1979), 391–97.

Polishuk, W. Z. et al., "Puerperal Endometritis and Intrauterine Adhesions," *International Surgery*, 60 (1975), 418–20.

PSRO Hospital Discharge Data Sets, January–December 1977. Professional Standards Review Organization, HCFA, DHEW. Washington, D.C., 1978–1979.

Ranney, B., "The Gentle Art of External Cephalic Version," *American Journal of Obstetrics and Gynecology*, 116 (1973), 239–51.

Ross, J. E., and B. W. Galliford, "Late Hemorrhage Following Cesarean Section," *American Journal of Obstetrics and Gynecology*, 119 (1974), 858–59.

Rubin, G. L. et al., "Maternal Death after Cesarean Section in Georgia," *American Journal of Obstetrics and Gynecology*, 139 (1981), 681–85.

Schrinsky, D. C., and R. C. Benson, "Rupture of the Pregnant Uterus: A Review," *Obstetrical and Gynecological Survey*, 33 (1978), 217–32.

Shearer, M., "Complications of Cesarean to Mother and Infant," *Birth and the Family Journal*, 4 (1977), 103–5.

Young, D., and C. Mahan, *Unnecessary Cesareans: Ways to Avoid Them*. Minneapolis: ICEA, 1980.

Wolter, D. F., "Patterns of Management with Breech Presentation," *American Journal of Obstetrics and Gynecology*, 125 (1976), 733–39.

Part Two

HOLISTIC HEALTH AND ORTHODOX MEDICINE: CHANGING CONCEPTS OF HEALTH AND DISEASE

Richard B. Miles

Since the early 1970s, two social movements have been developing in the United States along parallel paths. One is known as the "women's movement" and is focussed in such activities as the National Organization for Women and the Equal Rights Amendment. The other has been called the "holistic health movement," or health promotion, humanistic medicine, or other such terms descriptive of a shift in the public's perceptions about health care and the appropriateness of the services offered by orthodox medicine.

This article will explore some connections between these two movements, illustrating how both are examples of a larger social recognition of the role of personal responsibility, individual rights, a sense of control over self-destiny, and a sense of participation and choice in one's view of life, health, and well-being. A major connecting link between the two movements is their opposition to medical science's view of the world as reductionist, rational, and essentially physical. This view discounts the role of intuitive, emotional, and spiritual issues in health, illness, and healing. These attributes are seen as "feminine" in our society. Now that women are seeking the "right" to express their views, needs, emotions, and ambitions, conflict has arisen between women and orthodox medicine.

Mendelsohn cites case after case of discriminatory practices in medicine that demean women (1981). One simple example is that a gynecologist is considered a primary care physician for women, whereas a urologist is a specialist or secondary care provider for men. And hysterectomy is the "treatment of choice" for a number of gynecological problems, whereas prostate surgery or castration is hardly ever recommended for comparable problems for men, except in the most severe cases. In fact, the word *hysterectomy* implies that the operation is designed to remove the woman's "hysteria," in itself quite a comment about male medicine's view of women's health issues.

As another example, it should be noted that more than 70 percent of the individuals receiving electroshock therapy for emotional and mental disturbances are women (*Network against Psychiatric Assault* 1981). These instances, and many others, have led to alienation and hostility between women and traditional physicians.

Early in 1980, a number of women's organizations in New York City were invited to a meeting to discuss the question, "Is there an antidoctor feeling among women today?" The attending doctors were visibly upset by the women's comments about insufficient information provided, condescension and browbeating, lack of personal respect, misunderstanding of women's attitudes about ownership of their lives and bodies, and especially overprescription of mood-altering drugs to manage what could be considered normal emotional responses to everyday life situations (Aronson 1981).

As recently as 80 years ago, the family physician in our predominately rural society was a generalist, a close family friend, and aware of the spiritual, emotional, financial, and interpersonal dynamics of the patient's situation— all subjective factors in the evaluation of a health problem. Today, a woman patient in an urban area may undergo radical surgery performed by a specialist who has never met her in person, with all decisions based on laboratory tests, X-rays, read by a technician, without reference to objective data not related to the subjective dynamics of the patient's life.

Thus, as women seek advice, counsel, and service from the current medical "system," the need for emotional support, relief of anxiety, a sense of personal connection, and recognition of personal worth and dignity may be met with a sense of indifference or hostility from professionals who have not been trained to recognize the importance of these issues to all humans, and especially to women who feel that they have been too long unheard and unrecognized.

A direct example of this problem surfaced in a meeting held to explore the possibility of an "alternative" birth center. Parents interested in natural styles of birth were asked to attend an open house at a major medical facility. Obstetricians and other professionals joined them for an open forum. The comments of each group and the language they used illustrated their different views of the birth process:

> *Words the professionals used:* death, risk, control, protection, costs, proof, management, standards, efficiency.
> *Words the parents used:* family, love, bonding, feelings, anxiety, unhurried, quiet, meaningful, life ritual.

The words of the professionals were objective, rational, measurement-oriented, and mistrustful of the natural process. They indicated a deep *need to control* the event of birth. According to this view, natural processes left to their own devices would inevitably lead to disaster and death.

The words of the parents were subjective, emotional, caring-oriented, and mindful of natural relationships and family connections. They indicated a basic trust in the natural life process. In this view, natural events left to their own devices would most likely work out well if minimally interfered with and given their own time.

Almost all the professionals who spoke were men; most of the parents who spoke were women (Alternative Birth Center Open House 1977).

All of this indicates a growing awareness of a deep societal bias against the subjective, emotional, and "feminine" way of being in the world. In health care, women have begun to experience this bias as a threat to their sense of integrity and ownership of their bodies. In response, in a combination of the women's movement and the new health movements, such books as *Our Bodies, Our Selves* (1978) and *The Ms. Guide to Women's Health* (1979) have been written to improve women's knowledge and self-control.

TWO WAYS TO SEE THE WORLD

Since the historical beginnings of the study of human nature, there has been controversy about two perspectives of human nature, human perception, and human behavior. Which of these two perspectives will we be guided by:

1. That which is *out there*: objective, measurable, predictable, controllable, mechanistic, technical, rational (seen as masculine)?
2. That which is *in here*: subjective, symbolic, intuitive, emotional, artistic, unpredictable, nonrational (seen as feminine)?

The scientists, philosophers, and mystics have debated for centuries about whether either of these views is the "right" way to evaluate our perceptions of the world. We call our right hand *right* because it is functionally controlled by the dominant, rational, hemisphere of the brain/mind system. In contrast, that which is *left* (remaining, leftover) is the mystical, intuitive aspect of ourselves. This more subjective organization of perceptions and experiences has long been considered sinsister (from the Latin: omens from the left or unlucky side), demonic, and untrustworthy. (*Note:* The motor control of the body is governed by the opposite brain hemisphere; i.e., the right side of the body is operated by the left brain hemisphere, and the left side of the body is operated by the right brain hemisphere.)

Recent brain research has indicated that these two modes of human perception described above as "out here" and "in here" seem to be generated in the left (out there, rational, reductionist) and right (in here, subjective, symbolic) hemispheres of the neo-cortex (Ornstein 1972). Thus, both modes of perception are inherently human. Neither may be right, wrong, dominant, leftover, superior, or inferior. Therefore we should be exploring both modes and the relationship between them in human nature.

Within the past century, parallel to the development of laboratory science and industrial technology, America has taken as gospel the beliefs of objective, rational science and has foresaken much of the mystical and spiritual heritage of its original founders. A deep mistrust of the subjective, intuitive, and emotional aspects of human nature has become institutionalized, especially in the "hard sciences," including medicine.

HISTORICAL VIEWS OF THE ORIGIN OF DISEASE

Less than 100 years ago, there were three generally hypothesized origins of disease. The *divine theory* supposed that disease was punishment meted out by an angry God upon those who flaunted His wishes. The *demonic theory* suggested that disease was the result of possession by evil forces, most likely under the direct supervision of the Devil. The *miasmatic theory* grew from observation of the degenerative process of all living organisms when they are separated from their life environment, i.e., the apparently spontaneous emergence of worms and maggots in cast aside foods or vegetation. In this theory, the "miasma," or illness, was considered the result of invasion by, or the emergence of, these degenerative forces in nature.

When the microscope began to be widely used in scientific research in the late 1800s, many bacteria and viruses were "discovered" for the first time. Thus the miasmatic theory evolved into the *germ theory*. In 1858, Rudolph Virchow reported that disease is nothing but the reaction of the cells to the causative agent of the disease (Kaslow and Miles 1979).

Note that all these theories, which evolved into the germ theory that has dominated scientific medicine from the late 1800s until quite recently, assume disase to originate from forces of nature outside the human body and largely beyond human control.

Joseph Chilton Pearce has suggested that the basis of all technological development has been the assumption that the human role on Earth is to learn to master and dominate the forces of nature (1974). One need not look far in American scientific or popular literature to find support for this view of nature as a direct adversary to human existence. Everything from disease, the weather, other natural events, or even societal ills such as inflation or poverty is cast as an *enemy* to be militarily encountered as if in war. The experiencers of these events is regarded as a helpless *victim* in a world assumed to be out of control.

However, our views of the world, and of disease, are changing. Peter Drucker points out that in every discipline of study, the forward thinkers are challenging the basic assumptions upon which Western thought has developed since Biblical times (1976). In theoretical physics, child development, sociology, medicine, philosophy, and many other fields, books are appearing offering completely new views of the organization and function of natural systems.*

FOUR STAGES IN THE EVOLUTION OF THOUGHT

The evolution of thought in many fields can be compared to the "out there" and "in here" modes of thinking discussed earlier, progressing through four stages as outlined below. All four of these concepts have been discussed for centuries, but each has enjoyed a dominant role over time.

1. **Determinism** (out there)—Life is a series of clockwork events set in motion by forces beyond human destiny.

   Physics—Newtonian mechanics; religion—absolutist dogmatic systems; philosophy—determinism; medicine and psychology—illness is caused only be outside "agents" that need to identified and dealt with. A strictly cause-effect world.

2. **Chance** (neither out there nor in here)—Life is a series of accidental, random events without meaning or direction.

   Physics—relativity; religion—atheism and nihilism; philosophy—nihilism; medicine and psychology—behaviorism. A random "bell-curve" world measurable only by statistical probability.

3. **Free Will** (in here)—Life is a series of meaningful choices through which humans (and perhaps other life forms) choose their role in their own destiny.

   Physics—quantum mechanics; religion—mystical and revelatory systems; philsophy—free will and solipsism; medicine and psychology—humanistic and transpersonal.

4. **Cybernetic System Theory** (both out there and in here)—The entire universe is an interconnected series of interactions among dynamnic forces, self-regulating and self-directing.

   Physics—unified field theory; relgion—transcendence; philosophy—Huxley's perennial philosophy; medicine and psychology—holism.

*See titles listed under "Physics," "Child Rearing," "Alternate Futures," and "Health" in Suggested Readings at the end of this article.

RATIONAL, OBJECTIVE VIEWS BEING QUESTIONED TODAY

Rational, objective science as it has manifested itself in the past 50 years is essentially a random chance system based entirely on statistical probability. It has great difficulty with ultimate sources of creation, subjective experience, and intuitive or spiritual direction and meaning, not recognizing these aspects of life as directly significant in the physical events of the world.

In the 1950s, this rational, objective view became so dominant in America that religious organizations began to ask the question, "Is God dead?" Since then, many trends in society could be identified as attempts to reconnect our lives with natural and spiritual inspiration. The influx of Eastern philosophy, meditation, and gurus, the ecology movement, the development of cults, and the onset of the human potential and holistic health movements can all be seen as efforts to recapture some sense of meaning and purpose, and spiritual foundation, in a society losing that sense to a value system based on economic production, competition, and personal gain. All these new trends suggest that the secret of "the good life" is to be found inside the soul and in harmony with nature rather than in material success.

The rational, objective view that disease is an attack by, or an accident of, a random system of nature, is therefore, being questioned. If there is a possibility that the natural system is a cybernetic, interconnected, self-regulating organic whole, then disease would more likely be seen as a distortion or malfunction of that self-regulating system.

Our nature-as-enemy perspective of the last century spawned the germ theory and identified the infectious diseases. But it is interesting to note that these diseases ceased to be the primary causes of morbidity and mortality in the United States as long ago as 1920, long before the introduction of the miracle drugs and exotic surgeries (Glazier 1973). What we face now are the chronic disorders: cardiovascular disease, cancer, diabetes, arthritis, kidney failutre. However, we "attack" these problems, both in research and in treatment, as if they were infectious diseases, seeking to remove or eliminate the causative agent. Might it be more productive to look upon them as the consequence of overloads placed on the internal self-regulating systems of the human body?

FOUR APPROACHES TO HEALTH DISORDERS

Once we begin to ask this kind of question, several effective ways to approach the problems of illness and dysfunction emerge, ways that go beyond attacking the symptoms or causative agents of disease. The map of this territory in which we search for pathways to improved health might be divided into four possibilities:

1. Identify, then correct the (symptoms) of the disease

This approach is followed by most of the existing orthodox medical practices designed to "fix the problem." Included here are drug therapies, surgery, prescriptive diets, and radiation therapies. These traditional techniques are joined by some unorthodox medical practices such as intravenous chelation, hyperbaric oxygen tanks, colonic irrigation, and the rash of diet schemes available in the popular press. The basic assumption of these therapeutic concepts is that nature has made some awkward blunders, and we need clever science to outsmart her and fix these mistakes.

2. Restore, and rehabilitate, the body's natural capacity to obtain and maintain health; i.e., support the body's self-regulatory and homeostatic systems.

Homeostasis as a concept was first explored by the eminent French physiologist Claude Bernard in 1878. It is the essential tendency of the body to maintain "a state of equilibrium with respect to various functions and to the chemical compositions of the fluids and tissues; e.g., temperature, heart rate, blood pressure, water content, blood sugar (*Stedman's Medical Dictionary* 1981). Every organism is nature has an innate capacity to sense changes in its environment (both inner and outer) and to initiate responses that will maintain functional equilibrium. For example, when we become warm, we perspire for cooling; when we become cold, we shiver to generate heat.

Homeopathy supports homeostasis by prescribing "similars" (substances that foster symptoms which are similar to the disease), which are said to speed the body's homeostatic response and hence reinforce its inner wisdom. For example, osteopathy is based on a system proposing that muscular and bone alignment are necessary to the free flow of many body processes; therefore maladjustments of muscular alignment will foster homeostatic balance. Chiropractic medicine assumes a similar pose, but speaks instead of adjustments to assure proper alignment of neutral pathways to keep messages moving in the nervous system.

Each of these homeostatic-type systems has engaged in debate with orthodox medicine without a clear definition of any significantly different basis for action. These systems are designed to rebalance the body systems, not to "treat disease." If one tries to prove their effectiveness in "treating disease," this discrepancy of purpose prevents a clear comparison.

Eastern approaches such as meditation, acupuncture, and "body energy massage systems" (polarity, acupressure, jin shin jyutsu) are essentially based on the homeostatic premise of restoring appropriate balance and energy flow to the systems in the body.

In this perspective, the human body is looked upon as wise and sensitive. If we can evaluate our lives, and can get out of the way those factors that distort our natural capacity for self-regulation, the organism will heal itself. Here, nature is very wise, and science has become myopic.

3.　Seek out the environmental (societal, biological) patterns of interaction of the organism and investigate their possible role of illness.

From this view have come most of the major improvements in American public health in this country. Cleaner water, improved food production, sanitation, mosquito control, cleaner garbage and waste disposal techniques, and indoor plumbing—all have done far more for our societal health than medicines and surgery.

Unfortunately, as Ivan Illich points out, technology has the tendency to reach "paradoxical counterproductivity" (1976). Science starts down a pathway intending to improve the situation, but industry forgets the reason why. For example, improved food production techniques have led to processed foods that last forever on the shelf but have little nutritious value. Or the idea that we can "clean" water has led to wholesale dumping of toxic wastes into streams and rivers that, further downstream, are intake sources for drinking water. The cost of this is becoming excessive as we "take out" and "add to" water and foods that might better have been left alone.

The environment now offers us toxic waste disposal problems, air pollution, asbestos building materials, off-gassing from formaldehyde glues, PCB's, polymer plastics that are not biodegradable, nuclear radiation, and a seemingly endless list of health hazards. Our interference in nature to produce affluence and comfort seems to have a hidden price.

4. Consider the spiritual, ideological, attitudinal, and emotional congruity within the individual in regard to cultural belief systems, self-image, and family or ethnic symbols of meaning.

At the "primitive" end of this scale are voodoo, witch doctors, shamans, and tribal ceremonies. At a more contemporary level are the unorthodox practices of psychic and spiritual healing and the emerging psychologies of logotherapy (Victor Frankl), psychosynthesis (Roberto Assagioli), the collective unconscious (C. G. Jung), transpersonal psychology, and holistic health. In these perspectives, a person's beliefs about role of self, the meaning of life, and personal connection (or lack of connection) with higher orders of meaning, or God, all play an important role in the possibility of disease, disorder, and the maintenance of health. These concepts frame the universe as essentially purposive and supportive of human endeavor. Disconnection from the universal source of spiritual renewal and energy may result in desperation, disorder, and disease.

Perspectives #1 (identify and correct) and #3 (environmental) tend to be more outer and objective. Perspectives #2 (rebalance) and # 4 (spiritual) are more inner-directed and subjective.

DEFINITION OF "HOLISTIC"

The educational self-directive tools of holistic health are essentially predicated on rebalancing and spiritual redirection, with an acknowledged need for increased awareness of our interaction with the environment (essentially a spiritual issue).

It should be noted here that "holistic" as it is being used in this article is a perspective, or a system of thought. Its basis is in wholeness, integration, and trust in the natural order of the universe.

Thus, if a practitioner of any health modality claims to be holistic, he or she should espouse and manifest a holistic view of life. This would include a trustworthy professional-client relationship, disclosure of intent and direction, establishment of rapport and connection with the client, and willingness to explore the needs and interests of the client.

Many practitioners have begun to call themselves holistic without examining the inner system of belief the term implies. If you visit any practitioner of any discipline, you should ask yourself the following questions:

1. Do I trust this person?
2. Is she/he willing to listen to my needs and anxieties?
3. Is she/he willing to tell me what she/he is doing in a way that has meaning for me?
4. Does she/he acknowledge my integrity and offer me choice in my own process?
5. Does her/his personal view include a sense of connection with nature and spiritual guidance?

If the practitioner gives you short shrift and seems ready and willing to quickly fix your problem without your participation and with little recognition of your sense of balance or self-worth, then seek "holistic" care elsewhere because this person has yet to learn its meaning.

FACTORS THAT IMPROVE AND PROTECT BODY SELF-REGULATION

Recent research in scientific medicine has begun to make note of certain factors that tend to improve and protect your health.

Positive mental attitudes and a hopeful view of the future are significant retardants of aging and tend to diminish the incidence of coronary heart disease, cancer, emphysema, high blood pressure, and suicide (Vaillant 1979).

Attitudes and life outlook are primary factors in the body's metabolization and utilization of food value. People who enjoy foods in relaxed, friendly setting gain more nutritive value from their food, *regardless of content*, than careless eaters or people obsessed with food content (Baird and Schutz 1980).

Regular exercise improves the fibrinolytic (blood-clot dissolving) capacity of the blood, thus reducing the risk of stroke, pulmonary embolism and heart attack. This effect is in addition to exercise's ability to increase the body's high-density lipoproteins, the biochemical self-regulator of blood cholesterol (Williams 1980).

Simple fasting, or reduction of food intake, can bring about relief from symptoms of arthritis. Subjects who restricted food intake experienced a significant reduction in pain, joint swelling, and stiffness. When usual food intake was resumed, the symptoms reappeared, indicating a direct link between nutrition and disease episodes (Baird and Schutz 1980).

Through a growing number of similar studies, and with a fresh perspective about self-regulation and homeostasis, the central role played by attitudes, stress, nutritional imbalance, lack of exercise, and other subjective factors in the onset and continuation of disease becomes more apparent.

FACTORS THAT DISTORT BODY SELF-REGULATION

If we assume that the human organism is a self-healing and health-maintaining system, the question immediately must be asked, "Why do we become ill?"

The *U.S. Surgeon General's Report* (1979) stated that life-style factors such as nutrition habits, exercise, use of cigarettes and alcohol, and failure to observe simple safety precautions are far more significant causes of illness and dysfunction than any issues being actively researched today by scientific medicine.

Eight factors, as itemized below can be said to contribute to the distortion of the human body's natural capacity for self-regulation and self-healing. Long-term ignorance of these factors can result in the fatigue and collapse of the visceral and glandular systems that (a) maintain digestion and assimilation of foods, (b) repair and replace cells, (c) maintain muscular and nervous system function, (d) regulate body utilization of oxygen, and (e) maintain effective function of the immune system. The result of this fatigue and collapse is what we have come to call "chronic, degenerative disease."

1. Attitudes and Beliefs

The most important issues in disease causation here are the lack of connection with a higher order of meaning and purpose (feelings of separation, loss, and desperation) and learned helplessness (accumulated habit patterns of dependency and passivity).

The helpless "victim of nature" attitude we have held about disease, plus the secularization of our society, has left many people feeling totally powerless, with no God or source of spiritual inspiration to turn to in times of adversity. All the new movements, whether ecological, spiritual, political, or psychological, emphasize the need for a renewed sense of personal dignity and power. Thus the physically dysfunctional in our present society are deprived of any source of inner hope or volition and must wait passively for scientific breakthroughs to rescue them. Illich calls this "iatrogenic" (physician-caused) disease because the medical system promulgates a belief system that only science can find the answers to life (1976).

Once pain and dysfunction begin, the patient tends to build patterns of dependency and further passivity, frequently gaining the secondary benefits of care, attention, and control over others. These patterns become addictive, and eventually the person perceives him/her-self as "the problem." (I *am* an arthritic; I *am* an alcoholic). Once this image develops, it becomes increasingly difficult for the person to imagine life without the problem since most daily activity revolves around it. Resistance to change then becomes an inhibiting factor in the process of regaining health.

2. Unresolved Emotional Stress

The principal issues here are (a) accumulating, but unrecognized, stress from major life events, and (b) persistent conflict built into the life situation of the individual.

Major life events produce stress differently in each individual since the important factor is our attitude about, and response to, the event.

However, most of us are not aware of the cumulative impact of change and life events on our systems; hence we do little to identify and relax the resulting stress.

The Holmes-Rahe Significant Life Event Index lists 41 potential stressors, with the death of a spouse at the top with 100 points, and a minor traffic citation at the bottom with 10 points (1967). Not all listed events would be considered "bad," such as marriage, childbirth, job promotion, and buying a new home. However, these are also stressful events. The body experiences any change as stress, as we adapt to our new circumstances and environments. Hence, accumulated change can require increased attention to the development of relaxation skills. Holmes and Rahe report that individuals with an excess of 300 points in one year have a significantly higher risk of serious illness than someone with fewer major life changes (ibid).

Persistent conflict built into the everyday life pattern can keep the "fight-flight" arousal system in the body turned on most of the time, prepared for defensive action. And when the fight-flight system is "on," maintenance and repairs systems are diminished.

For example, a woman of age 35–50 with little or no work experience, children leaving home for lives of their own, and a failing marriage, has a high potential for conflict between needs of personal security and inner needs for self-image and self-esteem. Or a man who has made a large contribution to his company pension plan and has only a few years remaining until he can obtain his benefits, but hates his job and/or his co-workers, is gnashing his teeth each morning as he leaves for the office and is a prime target for ill health. This kind of daily, persistent inner conflict will rapidly fatigue the body and its natural self-regulating and immune systems.

3. Nutritional Imbalance

There are some 60 natural chemical elements needed by the human organism for regular function. Although we have studied the need for body energy (carbohydrates and fats) and the need for basic body building blocks (proteins), we have not clearly understood the third role of nutrition: supplying the vitamins, minerals, and trace elements so significantly involved in the self-regulatory, homeostatic systems.

American food habits in the past 50 years have swung away from fresh vegetables and fruits and too far into animals proteins, fats, and refined carbohydrates. Thus, our natural sources for vitamins, minerals, and trace elements have been diminished through diet choices.

4. Food Allergy and Sensitivity

There are thousands of substances on the planet that provide nutritional value. However, as a result of food production decisions, cultural traditions, and packaging and shipping convenience, today's supermarket may contain fewer than 300. A brief diet survey of most people's food habits will indicate than an individual may habitually eat fewer than 15 different substances (beef, corn, potatoes, eggs, etc.). Research is just now beginning to show us that if a person's food choices are limited to a narrow range of foods, and these foods do not provide the variety of chemical elements needed to sustain the body, then sensitivities or "allergies" may arise, causing eventual rejection of the habitual foods not wanted by the body. These are described as autoimmune responses and involve stimulation of white-cell scavengers in the bloodstream that harass weakened tissue systems. This may be the reason why the *Lakartidningen* article showed diminished arthritic symptoms when people fasted. A significant number of case studies have been accumulated illustrating this autoimmune relationship to food sensitivities (*Science News* 1979).

5. Environmental Contamination

A review of potential toxins in our environment can be somewhat overwhelming:

> In the workplace: asbestos, coal dust, dust metals, vapors, petrochemicals, heat, light, intense noise, vibration, radiation, and corrosives.
>
> In agriculture and gardening: insecticides, fertilizers, soil conditioners, fuel vapors, and herbicides.
>
> In building environments (home, offices): formaldehyde, glues, paints, fumes from burning plastics, sensitivity to artificial fabrics; or radiation from microwaves, televisions, fluorescent light fixtures, and cathode ray tubes for computers.
>
> Poor air quality, auto exhausts, industrial chimneys.
>
> Water contamination.

Maintaining a well-balanced and vital body can raise one's threshold for environmental exposure risks. However, this is a health issue that must be dealt with at a societal as well as a personal level. It is becoming more apparent that we cannot afford, economically, or for reasons of health, to introduce substances into our environment without a thorough consideration of their interactions with biological processes. This same consideration must also include both recreational and prescription drugs.

6. Movement Flexibility and the Body's Use of Oxygen

Persons who do not exercise regularly lose muscle tone and the optimum capacity to assimilate and transport oxygen. Since oxygen is a primary factor in almost every physiological event, diminished oxygen supply has a degenerative effect throughout the body. The body's regulating mechanisms will protect the brain, heart, visceral organs, and digestive systems, but will sacrifice the peripheral muscles and bones. Hence, "minimal oxygen deprivation" through lack of exercise may inevitable lead to loss of muscle power, weak bone structures in the joints, and restricted movement capacity. Unfortunately, this becomes a self-perpetuating spiral, and weakness and pain may further limit physical activity.

Fortunately, the body is self-regenerating and within certain limits, all the muscle power and oxygen use capacity can be redeveloped through appropriate movement and exercise.

7. Infectious Agents

Overwhelming presence in the body of bacterial, viral, or foreign entities can overcome the natural defense systems and produce disease. The person's capacity to respond productively to these agents, however, is determined by general physical condition and stress levels. Persons who work regularly with the above six factors are less likely to experience serious infections.

8. Traumatic Injury

Falls, auto accidents, burns, and other traumatic events place an extreme demand on the body's self-regulatory systems in their internal attempts to restore and maintain homeostatic balance.

NEW DIRECTIONS IN HEALTH CARE

Orthodox medicine has centered its attention on infectious diseases and the repair of traumatic injury, with some remarkable achievements and successes. This is essentially the result of the cultural view that disease is the result of outside natural forces. And these two areas are those in which scientific medical intervention is most likely to succeed. Unfortunately, medicine has endeavored to extend these approaches to cover almost all clinical situations.

Note that the first six factors discussed above, with some exception in regard to environmental issues, are under the direct control of the individual. See Figure A showing health influences under the control of the individual. Thus *health education* at the personal and family level will soon become a primary approach to many health problems. This can have a profound effect on how many women's health issues might be approached.

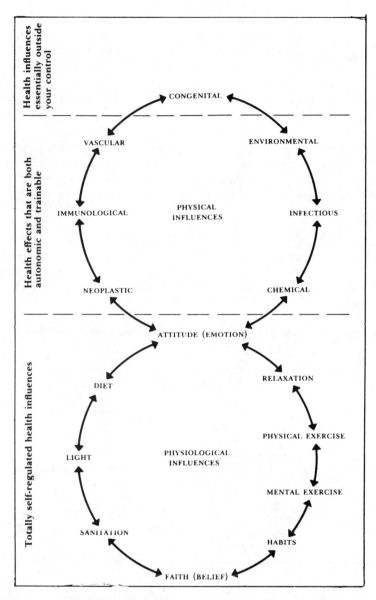

FIGURE A. "Health, Stress, Relaxation" chart by C. Norman Shealy. From *90 Days to Self-Health*. Courtesy of Dial Press.

For instance, many fairly regular occurrences in a woman's life—headaches, irregular menstrual periods, menstrual cramps, skin rashes, vaginal irritation and infection, weight concerns—are now seen as "diseases," and a whole pharmacopoeia of drugs is available to "treat" them; whereas, in all probability, these events are the result of homeostatic imbalances. The drugs only cause further imbalance and perpetuate the problem. A timely review of the six educational factors—attitudes, stresses, nutrition, allergies, environment, and exercise—may ameliorate the distortions in homeostasis, and the *problems will all clear up by themselves*. Many women have intuitively known this, but they have had no arena in which to explore their ideas.

It is also not too difficult to see that the introduction of birth control pills, which have a *consequential and essential* imbalancing effect (the reason why they are taken) on periodic female systems, is bound to create profound distortions of the rest of the body maintenance systems.

A COMPARISON OF VIEWS

If we look at a medical event, in this instance, childbirth, a comparison of the orthodox views and holistic views indicates why very different strategies are chosen in each case based on the perceived purpose of the strategies (see Table A).

TABLE A. A Comparison of Orthodox and Holistic Views Regarding Childbirth

	Orthodox Obstetrics	Holistic Health
Most important factor	Avoid death and risk Mistrust of nature	Promote love and family connection Trust of nature
Role of physician	Hero/rescuer Event manager	Advisor/supporter Experienced helper
Role of mother	Passive as possible Avoid pain and experience	Participant in a primary life ritual
Role of father	Excluded	Participant in a primary life ritual
Role of infant	Unconscious/prehuman	Highly sensitive and observant participant
Time factor	Organized for convenience of professionals	Allow nature to take its course
Most likely risk projected	Death of mother or infant	Damage to the essential connections and bonds for healthy growth and family development
Concern for the developmental potential of infant	Reduced to adequate physiological reactions—no concern for emotional or conscious experience of fear and pain	Paramount considerations of "welcoming" a new person into the world.
Most likely outcome	Fear, anxiety, stress, complications, which then appear to validate the need for rescue and intervention	Quiet, healthy, attentive, active infant

It is not difficult to see why communication between persons holding these significantly different world views is somewhat confused. They hardly speak the same language, and in a sense, don't live on the same planet.

In cancer therapy for women, a similar comparison chart could be made. Dr. Wallace Ellerbrook of Sunset Beach, California, is both a gynecologist and a psychiatrist. Hence, he "saw" both physiological and psychological emotional influences of disease in his patients. Noticing situational patterns in the cases of women coming to him with developing cancer, he identified "deep unexpressed anger" toward the spouse as a common issue among women with cervical cancer. Stepping into items one and two on our list of homeostasis distortion factors, Dr. Ellerbrook began to work with (a) the woman's sense of personal power and destiny, and (b) the dynamics of her relationship with her husband as factors in the cancer therapy. In a number of cases, as women gained a sense of power over their own destiny, and as their husbands joined in the counseling sessions and the long-held emotional issues surfaced, success in cancer therapies rapidly increased (Personal communication 1980).

Treating only the physiological measures of a disease or dysfunction is but a small part of what is going on in someone's life that can contribute to health failure.

SUMMARY

Most "women's problems" brought to health care professionals are most likely to be distortions of inner, self-regulating, and homeostatic body systems rather than diseases wrought by outside attackers. Hence, orthodox "treatment" approaches to them are rarely successful. Life style issues such as attitudes, stresses, nutrition, exercise, and environmental exposure are more likely to surface the "causes" of these problems.

Hence, women have been given short shrift by orthodox medicine because their approach to the world, and their problems, involve a different world view from traditional Western science. Newer, holistic, and educational approaches may prove both more comfortable and more productive for women's health issues (see Table B).

TABLE B. A Tabular Comparison of Orthodox and Holistic Health Medicine

Views of Orthodox Medicine	Views of Holistic Health
1. Nature makes many mistakes. Through scientific intervention we can fix the errors.	1. Nature is wise. In our lack of wisdom, we have interfered with the body's capacity to maintain natural health.
2. Disease is caused by invasion of the body by outside agents. These invasions are essentially beyond	2. Disease is caused by the distortion of the natural self-healing and self-regulating systems in the body.

Table B. (*Cont.*)

Views of Orthodox Medicine	Views of Holistic Health
human control unless effective immunizations are developed or the agents can be eliminated.	Infection can result in a "run-down" system.
3. The key to the management of disease is the control of, or elimination of, the effects (symptoms) of the disease.	3. The key to the alleviation of disease is the rebalancing and revitalization of the homeostatic balance in the body.
4. The purpose of diagnosis is to identify the causative agent.	4. The purpose of diagnosis (evaluation) is to identify those life factors that are contributing to distortion of homeostatic self-regulation.
5. The purpose of treatment is to modify, remove, or eliminate the symptoms and/or the causative agent.	5. The purpose of treatment (education) is to teach new patterns and motivations that will rebalance self-regulation systems and get the person on a productive health track.
6. Drugs and surgery are used to manipulate body structure and chemistry to suppress, eliminate, or modify symptoms.	6. Drugs and surgery are avoided except as last resorts since they are further distortions of homeostatic systems.
7. Patients expect a quick response from "rescue" tactics, based on previous experience with minor infectious diseases.	7. Patients realize that problems that have taken years to manifest may take some time to turn around.
8. The focus is on disease, disability, and limitations.	8. The focus is on health, positive future possibilities, and self-control.

References

Alternative Birth Center Open House, Stanford University Medical Center, 1977, meeting attended by the author.

Aronson, Shepard G., Associated Press article in San Francisco Chronicle, August 12, 1981.

Baird, Pamela, and Howard Schutz. "Life Style Correlates of Dietary and Biochemical Measures of Nutrition," *Journal of the American Dietetic Association*., Vol. 76, March, 1980.

Boston Women's Health Collective, *Our Bodies, Our Selves*. New York: Simon and Schuster, 1978.

Cooke, Cynthia W., and Susan Dworkin, *The Ms. Guide to Women's Health*. New York: Doubleday, 1979.

Drucker, Peter., *The Age of Discontinuity*. New York: Harper and Row, 1967.

Glazier, William, "The Task of Medicine," Scientific American, vol. 228 (April 1973).

Illich, Ivan, *Medical Nemesis*. New York: Pantheon Books/Random House, 1976.

Kaslow, Arthur L., and Richard B. Miles, *Freedom from Chronic Disease*. Los Angeles: J.P. Tarcher, Inc., 1979.

Lakartidningen (Swedish Medical Journal), quoted in *Science News*, July, 1979.

Mendelsohn, Robert S., *Male-Practice*. New York: Contemporary Books, 1981.

Network Against Psychiatric Assault, newsletter, San Francisco, 1981.

Ornstein, Robert E., *The Psychology of Consciousness*. Chapter 2, "The Two Sides of the Brain." San Francisco: W. H. Freeman & Company, 1972.

Pearce, Chilton Joseph, *Exploring the Crack in the Cosmic Egg*. New York: Julian Press, 1974.

Stedman's Medical Dictionary, 1980.

Vaillant, George, "Natural History of Male Psychological Health," *New England Journal of Medicine*, 1979 Dec. 6:301 (23) 1249–54.

Williams, R. Sanders, "Physical Conditioning Augments the Fibrinolytic Response to Venous Occlusion," *New England Journal of Medicine*, 1980 May 1: 302 (18) 987–81.

Suggested Readings

Physics:

Capra, Fritjof., *The Tao of Physics*. Berkeley: Shambhala Press, 1975.

Wolf, Fred Alan., *Taking the Quantum Leap*, New York: Harper & Row, 1981.

Zukav, Gary, *The Dancing Wu Li Masters*. New York: William Morrow & Co., 1979.

Child Rearing:

Berends, Polly Berrien. *Whole Child, Whole Parent*. Harpers Magazine Press, 1975.

Pearce, Joseph Chilton., *Magical Child*. New York: Dutton, 1977.

Pines, Maya. "Baby, You're Incredible," *Psychology Today*, vol. 16, no. 2., Feb., 1982.

Alternative Futures:

Ferguson, Marilyn. *The Aquarian Conspiracy*. Los Angeles, J. P. Tarcher, Inc., 1980.

Harman, Willis. *Incomplete Guide to the Future*. New York: Norton, 1976.

Schumacher, E. F. *A Guide for the Perplexed*. New York: Harper and Row, 1977.

Schumacher, E. F. *Small is Beautiful*. New York: Harper & Row, 1973.

Toffler, Alvin. *The Third Wave*. New York: Morrow, 1980.

Health:

Cousins, Norman. *Anatomy of an Illness*. New York: Norton, 1979.

Flynn, Patricia. *Holistic Health: The Art and Science of Care*. Bowie, Md.: Robert J. Brady Co., 1980.

Jaffe, Dennis. *Healing from Within*. New York: Knopf, 1980.

Kaslow, Arthur L., and Richard B. Miles. *Freedom from Chronic Disease*. Los Angeles: J.P. Tarcher, 1979.

Pelletier, Kenneth. *Mind as Healer, Mind as Slayer*. Delacorte Press, 1976.

Remen, Naomi. *The Human Patient*. New York: Anchor Press/Doubleday, 1980.

Listing of Holistic Health Organizations

American Holistic Medical Association
6932 Little River Turnpike
Annandale, VA
Director Jean Caywood

American Holistic Nursing Association
406 West Pacific
Telluride, CO

American Medical-Psychic Research
   Association
135 Madison Avenue NE
Albuquerque, NM 87123

Association for Holistic Health
P.O. Box 33202
San Diego, CA 92103

Berkeley Holistic Health Center
2640 College Avenue
Berkeley, CA 94704

California Institute of Integral Studies
3494 21st Street
Box NA
San Francisco, CA 94110

Center for Holistic Healing
569 Selby Avenue
St. Paul, MN 55102

Center for Integral Medicine
P.O. Box 955
Pacific Palisades, CA 90272

Center for Medical Consumers and
   Health Care Information, Inc.
237 Thompson Street
New York, NY 10013

Coalition for the Medical Rights of
   Women
The Women's Building
3543 18th Street
San Francisco, CA 94110

Committee for Freedom of Choice in
   Cancer Therapy
146 Main Street
Suite 408
Los Altos, CA 94022

Comprehensive Medical Service
93 Union Street
Newton Center, MA 02159

Consumer Coalition for Health
1751 N Street, NW
Washington, DC 20036

East-West Academy of Healing Arts
   Council of Nurse-Healers
P.O. Box 31211
San Francisco, CA 94131

East-West Center for Holistic Health
275 Madison Avenue
Suite 500
New York, NY 10016

East-West Foundation
359 Boylston Street
Boston, MA 02116

Florida Institute of Natural Health
1115 N. Main Street
Gainesville, FL 32601

Foundation for Alternate Cancer
   Therapies
P.O. Box 882
Dearborn, MI 48121

Foundation for Alternative Cancer
  Therapy, Ltd.
P.O. Box HH
Old Chelsea Station
New York, NY 10011

Heartspring Health Center
5A Bigelow Street
Cambridge, MA 02139

Holistic Health Center
1412 N. Broadway
Lexington, KY 40505

Holistic Health Center of San Jose
977 Asbury Street
San Jose, CA 95126

Holistic Health Organizing Committee
Village Design
1545 Dwight Way
Berkeley, CA 94703

Institute for the Study of Humanistic
  Medicine
1017 Dolores Street
San Francisco, CA 94110

Integral Health Service
245 School Street
Putnam, CT 06260

National Health Law Program (NHeLP)
University of California
10995 Le Conte Avenue
Room 640
Los Angeles, CA 90024

Rocky Mountain Healing Arts Institute
Box 4573
Boulder, CO 80306

School of Natural Life Therapy
The Kototama Institute
P.O. Box 1836
Sante Fe, NM 87501

Part Three

SELF-HEALING IN THE NINETEENTH CENTURY: A WOMEN'S MOVEMENT

Reprinted in part from *Medicine with Doctors: Home Health Care in American History*, ed. G. Risse, R. Numbers, and J. Leavitt (New York: Science History Publications, 1977).

Regina Markell Morantz

GROWING CRITICISM OF ESTABLISHED MEDICAL PRACTICE

"The time is passing," warned Ann Preston in her graduate medical thesis, "General Diagnosis," "when . . . the licensed graduate whose lancet is sprung for every head-ache and *heart-ache* that he may meet can obtain public confidence" (1851). Preston, soon to become dean of her alma mater, the newly established, Medical College of Pennsylvania, voiced what was by 1851 a lively public issue. Her fellow classmate, Angenette A. Hunt, echoed Preston's admonition when she observed in her own thesis, "The True Physician," that the present public criticism of the medical profession was well deserved: "The merit of the Physician," she declared vehemently, "is not now estimated by the quantity of medicines he prescribes, but by the effect produced, and the public throat is rebelling against swallowing nauseous drugs for the pleasure and profit of the doctors. What is more," continued Hunt, "public opinion is beginning to prove that there is a female side to *this subject*, as well as most others." She pointed out that women had natural abilities that made them peculiarly fitted for health care. With proper education, they could exercise their talents and move in the process to a higher sphere, "one not bounded by the kitchen and the nursery" (1851).

By midcentury, criticism of established medical practice had reached astonishing proportions; doctors had good reason to feel on the defensive. "The practice, or so-called *science* of medicine, has been little else than one of experiment," observed Marie Louise Shew in a scathing indictment. Standard medical therapeutics, she claimed, had hitherto been characterized by "uncertainty" and "chance." Little progress has been made in alleviating the sufferings of mankind (1844, pp. 22, 23). "Why," asked Mary Gove Nichols, "are we sick? Why cannot the doctors cure us?" Men, women, and society had sought a cure so long in vain that their began to distrust their doctors. "We are tired of professions and promises," said Mrs. Nichols. "We ask other help. Let woman be educated. Let her have healthy development . . ." (1846, p. 20).

Heroic methods were indeed painful and dangerous, and the American public, sick to death of bloodletting and calomel, rebelled. Occasionally, physicians themselves responded to the crisis with therapeutic nihilism. More often, sectarian practitioners, some with milder and more pleasant forms of treatment, competed successfully for public patronage.

HEALTH REFORM MOVEMENT—EMPHASIS ON PREVENTION AND SELF-HEALING

The health reform movement provided a different alternative to a dissatisfied public, and it flourished in the atmosphere created by vociferous debate between sectarians and regulars over more humane methods of treatment. In the early half of the nineteenth century, one begins to discern a gradual shift in attitudes. No longer was sickness to be tolerated with the stoicism of the colonials, who tended to leave such decisions in the hands of God. Slowly, the belief that man could be in greater control of his own destiny, that life and health could be improved through individual effort, replaced the silent resignation of previous generations. The health reform movement encapsulated this transition; the shift is apparent in its vocabulary, its imagery, even in its theory of the origin of disease.

Over and over again, health reformers argued that disease was *preventable*; that it was up to the individual to keep himself well. "Many people seem to think that all diseases are immediate visitations from the Almighty, arising from no cause but his *immediate* dispensation," Mary Gove Nichols observed in a book directed specifically to women (1920). "Many seem to have no idea that there are established laws with respect to life and health, and that the transgression of these laws is followed by disease" (1846, p. 20). Her mentor, Sylvester Graham, agreed. Before people attributed disease to a Supreme Being who supposedly loved them, he admonished his readers, they must prove that the cause lies not with their own bad habits (Applegate 1835, p. 23).

The causes of premature disease and death, declared Marie Louise Shew, wife of the prominent editor of the *Water-Cure Journal,* a popular health reform publication, were mostly within the control of mankind. It is "unwise, irrational, and unphilosophical to regard illness as the *infliction* of a Divine Providence. . . . It cannot be doubted," she continued, "that in accordance with the true designs of Providence, man was 'as a rule' designed to live in good health to a ripe old age" (1844, pp. 14–15). Recent sociologists have pointed out the important connection between the gradual abandonment of passivity and fatalism in the face of life's difficulties, including the willingness to manipulate oneself and one's environment, and the development of the modern personality (Broom 1972; Inkeles 1969).

Although health reform advocates came from all the several medical sects and the regulars, their shared theme was the prevention of disease through the teaching of the laws of physiology and hygiene. They accused the regulars of making "no effort to remove the causes of disease, while 'vainly' endeavoring to cure conditions while causes remain. We even have reason to believe," argued Dr. Ellen M. Snow, "that they have greatly multiplied disease by the use of poisonous drugs." In a chilling denunciation of the dependence of the people on physicians, she declared:

> They do not aim to enlighten mankind in regard to their physical well being, but rather seek to envelop their processes of cure in deep and impenetrable mystery. This mystery possesses a magic charm for the uninitiated and ignorant. You have only to look about you to become aware of the credulity and super- stition with which the Medical Profession is regarded. [Ibid.]

The concept of self-help was implicit in the health reformers' theory of sickness. Disease was the remedial effort of Nature to overcome or cast out of the body some impurity or poison that interfered with the functions of life (Nichols 1881; Bedortha 1858, p. 53). Since the natural condition of man was good health, to keep well he needed only to avoid unwise practices, such as eating the wrong foods and losing control of his "passions." Knowledge of his own physical nature would make man free. "People," announced Mrs. Shew, "must learn to think for themselves" (1844, p. iii). Ignorance could no longer be offered as an excuse for illness, agreed Mary Gove Nichols (1874, p. 80).

Health reformers deplored the complicated language of most medical journals. "Reader," warned the editor of the *Water-Cure Journal*, "if you cannot understand what an author is writing about, you may reasonably presume he does not know himself" ("Old School Medical Journals" 1850, p. 181). "I would have the *highest science,* clothed in words, that the people can understand," wrote Aurelia Raymond, in her graduate thesis at the Female Medical College of Pennsylvania. "I have studied medicine because I am one of the people . . . to enter my protest against that exclusiveness which sets itself up as something superior to the people" (1864).

WOMEN ASSUMING NEW LEADERSHIP ROLE

Health reformers emphasized in particular the central role of the wife and mother in supervising and directing the physiological regimen—itself a prerequisite to the higher spiritual life. This investment of woman with a special responsibility in the spiritual regeneration of her family, and by extension, of civilization as well, was a recurring theme in their literature.

Almost one-fourth of the members of the American Physiological Society were female, and the organization acknowledged the important role of women in the promotion of good health at its Second Annual Meeting, when the following resolution was passed:

> *Resolved,* That woman in her character as wife and mother is only second to the Diety in the influence that she exerts on the physical, the intellectual and the moral interests of the human race, and that her education should be adapted to qualify her in the highest degree to cherish those interests in the wisest and best manner. [Hoff and Fulton 1939, p. 701]

As a result, countless women took to the field as lecturers. In 1838, the newly formed Boston Ladies Physiological Society sponsored a successful and well-publicized series of lectures delivered by Mary Gove Nichols. Before long, similar societies appeared in Providence, Wilmington, Nantucket, Lynn, Bangor, New York, Oberlin, and numerous other towns and cities in the Northeast and West. Nichols, Paulina Wright Davis, Harriot Hunt, Lydia Folger Fowler, and Rachel Brooks Gleason were only a few of the better known of the dozens of women who traveled throughout New England and the West in these decades, teaching other women the "laws of life." Health reform struck a responsive chord in their enthusiastic female audiences. The lecture halls were filled with women eager for the knowledge that they hoped would ease their bewilderment with their increased responsibilities within the family—at a time when the home was plagued by pressures imposed from without, by a mobile, fragmented, and fast-changing society. The message of the health reformers seemed an answer, perhaps even a solution, to social instability.*

In the nineteenth century there emerged two competing images of the ideal nineteenth-century women, both of which drew strength from the culture that produced them. On the one hand, woman was described as weak, sickly, dependent, and ornamental. On the other, she was exalted as highly spiritual and morally superior—confined, for the most part, to the home, yet invested with genuine power and responsibility within her sphere. The health reformers, as well as the women's rights advocates, rejected the first and seized upon the second ideal—that of woman's moral power—using it effectively to explore significant and divergent outlets for female energies (Melder 1964; Lerner 1969).

Of particular concern was the state of female health. "If a plan for *destroying female health,* in all the ways in which it could be most effectively done, were drawn up," announced Catherine Beecher, "it would be exactly the course which is now pursued by a large portion of this nation, especially

---

*See sources listed in Suggested Readings list at the end of this chapter.

in the more wealthy classes" (1856, p. 7). Augustus K. Gardner, a prominent New York gynecologist, agreed that the present physical condition of women was deplorable (1860). Dr. James C. Jackson of the Dansville water cure unhappily confirmed Gardner's opinion. "American girls," he admitted, "are all sickly" (1867, p. 2). Mrs. S. M. Estee also wrote to the feminine readers of the *Water-Cure Journal,* "You are sick and have been for months, years, and some of you for your whole lives" (1858, p. 96).*

Health reform offered to countless women a means of coping with an imprecise, undependable, and often hostile environment. In a society in which women were expected to play an increasingly complex role in the nurture of children and the organization of family life, health reform brought to the bewildered housewife not just sympathy and compassion but a structured regimen, a way of life. In an era characterized by weakening ties between relatives and neighbors, health reform lectures, journals, and domestic tracts provided once again the friendly advice and companionship of the now remote kinswoman. Women were promised a means to end their isolation and to make contact with others of their sex. At lectures, study groups, and even through letters to the various journals, they shared their common experiences with other women. A deep sense of sisterhood was evidenced by the frequent use of the term. No longer must woman bear her burden alone.

Health reform was also a means by which many women articulated their feminism, and these reformers understood the importance of good health as a prerequisite for woman's place in the world. Health reformers were acutely conscious of the fact that woman was in the process of creating for herself a new role. "Woman . . . is a new element in society," wrote James C. Jackson, "just emerging from her hybernation . . . and so much better fitted to take to herself *new* ideas, and develop them" (1854, pp. 74). Good health was essential to woman's new self-expression, equality, and improved status. "Let mothers be educated in all that concerns life and health," insisted Mrs. Eliza de la Verge, M.D. *"Let them learn that knowledge gives the highest order of power"* (1855, p. 74—italics added).

Harriet Austin thought speculation on woman's sphere a waste of time. "It is her sphere," she insisted, "to do what she desires to do. . . . [and when] conscious of the divinity within her and of the mightiness of her power, she determines to elevate, not only her sex, but humanity, this too will be her sphere. But this work can never be accomplished while woman remains sick." Woman's sphere could not be expanded until she "learns and claims her first great right—the right to health" (1853, p. 57). Paulina Wright Davis admonished, "Women are answerable, in a very large degree for the

---

*Many well-known feminists, including Lucy Stone, Catherine Beecher, Elizabeth Smith Miller, Angelina Grimke, and Susan B. Anthony, were plagued by constant illness. Most of them were interested in health reform.

imbecilities of disease, mental and bodily, and for the premature deaths prevailing throughout society—for the weakness, wretchedness, and short- ness of life—and no remedy will be radical till reformation of life and practice obtains among our sex (1846, p. 29).

Such a psychological burden might well have been unbearable had not health reformers offered fellowship, moral support, and practical information. "I wish," wrote Mary Gove Nichols of her motives in becoming a health reformer, "to teach mothers how to cure their own diseases, and those of their children; and to increase health, purity, and happiness in the family and the home (1874, p. 14). For some women, at least, Mrs. Nichols and her fellow reformers achieved these goals. Numerous articles on cookery, bathing, teething, care of infants, childhood sexuality, cleanliness, and domestic economy carefully taught women how to manage their households properly. Itinerant physiological lecturers assaulted women's widespread ignorance of their bodies. Mrs. Nichols, for example, relied heavily on a discussion of anatomy and physiology in her lectures. She instructed her listeners in the formation of bone structure, the role of respiration and circulation, the anatomy and physiology of the stomach. The process of digestion was described in detail. The remainder of her course involved information on dietetics and the importance of physical education. Advice on the supervision of pregnancy and childbirth was surprisingly modern. Whereas regular physicians still treated pregnancy and childbirth as a dis- ease—often drugging both mother and infant—health reformers insisted that both be welcomed as natural events, urging exercise without fatigue, along with fresh air, proper diet, and cleanliness.

HEALTH REFORM—A SOURCE FOR SOCIAL CHANGE

Once the conception of woman as the moral arbiter of society gained an audience, the ideal itself became a potent source for social change. Involve- ment in health reform was one means by which countless women could widen their sphere by moving out into society. The most logical extension of the health reformers assessment of women's natural ailities was to teach women medicine. Indeed, the entrance of women into the medical profession grew out of the health reform movement. "In sickness there is no hand like a woman's hand," the *Water-Cure Journal* reminded its readers ("Woman's Tenderness and Love," 1848, p. 95). "The property of her nature, which renders her the best of nurses, with proper instruction, equally qualifies her to be the best of physicians. Above all is this the case with her own sex and her children" (Cornell 1853, p. 82). Enthusiastically, health reformers applauded the acceptance of women as medical students, chiding the regulars for their conservatism. "What," asked the editor of the *Water-Cure Journal*, "will our Allopathic doctors say to this? We pause for a reply. In the meantime, our women are buckling on the armor for a struggle which must ultimately prove successful" (Vol. 12, 1851). In time, these pioneer women physicians, who were attracted to medicine out of an ardent desire to fulfill their destinies as superior moral beings with natural abilities to cure, would be transformed into full-fledged professionals by their contact with an increasingly scientific and empirical discipline. They, as well as their system of values, would be permanently altered in the process.

CONCLUSION

The health reform movement flourished in the midnineteenth century largely because of the simultaneous occurrence of two historical events: (1) the failure of orthodox medicine to cure, and (2) the emergence of a modern personality type for whom such a situation was intolerable. Health reform was both cause *and* effect in the process, in the sense that it embodied the revolt against traditional authority in medical matters and the rejection of stoicism in the face of disease, while offering to individuals a temporarily viable alternative to the painful and dangerous therapeutics of the old school.

To women, health reform gave even more. Developing a coherent program designed to cope with both the physical and psychological burdens imposed by a society in transition, it held out to confused wives and mothers the prospect of improving the quality of life, not by changing the environment, but by gaining control of oneself. It promised women that they would raise their children healthy in mind and clean in body. It offered to them the possibility of keeping their husbands moral by cooking the right foods.

Furthermore, preaching sexual continence and physiological knowledge, health reformers helped legitimate the rights of women in sexual matters at a time when sexual contact was not necessarily a positive experience for many women. Health manuals aided women in dealing with sexuality in themselves, their husbands, and their children.

Emphasizing woman's essential role as teacher and spiritual arbiter within the family, health reform literature also contributed to the enhancement of woman's status at a time when cultural and economic changes had obscured her role and narrowed her usefulness. And although this investment of the womanly sphere with cosmic moral significance was only part of a broader cultural trend, shared by the society as a whole, health reformers, unlike many nineteenth-century thinkers, subscribed to the widest possible definition of woman's sphere. They understood full well that to purify society, women would indeed have to enter it.

Thus, for some brave, ambitious, and talented women, health reform provided an outlet and an escape from an intolerably narrow and confining role. Moving out into the world, women transformed society's conception of the duties and abilities of the female sex, while they themselves were also changed. Health reform marked a hitherto unexplored historical step on the tortuous road to full equality for women. How little did she divine the far-reaching implications of her words, when Mrs. S. M. Estee of the Petersburg Water Cure attempted to inspire her "sick sisters" with the following:

> Cheer up, ye sick and drooping! There is a panacea for your ills; it is not to be found in poisonous drugs, but in heaven's pure air, the soft, refreshing water that issues bubbling from the hill-sides, appropriate exercise, and proper diet; then cheer up, ye disconsolate ones! and be assured there is a balm in Gilead, and there are true physicians. [1858, p. 96]

REFERENCES

Applegate, William, *A Defense of the Graham System of Living*. New York: W. Applegate, 1835.

Austin, Harriet, "Women's Present and Future," *Water Cure Journal*, vol. 16 (1853).

Bedortha, N., article in *Water-Cure Journal*, vol. 25 (1858).

Beecher, Catherine, *Letters to the People on Health and Happiness*. New York, 1856, p. 7.

Brown, Richard D., "Modernization and the Modern Personality in America, 1600–1865," *Journal of Interdisciplinary History*, 2 (1972), 201–27.

Cornell, William M., "Woman the True Physician," *Water-Cure Journal*, vol. 46 (1853).

Davis, Pauline Wright, article in *Water- Cure Journal*, vol. 1 (1846).

de la Vergue, Eliza, article in *Water-Cure Journal*, vol. 20 (1855).

Estee, S. M., "To Sick Women," *Water-Cure Journal*, vol. (1968).

Gardner, Augustus K., as quoted in the *Water-Cure Journal*, 29 (1960), 21–22, 50–51. Reprinted from the *Knickerbocker Journal*.

Gove Nichols, Mary S., *Lectures to Women on Anatomy and Physiology*. New York: Harper and Brothers, 1846.

———, *A Woman's Work in Water-Cure and Sanitary Education*. London: Nichols, 1874.

Hoff, Hebbel E., and John F. Fulton, "The Centenary of the First American Physiological Society," *Bulletin of the History of Medicine*, vol. 5 (October 1939).

Hunt, Angenette A., "The True Physician," thesis for the Female Medical College of Pennsylvania, 1851.

Inkeles, Alex, "Making Men Modern: On the Causes and Consequences of Individual Change in Six Developing Countries," *American Journal of Sociology*, vol. 75 (1969).

Jackson, James C., article in *Water-Cure Journal*, vol. 15 (1854).

———, "Shall Our Girls Live or Die?" *Laws of Life*, vol. 10 (1867).

Lerner, Gerda, "The Lady and the Mill Girl: Changes in the Status of Women in the Age of Jackson," *American Studies Journal,* 10 (Spring 1969), 5–15.

Melder, Keith, "The Beginning of the Women's Rights Movement in the United States, 1800–1840," Ph.D. thesis for Yale University, 1964.

Nichols, Thomas L., *Eating to Live: The Diet Cure.* New York: M. L. Holbrook & Co., 1881.

"Old School Journals," *Water-Cure Journal,* vol. 9 (1850).

Preston, Ann, "General Diagnosis," thesis for the Medical College of Pennsylvania, 1851.

Raymond, Aurelia, "Thesis on the Human Brain," thesis for the Medical College of Pennsylvania, 1864.

Shew, Marie Louise, *Water-Cure for Ladies: A Popular Work on the Health Diet and Regimen of Females and Children,* revised by Joel Shew. New York: Wiley & Putnam, 1844.

"Woman's Tenderness and Love," *Water-Cure Journal,* vol. 5. (1848).

SUGGESTED READINGS

Library of Health 2 (1838): 70, 367: 6 (1842): 156 (1841): 40; Thomas L. Nichols, *Health Manual: Being Also A Memorial of the Life and Work of Mrs. Mary S. Gove Nichols* (London: Allen, 1887), p. 22; *WCJ* 1 (1846), 11 (1851): 29, 38, 93; 9 (1850): 90: 14 (1852): 56; 17 (1854): 46; 22 (1856): 131; 28 (1859): 57–58; 5 (1848): 83; *Graham Journal II* (1838): 37, 181, 288, 385; III (1839): 20, 37, 82; *The Lily III* (1851): 27. *The Una I* (1854): 206; II (1854): 263; *Boston Medical and Surgical Journal* 40 (1849): 107, 48 (1853): 443–444.

WCJ 12 (1851): 73–75; M.G. Nichols, "Woman, the Physician," *WCJ* 12 (1851): 73–75. "Female Physicians," *The Lily I* (1849): 94; II (1950): 39, 70, 77; "Female Physicians," *WCJ* 31 (1861): 84; Augusta R. Montgomery, "The Medical Education of Women," 1853, thesis, MCP Archives; *Godey's Lady's Book* 44 (1852): 185–189; 61 (1860): 270–271: 54 (1857): 371; 49 (1854): 80, 368, 456; *The Revolution I* (1868): 170, 201, 339; III (1870): 252, *WCJ* 13 (1852): 34–35, 86–87; 29 (1860): 45, 2–3; 31 (1861): 42; 28 (1859): 84.

ALTERNATIVE VERSUS ORTHODOX APPROACHES TO WOMEN'S HEALTH

Kay Weiss

In recent years, many consumers of health care have exchanged a once-abiding faith in Western technological treatments for a new faith in ancient and non-Western treatments. Alternative approaches are not necessarily antagonistic to traditional medical or psychological therapies; rather, they can be adjunctive. The technical achievements of our modern medical system will be integrated with the humanistic and psychosocial specialization of ancient systems to achieve the best of both worlds.

Many women consumers of medical services are coming to believe that alternative systems of health care are more adaptable than traditional medicine to the treatment of female diseases, diseases that typically arise during the normal life changes of women—at puberty, during reproductive life, or at menopause. The following chapters will illustrate some of these alternatives.

DISADVANTAGES OF WESTERN ORTHODOX APPROACH

In Western orthodox allopathic medicine, treatment (usually drugs or surgery) is normally given to suppress the symptom of the disease. And since the symptom of the disease, such as the fever accompanying a bacterial infection, is the body's way of curing the disease (as increased body temperature kills off bacteria), to the degree that we suppress the symptoms, we may actually prolong the illness. That is, suppression of the symptom, even if it results in a cure, will frequently ensure further episodes of the same disease. An example of this may be seen with vaginal infections (trichomoniasis). To the extent that the woman relies on anti-parasitic agents to destroy the infection, she neglects the opportunity to investigate and change the life habits that cause her to be susceptible to the pathogen.

Furthermore, in many instances, the obliteration of the symptom-causing pathogen requires drugs that are so poisonous to the system that they may result in greater eventual harm, for example, in the latent development of cancer.

In other instances, the effective obliteration of the symptom that was the body's avenue for the expression of its dis-ease will drive the dis-ease into deeper and more subtle levels of the organism, and finally become expressed as chronic disease. An example of this is the use of tranquilizers to treat mental dis-ease, resulting in the long-term depression of the immunosuppressive system and increased susceptibility to cancer and infectious diseases.

COMPARISON OF TREATMENT MODALITIES

Many ancient and modern medical systems compare allopathic medicine (in which the symptom of dis-ease is suppressed) and homeopathic medicine (the symptom of dis-ease is cooperated with because it is an expression of the body's wisdom as it reacts to cure its own dis-ease). In the West, the symptom—a headache, for example—is an annoyance that should be eliminated. In the East, it is a signal that the whole system needs realignment.

According to the concept of holistic health, the human being is made up of body, mind, and spirit. Dis-ease begins first in the spirit, as documented by Kirlian photography of the human aura,* then becomes a mental symptom, and finally manifests on the material level in the body as a physical symptom. In treating the physical symptom only, as in allopathic medicine, one does not affect the underlying dis-ease. To treat the dis-ease while it still exists on a mental level, as through meditation, is more effective. Finally, to identify and prevent dis-ease on a spiritual level ensures the continued health of the organism.

Central to all alternative health systems is the belief that body and mind are synonymous, that the body is the physical manifestation of the mind. This is in contrast to Western medical thought that views and treats body and mind as separate entities.

MODERN ALTERNATIVE MODES OF MEDICAL CARE

Modern alternative modes of medical care have their roots in ancient philosophical understandings of dis-ease. Most of these work by rebalancing the body, mind, and spirit of the organism. A balanced organism presents

---

*A method of photography showing an aura of energy emanating from animals and plants, which changes in response to physiological or emotional pressures.

a strong defense against external insults including bacteria, viruses, and trauma. Rebalancing efforts can be introduced through the body, mind, or spirit.

Systems like Polarity Therapy and Acupuncture seek to balance the electrical and magnetic energy of the body. Osteopathy, Chiropracty, Hatha Yoga, and Rolfing work by realigning the physical structures of the body. Indian and Chinese medicine have as their basis Ayurvedic and Macrobiotic diets, in concert with the belief that you are what you eat: foods are chosen not only for their nutritional value but also for their vibrational energies that match the particular needs of the individual. Herbal medicine has recently become popular as an alternative to pharmaceutical drugs for the treatment of certain symptoms. However, Chinese medicine has long recommended that disease be prevented on a daily basis by balancing the chemistry of the body (the microcosm) with properly chosen plants, herbs and vegetables from the individual's environment (the macrocosm).

Systems that address health on the physical level with the aim of affecting the mind are the psychophysical approaches such as massage, reflexology, acupressure, Rolfing, and movement approaches like bioenergetics, Tai Chi Chuan, Hatha Yoga, and aerobics.

Homeopathy works to dissolve dis-ease on the spiritual level even after its symptoms have become manifest in the body. Remedies are taken that contain infinitesimal amounts of an element that causes the symptoms of the disease when taken by a healthy person. These remedies are potentized so that their vibrational energy works in concert with the wisdom of the body in producing the symptom, thereby aiding the body in its efforts to counteract the disease.

Other alternative systems address health on the mental level (meditation, self-hypnosis, biofeedback). Important in these is the synchronization of the activity of the left and right hemispheres of the brain so that the analytical and emotional functions of the mind are in tune rather than in opposition and conflict. Since the body is the material manifestation of the mind, this coordination of the opposing spheres of the brain/mind results in coordination of the bodily systems.

Still other alternative modes of treatment are similar to allopathy in that they seek to suppress the symptom and reestablish health with nutritional or drug therapy. Nutritional correction of symptoms with megavitamin therapy is an example. In megavitamin therapy, the individual takes large doses of vitamins for a medicinal effect. In some instances, this may amount to a rebalancing, as when a person suffering from schizophrenia takes massive doses of a B vitamin (niacin) to counteract a genetically inherited deficiency of niacin. In other instances, the vitamins are being used as drugs to counteract a symptom in the belief that vitamins are safer alternatives than pharmaceutical drugs.

However, to the degree that these alternative modes of therapy address the disease problem rather than the healthy potential of the organism, they will be little more effective than allopathic medicine. For example, it is possible for an integrating and balancing system like acupuncture to be misused in a cookbook reductionistic way if it is used to cure symptoms rather than the underlying lack of ease in the body.

The value of alternative healing systems over orthodox medicine is that they seek to prevent disease rather than cure it, that they address the cause of disease rather than its symptoms, that they focus the responsibility of healing on the self rather than on a paid practitioner. These systems believe effective healing can only be accomplished by the person who cooperated in allowing the disease to begin.

Allopathic medicine is more effective for acute or episodic diseases, for example, traumatic injury or infectious injury: in this case, treatment is fast, aggressive, and goal-oriented; the responsibility for cure is on the practitioner. Holistic health systems, on the other hand, are more appropriate for treating chronic disease: here treatment focuses on prevention and is slow and process-oriented; the responsibility for cure is on the client.

The rise of self-care parallels the rise of chronic disease rates in Western society. Only four decades ago we lived in a world of curable disease, largely infectious, where professional intervention are both appropriate and effective. Now 80 percent of all disease is chronic, compared with only 30 percent 50 years ago.

The following chapters present a sampling of holistic or alternative modes of health care as they may be applied to women's health problems. In reading them, one must temper the Western mind's tendency to demand scientific proof of specific analytical details, in favor of the Eastern mind's acceptance that the whole person rather than the part (the presenting symptom) is of importance.

Although many of these systems are based on ancient philosophies, we will not go back to being Chinese or Indian classical physicians; rather we will go forward to a medical philosophy that reflects our current culture.

Central to the success of any therapy is the relationship between the practitioner and the client. The practitioner is sought, not to cure the disease, but to aid the client in health education, self-knowledge and self-care.

Chapter Nine

CHINESE MEDICINE AND WOMEN'S HEALTH

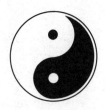

Angela Longo
Sandy Newhouse

> *Opening and closing the gates of heaven,*
> *can you play the role of woman?*
>
> [Lao-tse, Tao Te Ching, *Ch. 10*]
>
> *The valley spirit never dies,*
> *It is the woman, primal mother.*
> *Her gateway is the root of heaven and earth.*
> *It is like a veil barely seen.*
> *Use it; it will never fail.*
>
> [Lao-tsu, Tao Te Ching, *Ch. 6*]

The search for effective alternative medical treatment is a growing phenomenon. In a country that spends more than $100 billion annually on health care (Harmer 1975), the authors of this chapter feel that people deserve to know more about ancient systems of health care that treat the human being in a complete way. We present this article, based on our own experience and study, in the hope that medical practitioners and prospective patients alike will investigate Chinese medicine as a viable system to meet some of the complex health care needs existing today.

THEORIES OF YIN AND YANG AND THE FIVE ELEMENTS

Around three thousand years ago, the two fundamental guideposts of Chinese medical thought were put forth—the theory of yin and yang and the five element theory. Based on this philosophical framework, the prevention, diagnosis, and treatment of all disease can be understood.

The theory of yin and yang, originating in Taoist philosophy, espouses that all phenomena in the universe, including all processes and organs in the human body, demonstrate varying degrees of these two basic forces. Yin and yang are the two basic types of energy or *chi.* Yin is described as feminine and receptive and is associated with the qualities of coldness, wetness, darkness, the earth element, and nighttime. In the body, yin manifests as coldness, low blood pressure, paleness, chronic conditions, and parasympathetic nervous system symptoms. *Yang* is described as masculine energy and is demonstrated by heat, dryness, light, projection, day, and heaven. Yang energy manifests in the body as fevers, energy, acute conditions, high blood pressure, redness in the face, and other sympathetic nervous system symptoms. Most important is the understanding of the dynamic, ever-changing interplay of these two basic forces.

The *Tao Te Ching* (*The Way and Its Power*), written by Lao-tsu around 500 B.C., describes how from the yin and the yang arose all phenomena. "The five elements of water, fire, earth, metal, and wood encompass all the phenomena of nature" (Mann 1973, p. 77). Just like the forces of yin and yang, the five elements intricately depend on and respond to one another. This theory allows for an understanding of the human body and mind operating as an integrated holistic system. This integrated system is what allows the cause of illness to be known. And it is only through knowing the genuine cause that a cure can be properly effected.

Chinese medicine is a holistic system excelling in its ability to describe the interrelatedness of all aspects of the body, mind, and spirit. Dr. Kong (1976) tells the story of a person of little knowledge or experience being shown water for the first time and delighting in its wet, fluid nature. Later this same person is shown ice and notices how hard, cold, and different it appears. This person then sees some steam and experiences its gaseous, hot nature. Despite the appearance of three different entities, with some knowledge and experience the person comes to know that this is the same substance in three different forms. In the same way, the body, mind, and spirit can be seen as different expressions of the same entity. For example, mental problems can cause physical disease. Disease results from an imbalance of energy flow in the system.

In order to study and understand Chinese medicine, it is necessary to learn the traditional terminology of yin and yang and the five elements, for it is upon this base that the wealth of information amassed over the past three thousand years is organized.

Figure 9–1 explains the interrelationships of the five elements. The outer circle, called the creative circle or *chen* (in Chinese), can be understood as follows: fire creates ashes (earth); compression of earth creates metals; when water is placed on the earth, it gives birth to wood; and when wood is rubbed together to its kindling temperature, fire is born. This interplay of elements is called a mother-child relationship. Fire is said to be the mother of earth, and earth is the mother of metal. Wood is the child of earth, and fire is the child of wood, etc. A basic rule for treatment is to strengthen the mother organ when the child organ is energy-deficient; and if the child organ is excessive in energy, it is sedated directly.

APPLICATION TO WOMEN'S HEALTH PROBLEMS

Let us look at an example of this process of the interrelationships of the five elements. Gynecological health problems are generally caused by an overall weakness in the liver, kidney, and spleen meridians (energy pathways).

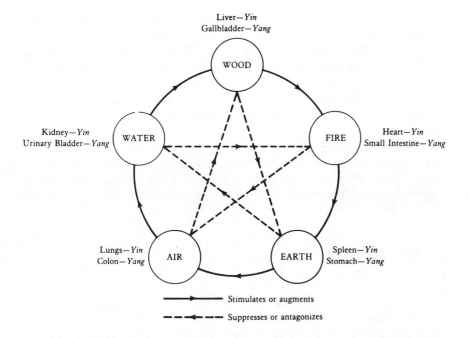

FIGURE 9–1. Relationships of the five essences and associated viscera. (From *Acupuncture in Medical Practice* by Louise Wensel. Reston, Va: Reston Publishing Company, 1980.)

Looking at Figure 9–1, you see that the liver is a wood element, the kidney a water element, and the spleen an earth element. Therefore, the mother organ of each of these elements is treated. Strengthening the heart, a fire organ, will directly strengthen the spleen, an earth organ, since fire is the mother of earth. Likewise, strengthening the spleen, an earth organ, will strengthen the lung, a metal organ. Next, strengthening the lung will directly strengthen the kidney, a water organ, since metal is the mother of water. And finally strengthening the kidney, a water organ, will strengthen the liver, a wood element. In this way, gynecological health problems can be treated.

FATHER, MOTHER, AND CHILD "ORGANS": ETIOLOGY OF DISEASE

The etiology of disease is understood on the basis of these two important relationships: the mother-child relationship and the father-child relationship of the five elements.

The nurturing mother-child relationship of Chinese medicine is complemented by a disciplining or controlling relationship: the father-child relationship. The inner star in Figure 9–1 demonstrates this relationship known as *ko*. Following the arrows in the diagram, we see that metal is the father of wood, wood is the father of earth, earth of water, water of fire, and fire of metal. When the fire element is too great in the body, the water element has the ability to control it. Likewise, earth contains and controls the water element.

These relationships can be observed in the natural world as well. If the father organ is overbearing and excessive in chi, then the child becomes weak. If the father organ is weak or debilitated, the child organ becomes wild and difficult to manage.

TRADITIONAL CHINESE MEDICINE

Written works describing gynecology and obstetrics date back to 300 B.C. The *Nei Jing*, an ancient Chinese medical classic (221 B.C.) consisting of 18-volumes with 162 chapters, describes the theoretical base of internal medicine (Zhang 1929). Later on in A.D. 610, Chao Yuanfang elaborated on the etiology of various gynecological disorders in the *Zhu Birg Yuan Hou Lun (Treatise on Etiology and Symptomatology)*. The importance of the study of obstetrics was also noted by Sun Si-mino in A.D. 625; he dedicated the first four chapters of his famous *Quian Jin Fang (Thousand Golden Prescriptions)* to the study of gynecology, obstetrics, and pediatrics. Three other important early texts on gynecology are: *An Encyclopedia of Useful Prescriptions for Women* by Ch'en Tze-ming (A.D. 1200), *Gynecological Prescriptions* by Fu Shan (A.D. 1650), and *A Collection of Gynecological and Obstetrical Prescriptions* by the Xiao Shan Monastery in A.D. 1770.

In order to understand the Chinese treatment of women's health problems, we must first explain traditional Chinese medical diagnosis and treatment. The four methods of medical diagnosis include observation (seeing), auscultation (hearing) and olfaction (smelling), questioning, and feeling the pulse. These methods gather information about the five elements (energy production and control), superficial parts of the body affected, types of weather that affect the condition, flavors of foods that affect it, etc.

In pulse diagnosis, external and internal symptoms are differentiated by distinguishing the floating pulse from the deep pulse. Cold versus hot symptoms are distinguished by a slow pulse versus a rapid pulse. "Substantial" and "insubstantial" symptoms are determined by the strength of the pulse. External and internal illnesses are recognized by comparing the pulses of the left and right wrists. It is known whether the illness is in the upper or the lower part of the body by comparing the pulses in different positions.

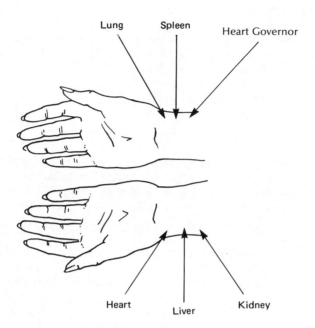

FIGURE 9–2. Location of major points used in pulse diagnosis.

Which of the five elements is imbalanced is determined by which of the six pulses on the two wrists is particularly strong or weak. Figure 9-2 illustrates the major points used in pulse diagnosis.

Tongue diagnosis is also a highly developed system. The tongue's skin color, coat, thickness, cracks, patches, and sores are all useful in diagnosis. Recently, numerous research studies have been conducted on the reliability of tongue inspection as a diagnostic method. The mechanism of tongue changes and their clinical significance are being cited in the literature. "Recent Investigations on Tongue Inspection," published in the *Chinese Medical Journal,* is a summary of Dr. Zelin's work in this area (1980). Eyes, hands,* and ears are also examined (Kushi 1979).

Contrary to the popular belief that Chinese medicine principally involves acupuncture, we point out that herbal treatment, moxibustion, and various techniques for traumatic injuries are also used. The discussion in this chapter will emphasize herbal treatment.

The goal of all treatment is to reestablish a balanced flow of energy in the meridians in the body. These meridians can be manipulated by pressure, massage, needles, and heat (moxibustion). There is one point on the body

*By studying the hands of children with diabetes, it can be predicted which sufferers are most likely to develop eye (blood vessel) disease and kidney failure, enabling preventive treatment, according to Janet Silverman in the *New England Journal of Medicine,* July 23, 1981, and other researchers at the University of Florida College of Medicine.

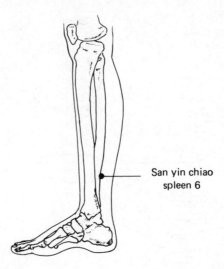

San yin chiao
spleen 6

FIGURE 9–3. Location of *San yin chiao,* meaning "three yin meeting place."

where the three yin meridians of spleen, liver, and kidneys meet that is most often treated for female disorders. *San yin chiao,* meaning "three yin meeting place" or spleen 6, is located on the inner side of the ankle, four client's fingers above the ankle, directly behind the fibula bone (see Figure 9–3). It is helpful to massage this point for menstrual disorders including cramping.

The *ren* and *chong* channels, originating in the uterus, are particularly important for women's health problems. The ren or conception vessel regulates the functioning of all yin organs and nourishes the fetus. The chong channel regulates the chi and blood of the twelve regular channels.

> The chi and blood of the twelve regular channels pass into the uterus through the ren and chong channels, affecting the menstrual flow and its cycle. [*Essentials of Chinese Acupuncture* 1980, p. 30]

Moxibustion is more of a yang technique than needling. If a period comes too early, for example, this connotes an excess in yin energy, and moxibustion would be used instead of needles. Also, when there is cramping, if the body is cold, moxibustion would be the preferred treatment choice.

Ear acupuncture is a complete system within itself and is quite powerful for balancing the hormones and overall energy of the body.

HERBAL MEDICINE

Herbal medicine is an important type of treatment. In Chinese medicine, the same herb can be used for many different disorders. Likewise, the same disease in different individuals will be treated with different medicines, depending on the unique needs of the individual patient. In this way, Chinese medical theory and practice provide a very flexible system. See Table 9–1 on functions of some common Chinese herbs.

Chinese herbs can be classified as to whether their energy effect on the body produces heat or cold, warmth or coolness. Herbs can be of one or a combination of flavors including sweet, spicy, sour, bitter, salty, or neutral. Herbs with the same energy effect or flavor have some of the same therapeutic properties.

Different flavors in foods and herbs correspond to the different elements (earth, fire, wood, metal, water). According to their flavors, herbs affect different meridians. In general, sweet herbs influence the spleen and stomach meridians, spicy herbs affect the lung and large intestine meridians, bitter herbs affect the heart and small intestine meridians, salty herbs affect the kidney and bladder meridians, and sour herbs act on the liver and gallbladder meridians.

TABLE 9–1. Functions of Some Common Chinese Herbs

Polypodium lingua Sw. (polydiaceae)—Astringent and diuretic for gonorrhea, menorrhagia, urethrorrhagia cystitis.

Lygodium japonicum SE. (schizaeacae)—Antiphlagistic and diuretic for cystitis, urethritis, hematuria of gonorrhea, urinary calculus.

Cyperus rotundus L. (cyperaceae)—Aromatic for nervous gastralgia, dyspepsia, diarrhea, emmenagogue, sedative, and analgesic for dysmenorrhea, amenorrhea, chronic metritis.

Evonymus alatus regel (celasthroaceas)—Analgesic emmenagogue and purgative for female disorders.

Kochia scoparia schrad (chenopodiaceae)—Diuretic, astringent, and antiphlogistic for disorders of the urinary tract.

Carthamus tinctorius L. (compositae)—Uterine astringent for dysmenorrhea.

Echinops dahuricus fisch (compositae)—Hemostatic for treatment of abscesses, mastitis, boils, and contusions.

This list extracted from pp. 50–85 of the *American Journal of Chinese Medicine* in an article by L. S. Chuang and W. Y. Chui of the Chinese University of Hong Kong: "The 14-MeV Neutron Activation Analysis of Chinese Medicines for Protein, Phosphorus, Potassium, and Magnesium Contents (II)," Spring-Summer 1980.

The *Nei Jing* discusses the relationship between the tastes of the herbs and their directions of movement within the body:

> The spicy and sweet flavors disperse upward and are yang. The sour and bitter flavors flow downward and are yin. The salty flavor flows downward and is yin. The mild flavor leaks and flows and is yang. [Zhang 1929, p. 49]

Herbs can move upward or downward, and they can float as opposed to sinking. So it follows that herbs with a tendency to move upward are in control of the upward and outward tendencies of the body, and they tend to build up the yang, remove dampness and congestion in the upper regions, and disperse cold. On the other hand, herbs with a tendency to move downward and to sink are in control of the downward and inward tendencies of the body, and they tend to decrease the yang or "heat" element, draw energy together, and remove congestion in the lower regions.

A herbal prescription can be small (containing one-to-three herbs), medium (four-to-six herbs), or big (eight-to-ten herbs), depending on what the doctor feels would be best for the patient. The major problem is always the target of treatment; minor problems will be cleared up when the major problem is treated. Sometimes the most complicated problems will only require a small prescription. This depends totally on what the doctor feels will be best, based on his prior study and experience with other patients.

Dang qui or *radix angelica sinesis* is an herb fairly well known in the West and is extremely important for women's health problems. It nourishes new blood, dissolves congested blood and clots, and relieves certain types of pain. The tail or root of this herb stimulates blood, while the head, which is the thicker, larger portion closer to the surface of the soil when cultivated, is used to produce new blood. Often the head and tail are used together. Dang qui is often used in anemia, to increase the amount of blood for menstruating and lactating women. In doing so it also increases general vitality and relieves the symptoms of palpitations, insomnia, and dizziness. It is used in cases of amenorrhea due to blood congestion and in dysmenorrhea when there is scanty blood flow. In addition, it is used to increase circulation in rheumatism and in injuries that involve blood congestion.

The energy effect of this herb is hot and it acts on the heart, liver, and spleen meridians. Contraindications for dang qui are an excess yang nature or when there is a "hot" condition in the body. Under such circumstances, dang qui can only be used if it is properly balanced with other herbs.

TREATMENT OF SPECIFIC FEMALE CONDITIONS

The female organs are governed by the energy of the three yin organ systems: kidney, spleen, and liver. The kidney meridian governs the ovaries and helps the spleen meridian to generate blood. The spleen meridian governs the blood, its circulation, digestion, and lymph, and has a special relationship to the breasts. The liver meridian regulates energy and blood flow in the body. It also governs the uterus, the nervous system, and the emotions. The interrelationship between the liver and the emotions is highlighted by the following quotation:

> The liver is related to emotional activities, especially depression and anger. Prolonged mental depression or a fit of anger may weaken the liver so that it is unable to promote the unrestrained and free flow of chi. Conversely, dysfunction of the liver is often accompanied by emotional changes such as mental depression and irascibility. [*Essentials of Chinese Acupuncture*, p. 24]

Women's health care needs that Chinese medicine addresses include: proper care of the woman before and after pregnancy, sterility and miscarriage, menstrual problems, vaginal and bladder infections, breast tumors, dysplasia, and ovarian cysts.

Pregnancy

Several classic herbal prescriptions are used for the benefit of the mother and fetus during pregnancy. Acupuncture is rarely used during this time due to its yin nature. *Soppyee tai bo*, a 12-herb prescription is given at 3 months, and *sapp sam tai bo* is prescribed after 6 months and after 13 months. During pregnancy, the woman's chi is built up by eating Chinese black beans cooked with red dates. The beans are especially good for the kidneys and spleen; the red dates for the heart, blood, and circulation. Black beans and red dates are also useful to stop spotting during pregnancy. Two and one-half weeks after the birth, there is cleansing prescription to be taken that is said to heal any problems incurred during pregnancy.

The sex of the fetus can be determined by pulse diagnosis. The strength of the deep pulse of the mother is compared with the strength of her superficial pulse. If the deep pulse is stronger, it is probably a girl; and if the superficial pulse is stronger, it's a boy. This can be confirmed by comparing the pulse of the middle finger position on the mother's right hand with the middle finger's position on her left hand. If the right is stronger, it's a girl; and if the left is stronger, it's a boy.

Sterility and Miscarriage

The reason why a woman is not conceiving must always be determined first. Generally the overall body energy is low. This may be due to a chronic infection that results in a blockage in the uterine tubes, and is mainly related to the kidney meridian, although the spleen and liver meridians are also involved. In other cases, the problem is due to a "cold uterus." In this case, the lower abdomen will feel very cold, indicating low energy. Under these circumstances, the ora are not able to function properly. Moxibustion will often be the preferred treatment in such a case. If ova are not being made, the herbal prescription *quai pei tong* is the preferred treatment.* If the failure to conceive or a miscarriage is due to having had many abortions, an herbal cleansing is required. *Angelica sinesis, lingustis* and *leonurus*, together with some neutral herbs, are prescribed.

Miscarriage can be due to a number of different problems. Sometimes the energy of the kidney meridian needs to be built up in order to make the uterus strong enough to carry the fetus. At other times, the energy of the spleen meridian must be increased in order to stabilize the blood and improve the digestion and assimilation of nutrients.

Menstruation and Blood Problems

Medicinal herbs are used for the regulation of blood, an important aspect of many diseases. There are herbs to produce blood, activate blood, stop bleeding, and remove blood congestion.

Menstrual cramps are seen to be related to a problem with the central nervous system. If the nervous system is strengthened, the blood will be healthier; and similarly, if the blood is made stronger, the nervous system will function better. Menstrual problems can be caused by internal or external sources, including accidents. Internal causes are often due to weaknesses in the liver and spleen meridians. The consistency and color of the blood as well as the length of the period are highly diagnostic for female problems. If the period comes too early, an overall body energy weakness is indicated. If the period arrives late, this means the blood has excess heat, indicated by darker blood (excess yang energy). When poor circulation accompanies this condition, ovarian cysts and breast growths are sometimes present. This is discussed further in the section on growths.

Some examples of Chinese herbs used for menstrual disorders include *rhizoma corydalis, radix rehmanniae* (untreated), *atractylodis alba, salviae miltiorrhizae, rhizoma coptidis,* and Chinese rose blossoms. Often as many as six to ten different herbs will be combined to treat this problem. The patient is instructed to boil these herbs down to make a cup of tea; then she should drink a half-cup in the morning and a half-cup at night. After three days, a new bag of herbs may be used.

Quai pei tong is translated as the prescription to restore spleen function.

Vaginal and Bladder Infections

Infections of the vagina and bladder are basically caused by an overall low energy in the body. Vaginal infections are diagnosed on the basis of the body energy and the discharge's color. White discharges are related to a weakness in the metal energy and low chi; yellow discharges are related to the earth energy, specifically the spleen; green discharges are due to the liver; and red discharges are related to the fire energy and are specifically connected to the blood. Vaginal infections arise from a condition known an "yin fire," which involves "excess yang in the yin." Diagnostically, one sees that these problems are preceded or accompanied by symptoms of great thirst, feeling hot but with no measurable fever, canker sores on the tongue or lips, and a feeling of being burnt out.

Symptoms of dark menstrual blood, itchy red skin rashes, pain in the joints, nervousness, and restlessness are some other symptoms sometimes seen. The pulse is usually light and rapid. The herbal treatment is given on the basis of which yin organ system has the heat. The herbs clear out the yin fire, allowing the real chi to arise. Although there are herbal douches to help with the symptoms, the yin fire must first be cleared and the overall body chi built up in order for the problem to be really cured.

Bladder infections are usually caused by "yang fire" and arise from small intestine heat. The herbal prescription given includes *glechoma longituba* and *fructus conni*, which clear the heat from the small intestine and heart. If it is a chronic problem, *semen coicis* (pearl barley) and red dates are added. In one such case treated, a 26-year-old woman with chronic bladder infections, constipation, a bloated feeling, and foggy thinking received relief from her symptoms, and the bladder infection was cured after four treatments of acupuncture and one month of herbal medicine.

Cervical Dysplasia

The principal cause of dysplasia is a liver imbalance. The kidneys and spleen meridians are also weak. The following case study illustrates this problem and the treatment used.

Marla is a 25-year-old woman who had been diagnosed with cervical dysplasia by her gynecologist two and one-half years prior to seeking out Chinese herbal medicine and acupuncture. She was monitored with colposcopies every three-to-six months after several abnormal class II Pap smears and a benign biopsy. The condition had grown worse at her last gynecological exam, prior to seeking Chinese medical treatment. Her initial Chinese diagnosis was a weakness in the liver, kidney, and spleen meridians, as well as weak blood and overall low chi. After eight weeks of treatment—seven weeks of Chinese herbs and six acupuncture treatments—for the first time in three years her colposcopy exam indicated no traces of dysplasia. Herbal treatment in this case included *angelica sinesis, lingustici wallichii, cyperus rotundus, paeonia alba, semen amoni,* Chinese rose blossoms, and cardamom.

This clinical picture of a weakness in the liver, kidney, and spleen meridians together with weak blood and overall low chi is characteristic of many women's health problems. Diagnosed through the pulse and by examining the tongue, this problem can be treated by rebuilding the energy of these meridians through the use of an intricate combination of herbs. Carefully chosen and combined, certain herbs can rebuild the energy in specific meridians. Likewise, there are herbs that perform the function of cleaning and strengthening the blood. It must be especially noted that the correct use of Chinese herbs is a precise and complex science that takes more than 20 years to master.

Breast Tumors, Uterine Tumors, and Ovarian Cysts

Cysts and tumors often accompany menstrual problems. These growths are seen to be caused by poor circulation resulting in the stagnation of blood as evidenced by an increase of heat. These conditions are seen as "yin fire" problems. With the use of herbs, acupuncture, and specific nutritional guidelines, the circulation can be improved, resulting in increased menstrual flow. The improved circulation and nutrition cleanse the blood, releasing the stagnation of blood and chi. In this way, the cysts and lumps are released.

If the blood is not flowing due to an overall weakness resulting in poor assimilation of nutrients, then the famous ancient prescription for strengthening the kidneys, liver, and spleen is used: *Se mut tong* or the "Four Substance Prescription" consists of *Angelica sinesis, rhizoma ligustici wallichii, radix paeoniae alba,* and *radix rhemaniae* (treated). The specific proportions of each herb used in this prescription are what makes it so effective.

In cases of uterine tumors, the stronger herb of *leonuris* is used; this herb acts directly on the uterus, causing increased circulation and cleansing. When there is pain resulting from poor blood circulation, corydalis would be added. The treatment here is to first cleanse the body, then build up the body's energy. Three packages of these herbs will be given a week for two weeks, then two packages a week for two weeks, after which other herbs will be added to build up the chi. Acupuncture and moxibustion may be weekly or biweekly. In general, the length of the healing period is proportional to the length of time the condition persisted prior to treatment.

The following case studies illustrate the effectiveness of the above described forms of treatment.

A dramatic case is that of Patty, a 24-year-old college student who exercised daily and had had no period for three years and a benign breast tumor on her right breast. The tumor had been surgically removed one year earlier but had grown back. The tumor, two inches long, one inch wide, and one-half inch thick, was attached to the skin of her breast. After one acupuncture treatment, her period began. After three months of herbs, moxibustion, and weekly acupuncture treatments, the tumor went away. Follow-up exams at six-month intervals for two years showed no reoccurrence of her problems.

Paula, a 29-year-old medical lab technician, had a scanty, dark-colored menstrual flow, as well as a small tumor on her breast. In this case, eight months of weekly acupuncture treatments, herbs, and moxibustion were required before the tumor remitted. This patient did not exercise as frequently as the previous case.

Judy, a 28-year-old woman, had a painful ovarian cyst, the size of a golf ball. After two and a half months of acupuncture and herbal treatment, the cyst disappeared, which was subsequently verified by a pelvic exam.

A 32-year-old single woman by the name of Sally was bleeding at ovulation. Her gynecologist could not determine the problem. She was treated with intensive acupuncture and herbs. A small pedunculated fibroid tumor was passed after two weeks. This tumor was biopsied as a uterine tumor. The bleeding at ovulation ceased.

The next patient, Jana, a 35-year-old mother, had a dark-colored menstrual flow, considerable pain in the lower abdomen, and a slightly larger than golf-ball size uterine fibroid tumor diagnosed by her gynecologist. After six months of treatment, the pain went away, the fibroid tumor disintegrated, and her general energy improved.

One final case is that of Karin, a 40-year-old patient who had a spherical breast lump one inch in diameter, which appeared suddenly and easily moved around. After one treatment of acupuncture and two weeks of herbs over a month's time, the lump went away.

Mastitis

Chinese medicine says that the causative factor of acute mastitis is retention of milk in the breast caused by mental depression. This depression affects the chi of the liver, resulting in stagnated toxic heat in the stomach channel. Symptoms of this condition include heat and pain in the breast, swelling, and redness accompanied by chills, fever, nausea, irritability, and thirst. The pulse is wiry and rapid. To cure this condition, the chi of the liver and stomach channels must be regulated. This is accomplished by relieving the depression and eliminating the heat by decreasing the energy in the liver, stomach, and gallbladder meridians. Moxibustion is sometimes used in addition (*Essentials of Chinese Acupuncture* 1980, p. 386).

CONCLUSION

We hope that the theory and cases presented in this article have intrigued readers to investigate Chinese medicine further. In seeking a doctor, it is of course most important to locate a competent one. We must caution our readers that proper use of herbs and acupuncture takes numerous years of study under the supervision of a skillful teacher. See Table 9–2 at the end of this chapter for the use of acupuncture for female disorders.

  This article is a first step. Reviewing the current literature on Chinese medicine demonstrates the overwhelming need for further research. There exist very few articles on Chinese medicine for women's health problems. It is our hope that research funds will be obtained to document the impressive results of traditionally trained Chinese medical practitioners. Proper scientific research will enable this rich tradition to be recognized and utilized more fully in Western society. Our deep gratitude is extended to our doctor and teacher—Dr. Lam Kong—we could not have written this article without his invaluable help.

> *Something mysteriously formed,*
> *Born before heaven and earth,*
> *In the silence and the void,*
> *Standing alone and unchanging,*
> *Ever present and in motion,*
> *Perhaps it is the mother of ten thousand things*
> *I do not know its name*
> *Call it Tao*
> *For lack of a better word, I call it great.*
>
> [*Lao-tsu*, Tao Te Ching, *Ch*. 25]

TABLE 9–2. The Treatment of Female Disorders with Acupuncture

IRREGULAR MENSTRUATION

1. *Cause of Disease*
Blood Hot, Fire Brilliant. Due to too many hot spicy foods; excessive anger.

Symptoms
Period comes early; large amounts of blood, colored purple and lumpy; heart troubled; head dizzy; the Five Hearts are troubled and hot.

Diagnostic Features
Pulse rapid and strong; tip of tongue red, with thin yellow coat.

*Treatment—Accupuncture Points**
P6—Quiets the heart; regulates the chi; all extra meridians meet here.
CV4—Builds up Kidney; adjusts the chi; disperses fire or yang.
SP6—Opens up or softens the liver, so does not create fire. Strengthens spleen; benefits Kidney, Spleen, Liver.

IRREGULAR MENSTRUATION

2. *Cause of Disease*
Blood Hot, Chi Empty.

Symptoms
Period comes early; small amounts of pale blood; dyspnoea; body weary.

Diagnostic Features
Pulse deep and slowed down and without strength; tongue not furred but red flesh, little saliva.

*Treatment—Accupuncture Points**
To disperse heat of blood treat:
SP6—can cool heat in 3 lower yin meridians.
SP10—can disperse heat in blood.
LV2—disperse LV fire.
CV4, CV6, to tonify chi.

IRREGULAR MENSTRUATION

3. *Cause of Disease*
Blood Cold and Empty. Due to too much cold food; living in damp climate.

Symptoms
Period comes late; small amount of pale blood; pieces in abdomen like cyst; pain better by pressure and with hot water bottle.

Diagnostic Features
Pulse slowed down.

*Treatment—Accupuncture Points**
CV3—tonify uterus, use moxa.
CV4—tonify Kidney and Chi.
SP10—tonify sea of blood.
ST36—tonify whole body.
ST29—moves blood, increases period.

IRREGULAR MENSTRUATION

4. *Cause of Disease*
Blood Cold and Chi empty. Unable to strengthen lower warmer. Body weak, anemia.

Symptoms
Period comes late—over 40 days; large amounts of blood, which cannot be stopped.

Diagnostic Features
Pulse deep and weak.

*Treatment: Acupuncture Points**
CV6—makes chi move properly.
ST36—tonifies body.
SP1—moxa; strengthens spleen; adjusts blood, holds blood in meridians.

IRREGULAR MENSTRUATION

5. *Cause and Disease*
Liver and Kidney depressed.

Symptoms
Periods irregular, may come early or late.

Diagnostic Features
Pulse wiry.

*Treatment: Acupuncture Points**
BL17—Meeting point of blood; nourishes and regulates blood.
BL18—Bladder associated point of the Liver.
CV3—Tonify uterus.
SP8—Adjusts uterus; regulates period; disperses stuck blood.

---

*See *Acupuncture in Medical Practice,* Louise Wensel. Reston Publishing Company. Reston, Va., 1980, for explanation of acupunture points.

DYSMENORRHOEA

1. *Cause and Disease*
   Blood Hot, Chi Depressed; dead blood blocked and congealed.

   Symptoms
   Period comes early; lower abdomen painful; blood purple and lumpy.

   Diagnostic Features
   Pulse wiry.

   *Treatment—Acupuncture Points**
   BL17—regulates blood, expels heat.
   CV6—Tonifies Chi.
   LV14/Mu point of LV. Transforms stuckness.

DYSMENORRHOEA

2. *Cause of Disease*
   Chi and Blood Empty and **Deficient;** water does not submerge Wood.

   Symptoms
   Period comes late; lower abdomen painful.

   Diagnostic Features
   Pulse slowed down.
   Treatment—Acupuncture Points*
   BL23—Strengthens KD
   L7—moves Ren Mo master point.
   KI1—wood point on Kidney meridian use moxa.
   SP6

DYSMENORRHOEA

3. *Cause of Disease*
   Blood Empty and **Cold.**

   Symptoms
   Lower abdomen painful during period; dragging pain in both sides; limbs aching and tired.

   Diagnostic Features
   Pulse deep.

   *Treatment—Acupuncture Points**
   CV3—Tonify uterus.
   CV4—Tonify KI and Chi.
   SP10—sea of blood tonify.
   ST36—Tonify whole body.

AMENORRHOAE

1. *Cause of Disease*
   Blood Obstructed; caused by Cold Chi.

   Symptoms
   Menses cease; lower abdomen swollen and hard, becoming larger daily as though pregnant.

   Diagnostic Features
   Pulse deep and tight.

   *Treatment—Acupuncture Points**
   CV—tonify uterus.
   L14—and **SP6**—used together they move blood and move uterus, remove stuckness.

AMENORRHOEA

2. *Cause of Disease*
   Blood deficient; Grief injures Heart and Spleen.

   Symptoms
   Menstruation ceases; appetite decreases rapidly; skin and flesh dry and emaciated; Shen tired; body lethargic.

   Diagnostic Features
   Pulse deep.

   Treatment
   BL38—neurasthenia, regulates emotions.
   BL20—Spleen associated point.
   H8—Quiets spirit.
   CV4

AMENORRHOEA

3. *Cause of Disease*
   Blood Withered; bearing and/or suckling large number of children; excessive sexual intercourse; Jing exhausted.

   Symptoms
   Menses cease, little appetite; skin dry and withered; incessant coughing.

   Diagnostic Features
   Pulse deep.

   Treatment
   BL23
   CV4
   ST36
   B17

VAGINAL DISCHARGE

1. *Cause of Disease*
   White discharge; spleen meridian not protected; Damp Evil sinks downwards.

   Symptoms
   White discharge like saliva or mucus, if chronic is foul smelling.

   Diagnostic Features
   Pulse slowed down and slippery.

   Treatment
   BL20—
   GB26—removes damp heat from lower warmer enables blood to enter Dai Mo.
   CV3
   SP6
   SP0—transforms stuck dampness; benefits lower warmer.

VAGINAL DISCHARGE

1. *Cause of Disease*
   Green discharge: liver meridian Damp and Hot.

   Symptoms
   Discharge like green bean juice, thick and glutinous; foul-smelling.

   Diagnostic Features
   Pulse wiry, slippery, weak, and floating.

   Treatment
   BL18—Liver associated point.
   LV13—removes heat and dampness, Spleen Mu point.
   CV3—adjusts uterus.
   SP6—
   LV2—disperses fire of liver, moves stuck Chi.

VAGINAL DISCHARGE

3. *Cause of Disease*
   Black discharge: Fire very hot and abundant.

   Symptoms
   Discharge like black-bean juice; foul smelling; lower abdomen painful; pain in bladder as though pierced with a knife; vagina swollen; face red.

   Diagnostic Features
   Pulse slow, weak, and floating.

Treatment
BL23
GB26
CV3
SP6
K3—clears Heat

VAGINAL DISCHARGE

4. *Causes of Disease*
   Yellow discharge: Damp Evil in Vessel of conception.

   Symptoms
   Discharge like the thick juice of yellow tea and foul-smelling.

   Diagnostic Features
   Pulse weak and floating.

   Treatment
   GB26
   CV4
   LU7—master point Ren Mo.
   K6—coupled point
   SP6

VAGINAL DISCHARGE

5. *Cause of Disease*
   Red discharge: Damp and Heat; injures the blood.

   Symptoms
   Discharge red like blood but is not blood; slight continuous discharge.

   Diagnostic Features
   Pulse deep.

   Treatment
   BL15
   BL17
   CV3
   SP6
   SP10

From NCNM, The National College of Naturopathic Medicine, 510 SW Third Avenue, Portland, Oregon.

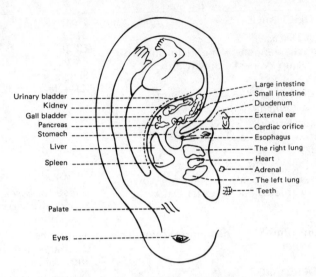

FIGURE 9–4. The ear, simulating a fetus within the womb in an upside-down position. The organ locations shown here illustrate common acupuncture points.

REFERENCES

Essentials of Chinese Acupuncture, 1st ed. Collated by Beijing College of Traditional Chinese Medicine, Shanghai College of Traditional Chinese Medicine, Janjing College, and Acupuncture Institute of the Academy of Chinese Medicine. Beijing, China: Foreign Languages Press, 1980.

Harmer, Ruth M., *American Medical Avarice.* New York: Abelard-Shuman, 1975.

Kong, Lam et al., "Potential Anti-Fertility Plants from Chinese Medicine," *American Journal of Chinese Medicine,* vol. 4, no. 2 (1976).

Kushi, Michio, *Oriental Diagnosis: What Your Face Reveals.* Boston: East-West Foundation, 1979.

Lao-tsu, *Tao Te Ching.* New York: Vintage Books, 1972.

Mann, Felix, *Acupuncture, The Ancient Chinese Art of Healing and How It Works.* New York: Vintage Books, 1973.

Zelin, Chen, "Recent Investigations on Tongue Inspection," *Chinese Medical Journal,* vol. 93, no. 6 (1980).

Zhang, Jin-an, *Huang Di Nei Jing (The Yellow Emperor's Classic of Internal Medicine).* 2600 B.C. Reprinted from the edition of *Si Bu Bei Yao.* Peking: Zhong Hua Book Co., 1929.

SUGGESTED READINGS

American Journal of Chinese Medicine, Garden City, N.Y., 1980.

Kushi, Michio, *Oriental Diagnosis: What Your Face Reveals.* Brookline, Mass., East-West Foundation, Brookline, Ma. 1980.

Wallnoffer, Heinrich, and Anna von Rottauscher, *Chinese Folk Medicine*. New York: Mentor Books, 1965.

The Yellow Emperor's Classic of Internal Medicine, trans. Ilza Vieth. Berkeley, Calif.: University of California Press, 1972.

Chapter Ten

ACUPUNCTURE FOR WOMEN'S HEALTH

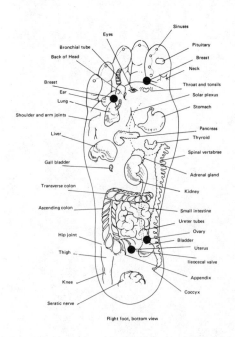

Right foot, bottom view

Louise Wensel

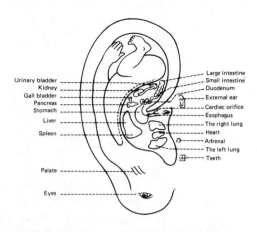

Urinary bladder	Large intestine
Kidney	Small intestine
Gall bladder	Duodenum
Pancreas	External ear
Stomach	Cardiac orifice
Liver	Esophagus
Spleen	The right lung
	Heart
	Adrenal
	The left lung
Palate	Teeth
Eyes	

The ear, simulating a fetus within the womb in an upside-down position.

THEORETICAL BACKGROUND

Thousands of years before American and European scientists discovered atoms, electrons, and electricity, the Chinese developed a concept of the entire universe as being in balance between yin and yang energy factors. *Yin* and *Yang* may be roughly equated with negatively and positively charged electricity, but these concepts are elaborate and difficult to define in English (Wensel 1980).

The ancient Chinese regarded the body as a microcosm that required a balance of yin and yang body energy to enjoy good health (*Huang Ti Nei Ching Su Wen* 1949). Each part of the body was also thought of as an individual microcosm that required its own balance of yin and yang energy to function properly. Thus disease symptoms were caused by an imbalance of yin and yang in some part of the body. Such imbalance could be caused by injury or bacterial invasion. The goal of acupuncture was to restore the balance of yin and yang in the afflicted part and in the body as a whole.

The practice of acupuncture is based on theories of energy flow in the body and can be described as external treatment of internal disorders. The Chinese developed these theories and diagrammed meridians of energy transmission to and from vital organs of the body thousands of years ago. Like low-voltage electricity, these major channels of body energy transmission are invisible and are not present in cadavers. When Americans do electrocardiograms or electroencephalograms, however, they are employing the concept of body energy transmission, which is not entirely dependent on nerves or blood vessels.

During many years of experimenting, the Chinese discovered that inserting sharp objects superficially at certain points on their meridians of energy transmission could relieve pain or improve the function of other

183

specific parts of the body at some distance from these points. They observed that needles inserted into these points produced a special sensation called *Te-Chi* or "energization" whereas needles inserted into adjacent areas of the skin did not produce this sensation.

Our observations of referred pain transmitted along nerve pathways are consistent with acupuncture theory, but Americans are just beginning to acknowledge that bioelectricity is not entirely dependent on nerve fibers for its transmission. Modern knowledge of embryology helps explain why parts of the body that appear completely separate from each other after birth have a history of common derivation in embryology and, therefore, a relationship that is not evident in an ordinary physical examination.

Modern electronic instruments enable us to locate acupuncture points precisely where the ancient Chinese showed them to be on their diagrams. These instruments measure electric resistance, which is lower at the acupuncture points than on the surrounding tissues. Some American chiropractors use these instruments to give electric stimulation at acupuncture points and call this practice "electro-acupressure."

SCIENTIFIC BASIS

Many Americans suspect that acupuncture is mainly a type of hypnosis or faith-healing. However, there is good scientific evidence to the contrary (Collison 1974 et al.). Furthermore, acupuncture is effective for treating animals not susceptible to hypnosis or faith healing (Freeman 1974; Kao and Kao 1974). One does not have to believe in acupuncture to be helped by it.

Research by American and European scientists led to the discovery of endorphins and enkephalins in 1975. These endogenous biochemicals have been found in the brain, endocrine glands, and various other parts of the body. Their actions include relieving pain, allergies, and depression (Mendelson 1977). They also promote healing, restoration of function, and homeostatis—the body's tendency to regulate its functions for good health. Acupuncture has been shown to cause a significant increase in the levels of endorphins and enkephalins in the body, thereby explaining scientifically why acupuncture relieves pain and is effective treatment for many medical disorders (Miller 1979).

Biochemists have tried to synethesize various endorphins, and psychiatrists are experimenting with them in the treatment of mental illness. None of these synthetic endorphins, however, seems to be as effective as acupuncture in increasing natural endorphin levels (Snyder 1978).

WHY NOT RECOMMENDED BY MORE AMERICAN PHYSICIANS

Physicians tend to treat their patients with what they have been taught is appropriate methods and the best available for any given condition. They are hesitant to prescribe something that is not considered "standard treatment." Unfortunately, most American physicians have not been taught much about the effectiveness and safety of acupuncture, so acupuncture has not yet been accepted as "standard treatment." Most American physicians still define "treatment" as drugs or surgery and are unaware of the scientific basis for acupuncture. They are unlikely to be able to perform it themselves and may not know anyone they trust to perform it with skill and asceptic technique.

INDICATIONS AND CONTRAINDICATIONS

Acupuncture should not be used to relieve excessive bleeding, vaginal discharges, or undiagnosed pain, any of which might be a symptom of some disorder requiring prompt surgery or antibiotics. It also should not be used as treatment for cancer or any kind of infection. Nor should it be used during pregnancy, except for delivery, because it may initiate abortion or premature labor.

Besides being useful for relieving pain, acupuncture can be a safe and effective alternative to drugs or surgery for many gynecologic disorders. It is also the safest anesthesia for childbirth, even Cesarean sections.

Acupuncture can be especially helpful for menstrual and menopausal problems, endometriosis, and sexual dysfunctions. It may also be effective and much safer than psychotropic drugs for relieving depresison, anxiety, and insomnia.

Since acupuncture by a competent acupuncturist has no undesirable side effects, it is safer than drugs or surgery for many chronic conditions, including those discussed in this chapter. In some cases it may not be effective, but there is no danger that it will make any condition worse or interfere with chemical treatment such as drugs for diabetes, heart disease, epilepsy, or hypertension. If many acupuncture treatments are taken, however, the need for drugs to lower blood sugar or blood pressure may be decreased. Acupuncture may also reduce the need for drugs to control seizures, but it is dangerous to discontinue such drugs suddenly without consulting a physician. If a person has been taking cortisone or one of its derivatives, withdrawal may be so difficult that the drug has to be continued long after acupuncture has relieved the symptoms for which the drug was prescribed.

Many women submit to unnecessary and mutilating surgery or take drugs with dangerous side effects because they are unaware that acupuncture could, in many cases, relieve their symptoms and correct the pathology causing them. The situations discussed in the following pages of this chapter are of special interest to women, but these are not the only circumstances for which women might benefit from acupuncture treatments.

SITUATIONS THAT MAY BE HELPED BY ACUPUNCTURE

Dysmenorrhea (Menstrual Pain)

Pain just before or during menstruation can usually be relieved by acupuncture unless there is some anatomic blockage of the menstrual flow. If acupuncture is going to relieve menstrual pain and cramps, six treatments should be enough for lasting relief unless the pain is from endometriosis, which requires longer treatment.

Endometriosis

Severe menstrual cramps and sometimes frequent and excessive menstrual bleeding may be symptoms of endometriosis. It is a condition in which some of the menstrual discharge goes into the abodminal cavity instead of being normally excreted through the vagina. This discharge can become attached to various parts of the pelvis and lower abdomen, causing them to malfunction. Although endometriosis decreases fertility, it may be relieved by pregnancy. In some cases, progesterone treatment may relieve endometriosis, but hysterectomy is often required.

It is so difficult to believe that acupuncture could relieve the symptoms of endometriosis that the American physicians at the Washington Acupuncture Center would not let the Chinese acupuncturists treat patients for this condition during the first five years of operation of the Center. Then one of the secretaries, who had been told by two gynecologists that she had endometriosis and needed a hysterectomy, talked with one of the Chinese acupuncturists about it and persuaded the Center to let him try treating her. He gave her a series of six treatments a month for several months. Much to everyone's surprise, all of her symptoms were relieved. Since then, other women have been treated by acupuncture for this condition with good results.

Amenorrhea

Absence or infrequency of menses is a symptom that seldom requires medical intervention unless it is associated with abdominal pain or an indication of pregnancy. Taking hormone pills or injections may establish regular menstrual periods, but this will suppress the body's natural ability to produce these hormones.

Acupuncture can stimulate the endocrine glands to produce more of the hormones needed for normal development and functioning of reproductive organs, breasts, and other characteristics associated with femininity. Needles should never be inserted into the breasts or genitalia. Instead, they are inserted superficially into other areas as indicated in Figure 10–1.

Mental illness and the drugs given to treat it may cause amenorrhea or infrequency of menses. Acupuncture is an effective substitute for such drugs. Since poor nutrition may be a cause of amenorrhea, nutritional therapy should be given along with acupuncture.

Infertility

If a woman and her mate have had thorough examinations to rule out the organic causes of infertility, acupuncture may be helpful. It can help induce ovulation in cases of anovulatory syndrome. Nutritional therapy should be given along with acupuncture and continued after a series of ten acupuncture treatments have been completed. Acupuncture treatments should be given on a daily basis starting three or four days after the beginning of a menstrual period. Acupuncture should not be given after a pregnancy has begun because of the possibility that it might cause abortion. Acupuncture can also be effective in increasing male sperm count and sexual potency.

Induction of Labor and Abortion

There are several acupuncture points that can be effective for inducing labor and stimulating the uterus to contract more forcefully. Acupuncture at these points may cause abortion early in pregnancy. This would be safer and less unpleasant than a surgical abortion, but using acupuncture in this way is not a dependable method of contraception. The further advanced the pregnancy is, the more likely it is that acupuncture will initiate uterine contractions.

Some of the acupuncture points used most frequently to treat other conditions are the same as those used to induce uterine contractions. For this reason, it is not advisable to use acupuncture during pregnancy unless one wants to terminate it.

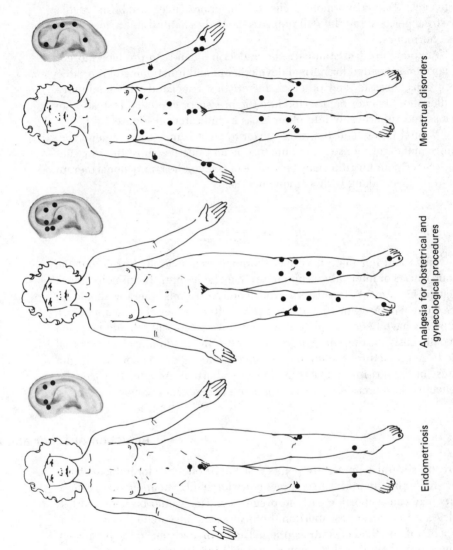

Endometriosis

Analgesia for obstetrical and
gynecological procedures

Menstrual disorders

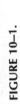

FIGURE 10–1.

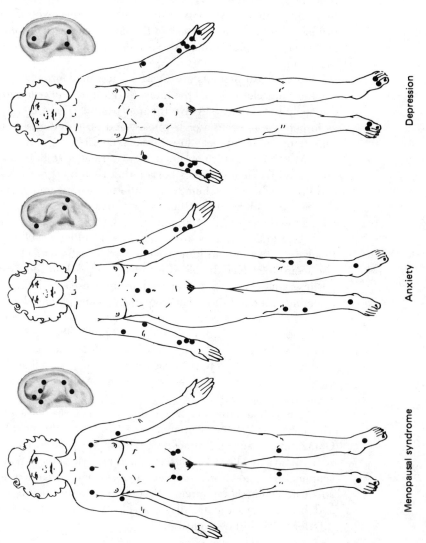

Depression

Anxiety

Menopausal syndrome

FIGURE 10–1. (Continued)

Anesthesia or Analgesia

The English words *anesthesia* and *analgesia* are misleading when used to describe the freedom from surgical or obstetrical pain that can be produced by acupuncture. Acupuncture does not alter the level of consciousness or produce numbness of any part of the body. The patient under acupuncture analgesia remains able to converse and cooperate with the surgical or obstetrical team.

Obstetrical patients are aware of uterine contractions and are able to use their muscles to expel the fetus. Surgical patients can tell when incisions are made but do not perceive them as painful. There is no loss of memory, as in general anesthesia or hypnosis, and no parethesia comparable to the sensations following local anesthesia (Wen 1977).

Most operating room deaths and cardiac arrests in the United States are caused by chemical anesthesia rather than by surgery (Gordon, Larson, and Prestivich 1976). Chemical anesthesia given to a pregnant woman affects the baby as well as the mother and may result in permanent damage to the baby's nervous system. Acupuncture does not have this same danger.

Acupuncture can be used to induce a feeling of well-being or calmness to allay the fear and apprehensiveness most patients feel before surgery. It also seems to reduce the bleeding during surgical procedures. Furthermore, postoperative patients are spared from nausea and the difficulties with urinating and defecating that frequently follow chemical anesthesia.

The success of acupuncture analgesia depends mainly on the skill of the acupuncturist. Although there are few skilled acupuncturists in the United States at present, it takes less time to train a physician, nurse, or medical technician to perform acupuncture analgesia than to teach her how to give acupuncture treatments for chronic diseases or to give chemical anesthesia or analgesia.

The actual induction of acupuncture analgesia takes about 20 minutes. The more skilled the acupuncturist, the fewer the needles required. In China, major surgical procedures have been performed with only one acupuncture needle as analgesia without electric potentiation. The beginning acupuncturist, however, may need to insert more than ten needles to obtain adequate analgesia for surgery. Using acupuncture points on the ears, feet, and hands keeps the needles and electro-acupuncture instruments from interfering with the surgical field.

Menopausal Syndrome

Acupuncture is much safer and often more effective than estrogen for controlling the hot flashes, depression, and other unpleasant symptoms many women feel a few years before and after the cessation of their menstrual periods.

Until recently, physicians routinely prescribed estrogens for women past the age of 35 who complained of hot flashes or depression. Unfortunately, many women have had their chances for developing cancer, thrombophlebitis, strokes, and heart attacks increased by this practice. Now that physicians are aware of this danger, they are likely to prescribe psychotropic drugs instead. But these may damage the heart muscle or the basal ganglia of the brain, causing dyskinesia with impaired coordination and tremors.

A series of ten acupuncture treatments, along with nutritional therapy to be continued afterwards, will usually relieve hot flashes, depression, and other menopausal symptoms. Acupuncture will promote a feeling of well-being and self-confidence, which will enable a woman to cope more effectively with her life situation.

Depression

There are basically two types of depression—exogenous and endogenous. Exogenous depression results from factors in the external environment, such as loss of a loved one. Endogenous depression is caused by biochemical factors within a person's body and may be independent of one's life situation.

Some researchers have found deficiencies of the biochemicals serotonin and dopamine in depressed patients and have, therefore, concluded that endogenous depression is a symptom of biochemical deficiency, which can be corrected by drugs. As a result, many drugs have been developed to treat depression. Most of these drugs are at least somewhat effective but have serious side effects. It cannot be determined, however, whether the biochemical deficiencies in depression result from the patient's attitude toward life, or whether the biochemical deficiencies occur for other reasons and cause the attitudes and thinking patterns characteristic of depression.

Acupuncture will not replace the biochemical deficiencies found in some endogenous depressions, but it does promote normalization of body metabolism and stimulates the patient's body to produce optimal amounts of the biochemicals it needs for good health. Since acupuncture does not have the side effects of antidepressant drugs, electric shock, or hormones, it is much safer and usually is at least as effective.

By causing an increase in the body's production of endorphins and enkephalins, acupuncture can give a person a feeling of well-being, which relieves depression. Usually a person feels less depressed after the first acupuncture treatment, but at least six treatments should be taken for lasting relief.

Anxiety

Feelings of restlessness and apprehensiveness complicate many illnesses and may precede their development. People suffering from anxiety may appear acutely ill and fear that death is imminent, or they may appear outwardly calm but have psychosomatic symptoms. Anxiety may accompany pain and intensify it.

Too many people take tranquilizing drugs or alcohol to relieve anxiety. These can have serious undesirable side effects and can lead to addicion or fatal overdoses.

Traditional Chinese medicine considers anxiety a symptom of imbalance between the *yin* and *yang* aspects of vital energy. In many cases, it can be effectively relieved by acupuncture. The points used for treating anxiety are included in the treatment of many types of illness, especially for the relief of pain that may accompany them.

Some people can even learn to control their own anxiety symptoms by applying finger pressure to some of the acupuncture points. (See Figure 10–1 for points on front of body and ears.)

Allergies

Allergies are excessively adverse reactions to certain substances that a person is exposed to by skin contact, inhalation, ingestion, or injection. Hay fever, bronchial asthma, angioneurotic edema, many skin rashes, and some cases of nausea and vomiting are allergic reactions. Even some cases of arthritis, colitis, and hyperactivity are thought to have an allergic component.

The substance to which the person is allergic is called the *antigen,* and the blood components produced in response to antigens are called *antibodies*. Much research is being done on antigen-antibody reactions in relation to the body's immune mechanisms. The Washington Acupuncture Center has engaged in such research with the Microbiology Department of George Washington University Medical School to evaluate the regulatory effect of acupuncture on this body process.

Any drug is a potential allergen that may produce a life-threatening allergic reaction. Even antihistamines produce severe allergic reactions for some people. Acupuncture can reduce a person's allergic responses to most common allergens—enough to relieve and prevent hay fever, asthma, some cases of dermatitis, indigestion, and diarrhea. It can also be used as an alternative to potentially allergenic drugs for relieving pain and treating many diseases. Acupuncture, however, should not be depended on as the only treatment for severe allergic reactions to drugs or for anaphylactic shock.

Although allergies may be classified as respiratory, food, drug, or dermatologic, people with severe allergic diatheses may show allergic symptoms in many different parts of their bodies. Instead of treating specific allergic symptoms, acupuncture can be used to reduce a person's general tendency to react allergically.

OTHER CONDITIONS AMENABLE TO ACUPUNCTURE

There are many other medical problems for which acupuncture may be the most effective as well as the safest treatment. These include various types of arthritis, Raynaud's syndrome, psoriasis, colitis, hiccups, whiplash injury residuals, spinal disc disorders, bursitis, tendonitis, muscle strains and spasms, amnesia, insomnia, neurogenic hearing loss, tinnitus, multiple sclerosis, Bell's palsy, cerebral palsy, paresis, stroke residuals, dyskinesia, urinary and fecal incontinence, trigeminal neuralgia, herpes zoster, various types of headache, anorexia, insomnia, obesity, drug addiction, alcoholism, hyperactivity, autism, and schizophrenia.

Acupuncture treatment of these conditions (along with diagrams and precise anatomical locations of acupuncture points for treating each of them) is discussed and described in a book by this author entitled *Acupuncture in Medical Practice* (Wensel 1980).

SPECIFIC POINTS FOR SPECIFIC CONDITIONS

Prescriptions for specific acupuncture points to use for specific conditions are given in the above-mentioned books and in Chinese acupuncture textbooks. These prescriptions, however, should be used as guidelines rather than as specific formulas to be used for each treatment.

These points may be used bilaterally or unilaterally. Not all of them need to be used for each treatment for each person being treated. They can be supplemented with other points to be determined by evaluation of a person as a whole and according to past experience. Skilled acupuncturists seldom insert more than ten needles per treatment, even if they are treating someone for more than one ailment. Often the same basic acupuncture points are included in the standard points for treating many different disorders.

The diagrams shown in Figure 10–1 illustrate the general location of the acupuncture points used most frequently to treat some of the conditions described in this chapter.

REFERENCES

Collison, D., "Acupuncture and Hypnotherapy," *Medical Journal of Australia*, vol. 2, no. 3 (1974).

Freeman, A., "Veterinary Acupuncture," *Journal of the American Veterinary Medicine Association*, 164, no. 5 (1974), 446–48.

Frost, E. A., "Acupuncture and Hypnosis: Apples and Oranges," *New York State Journal of Medicine*, 78, no. 11 (1978), 1768–72.

Gordon, T., C. P. Larson, Jr., and R. Prestivich, "Unexpected Cardiac Arrest during Anesthesia and Surgery," *JAMA*, 236 (1976), 2758–60.

Huang Ti Nei Ching Su Wen (The Yellow Emperor's Classic of Internal Medicine). Compiled circa 221 B.C. and translated by Ilza Veith. Berkeley: University of California Press, 1949.

Kao, F. F., and J. J. Kao, "Veterinary Acupuncture," *American Journal of Chinese Medicine*, 2, no. 1 (1974), 89–102.

Mac Hovec, F. J., and S. C. Man, "Acupuncture and Hypnosis Compared: Fifty-Eight Cases," *American Journal of Clinical Hypnosis*, 21, no. 1 (1978), 45–47.

Mendelson, G., "The Role of Enkephalin in the Mechanism of Acupuncture Analgesia in Man," *Medical Hypotheses*, 2, no. 4 (1977); 144–45.

Miller, Richard J., "The Potential of Endorphins," *Behavioral Medicine*, May 1979, pp. 30–33.

Nemerof, Henry, and Irwin Rothman, "Acupuncture and Hypnotism," *American Journal of Clinical Hypnosis*, 16, no. 3 (1974), 156–59.

Snyder, Solomon H., "The Opiate Receptor and Morphinelike Peptides in the Brain," *American Journal of Psychiatry*, 135, no. 6 (1978), 645–52.

Wen, W., "Acupuncture Anesthesia in China," *Comparative Medicine East and West*, 5 (Summer 1977), 185–88.

Wensel, Louise O., *Acupuncture in Medical Practice*. Reston, Va.: Reston Publishing Company, Inc., 1980.

SUGGESTED READINGS

Academy of Traditional Chinese Medicine, *An Outline of Chinese Acupuncture*. Peking: Foreign Language Press, 1975.

American Journal of Acupuncture. Felton, Calif: 1980.

Chang, Stephen, *The Complete Book of Acupuncture*. Millbrae, Calif.: Celestrial Arts, 1976.

Connelly, Dianne M., *Traditional Acupuncture: The Law of the Five Elements*. Columbia, Md.: The Center for Traditional Acupuncture, Inc., 1979.

Huang, Helena, *Ear Acupuncture*. Emmaus, Pa.: Rodale Press, 1974.

Leges, J.P., *The Little Red Book of Acupuncture*. Wellingborough, England: Thorsons, 1978.

Journal of Acupuncture and Electrotherapeutics Research. Elmsford, N.Y.: Pergamon Press, Inc., 1980.

Manaka, Yoshio, and Ian A. Urquhart, *The Layman's Guide to Acupuncture*. New York: Weatherhill, 1972.

Mann, Felix, *Acupuncture: The Ancient Chinese Art of Healing and How It Works Scientifically* (revised ed.). New York: Vintage Books, 1973.

Wexu, Marió, *The Ear: Gateways to Balancing the Body. A Modern Guide to Ear Acupuncture*. New York: ASI Publishers, 1975.

ORGANIZATIONS FOR ACUPUNCTURE

Acupuncture Center of New York
426 East 89th Street
New York, NY 10028

Acupuncture Project
Franz Hall A-181
University of California School of
   Medicine
Los Angeles, CA 90024

Acupuncture Research Institute
P.O. Box 7534
Long Beach, CA 90807

Acupuncture Research Institute
9375 Fernando Road
Sun Valley, CA 91352

Acupuncture Wholistic Center
822 South Atlantic Boulevard
Monterey Park, CA 91754

The Center for Traditional Acupuncture,
   Inc.
The American City Building
Columbia, MD 21044

Emory University
Acupuncture Research Project
School of Dentistry
1462 Clifton Road, N.E.
Atlanta, GA 30322

Institute of Pneumology
5524 MacArthur Boulevard, N.W.
Washington, DC 20016

Massachusetts General Hospital
   Acupuncture Research Project
32 Fruit St.
Boston, MA 02114

National Acupuncture Association
P.O. Box 24509
Los Angeles, CA 90024

National Acupuncture Research
   Society
1841 Broadway
New York, NY 10023

Nevada Board of Chinese Medicine
201 South Fall Street
Carson City, NV 89701

New England School of Acupuncture
5 Bridge Street
Watertown, MA 02171

Ryodoraker Research Institute of
   North America, Inc.
8133 Wornall Road
Kansas City, MO 64114

United Acupuncturists of California
125 Quincy Street
St. Mary's Square
San Francisco, CA 94108

Chapter Eleven

HOMEOPATHY AND WOMEN'S HEALTH

Jennifer Jacobs

Homeopathy, a 200-year-old form of natural healing, offers much in the area of women's health. Homeopathy is one of several healing disciplines that recognizes the body's own innate ability to heal itself. The purpose of treatment is not merely to attack germs that are invading the body or to suppress the symptoms that the body has produced as a reaction to illness; rather, the purpose is to strengthen the body's own defense mechanisms so that it can heal itself.

THE PRINCIPLE OF SIMILARS

Homeopathy was developed by a German physician, Samuel Hahnemann (1755–1843). While working as a medical translator, Hahnemann became interested in the properties of quinine to cure malaria and decided to test the drug on himself. Surprisingly enough, after taking large doses of quinine, he developed periodic chills and fever that were very similar to the symptoms of malaria itself.

He remembered the writings of Hippocrates, who in 400 B.C. had said: "Through the like, disease is produced and through the application of the like, it is cured" (Panos and Heimlich 1980, p. 11). From this he developed the *principle of similars*, or "like cures like," which forms the basis of homeopathy. According to the principle of similars, a substance that causes disease symptoms in a healthy person will cure the same symptoms in someone who is sick.

An example of this is the substance Ipecac, which is one of the home-opathic remedies. As many people know, a large dose of Ipecac can cause severe nausea and vomiting. However, in a woman who is experiencing nausea and vomiting of pregnancy, a small dose of the remedy Ipecac can often cure these symptoms.

The name *homeopathy* was derived from the Greek words, *homeo*, or "like," and *pathos*, which means "suffering." In homeopathy we use medicines that produce symptoms *like* the illness. In contrast, we refer to modern Western medicine as *allopathy*, from the Greek word for "other" and "suffering," since medicines are given that produce opposite effects from the illness.

Aspirin for fever is a good example of allopathic prescribing. The body, in response to illness, produces a fever as part of the healing process. Many viruses are known to be unable to survive high temperatures and many people have experienced that once their fever breaks its peak they feel much better. So taking aspirin to artificially control the fever is opposing the body's normal healing mechanism, dealing only with the symptoms of fever, rather than the illness itself.

In homeopathy, we often give the remedy Belladonna for someone with a high fever. Belladonna, or Deadly Nightshade, when given in large doses causes heat, redness, throbbing, burning, even delirium. But a small amount of Belladonna can actually alleviate these symptoms. We see this as a mechanism by which the body's own healing is enhanced and stimulated to come to completion.

HOMEOPATHIC REMEDIES

The remedies that are used in homeopathy are naturally occurring substances—plant, animal, or mineral in origin. They have been specially prepared by the processes of serial dilution and potentization to become active on the deepest energetic level. In *serial dilution* the substances are first dissolved or suspended in a water/alcohol mixture that is known as a *mother tincture*. One drop of tincture is then mixed with 10 drops of water/alcohol, then one drop of that mixture with 10 drops of water/alcohol, and so on. The process is repeated hundreds or thousands of times depending on what potency of remedy is being prepared. The potency 200, which is often used, means the mother tincture has been diluted by a factor of 1 in 10 for 200 times, equivalent to 10^{-200} in scientific notation. Other common potencies in use are 30, 1000, and 10,000.

Hahnemann found that remedies became stronger as they were more dilute. He also found that they became more potent by shaking the vials containing the mixtures several times between each dilution. This process, known as *potentization*, is thought to release the electromagnetic energy contained in the substances.

HOW DOES HOMEOPATHY WORK?

Twentieth-century physics recognizes the existence of particles smaller than atoms as well as electromagnetic fields associated with all matter. Through Kirlian photography, the aura or electromagnetic field surrounding a substance or person is visualized. It is thought that by matching the vibrations of the electromagnetic field of a person with the vibrations of a remedy, that person's field will be strengthened and healing will result. The symptoms that a person is manifesting in an attempt to heal are used as clues to find a remedy with similar symptoms, as well as similar vibrational energy.

THE NATURAL HEALING PROCESS

A healing crisis can sometimes occur after taking a homeopathic remedy. By this we mean that symptoms can sometimes become worse temporarily as they surface and are eliminated by the healing process.

There are certain natural laws of healing that are merely augmented by the remedies. The fact that healing occurs from within outward is the most fundamental of these "laws." The total body-mind-person is seen as a hierarchy, with the deepest level being the mental and spiritual, the emotional layer next, and the physical body as the most superficial layer. Within the physical level the hierarchy continues from the vital organs such as the brain and heart, out to more superficial organs such as the skin and body orifices.

We often notice that people will develop bodily eruptions and/or discharges after being treated homeopathically. This is indicative that healing is occurring, that some imbalance within the body is coming out to the surface.

For this reason, illnesses such as herpes or vaginal infections are difficult to treat homeopathically since they are seen as surface manifestations of a deeper, positive healing mechanism that is happening. People are often advised to be patient and allow these things to occur since it is also felt that to suppress these symptoms might push the illness back down to a deeper level. We usually suggest palliative measures, such as vinegar and garlic douching for vaginitis or Vitamin E oil for herpes. The idea is to diminish the uncomfortable aspects of these symptoms while letting them run their course.

INTEGRATED APPROACH BENEFICIAL FOR WOMEN'S HEALTH

Homeopathy is a wonderful system of healing for many women's health problems. This is because in homeopathy we look at the picture of the whole person—all of the symptoms someone is having on a physical level, as well as certain general factors about that person. Sleep, appetite, body temperature, moods, temperament, and personality are all inquired about in the course of a homeopathic interview. Since many women's health problems have elusive causes and are often attributed to psychosomatic or hormonal imbalances by allopaths, this integrated approach is very successful. In homeopathy we do not care so much what the "cause" of an illness is. The holistic approach recognizes that a multitude of factors such as poor nutrition, emotional disturbance, and environmental stress all contribute to illness. We simply look at the symptoms a person is having and choose a remedy to match those symptoms.

Historically, homeopathy has always appealed to women, and even today there is a much larger percentage of women homeopaths than in other fields of medicine. Margery Blackie, a famous British homeopath, is the personal physician of Queen Elizabeth II. Homeopathy has always been popular with women because of its noninvasive nature, easy accessibility, and excellent application to childhood and other acute illnesses. Since women are often the healers and nurturers in a household or community, homeopathy is a powerful tool for them to use. At the turn of the century, "homeopathy won the support of large numbers of American women, who constituted approximately two-thirds of its patrons and who were among its most active propagators" (Risse et al. 1977).

HOMEOPATHY IN PREGNANCY AND CHILDBIRTH

The pregnant woman has a real friend in homeopathy. For not only is homeopathy safe and effective, it also has no unpleasant side effects and cannot harm the unborn child. Nausea of pregnancy, threatened miscarriage, water retention, and emotional changes can all respond well to homeopathic treatment.

There is no specific remedy that will treat any one of these conditions. Ten different women with the same presenting complaint, such as nausea, may each be treated with a different remedy, depending on the *totality of symptoms*. Is the nause worse in the morning or evening, before or after eating? Is it worse indoors or out? Is the woman chilly? Is she drinking more or less fluids than usual? How are her appetite and moods? Is she feeling irritable, moody, or crying easily? These are some of the factors that are considered in the choice of a remedy. As one can see, homeopathy is much more complex than just prescribing an antinausea pill. This concept of totality of symptoms underlies all of homeopathic treatment. The *person* is treated, not the disease. So no matter what illness someone is suffering from, the same factors are considered, and a remedy is chosen based on that person's total symptoms.

Homeopathy is particularly helpful in childbirth. Remedies can often be given to ease a difficult labor or hasten delivery. After the birth, homeopathic first-aid remedies, such as arnica for bruising, can help reduce swelling and promote speedy recovery. Postpartum depression, or "baby-blues," can also be treated, as well as problems with breast feeding.

For the infant, dramatic results of homeopathy have been reported. For an infant who is slow to breathe or has poor color shortly after birth, aconite, a first-aid remedy for shock, will often counteract the effects of a difficult birth. Chamomilla is a wonderful children's remedy, both for colic and for teething problems. But Chamomilla will not help all infants with colic or teething problems. The Chamomilla child is peevish, thirsty, wants to be carried all the time, often has one cheek red, the other pale, and is usually worse in late afternoon to early evening. If the child has these, as well as other Chamomilla symptoms, the remedy will help the colic.

FIRST-AID, ACUTE, AND CHRONIC PRESCRIBING

It is important to know the differences between various types of homeopathic prescribing and the limitations of home treatment. *First-aid* treatment refers to accidents and injuries for which there are a limited number of remedies that can usually be used in all cases. Arnica, when given immediately after almost any injury, can greatly reduce the amount of suffering due to swelling, inflammation, and bruising. Hypericum for puncture wounds, rhus tox for strains, and calendula for topical treatment of skin abrasions should all be kept in the well-stocked homeopathic home medicine chest, and can be used by anyone with a beginning knowledge of homeopathy.

However, one must be careful with home treatment of acute or chronic illnesses. An *acute illness* is one that has suddenly occurred, will usually reach a peak, and then subsides. Colds, sore throats, bladder or breast infections, stomach flu, and food poisoning are all examples of acute, self-limited illnesses. These can often be "nipped in the bud" by proper homeopathic treatment early in the course of the illness. A thorough knowledge of homeopathy is necessary to treat these kinds of illnesses, however, as the totality of symptoms applies, and choice of a remedy can be difficult.

Chronic illnesses are those that tend to recur over a period of time in a person's life. Asthma, eczema, colitis, high blood pressure, infertility, menstrual cramps, and migraine headaches are chronic illnesses commonly treated by homeopathic remedies. These are the most frustrating and difficult cases for the homeopath, but many people have been able to discontinue their allopathic medications for these conditions after several months of homeopathic treatment. However, no one should attempt to treat chronic illness without being fully trained as a homeopath.

Most common women's health problems will fall into either the acute or chronic category of homeopathic treatment. Particular success can be found for the treatment of functional disorders, those for which there is no organic or anatomic abnormality found on examination.

Difficulties with menstruation, such as severe cramps, irregular periods, and too much bleeding, will often fall into the functional category. The allopathic physician usually examines a woman with these kinds of symptoms and says, "Well, the exam is normal, so it must be hormonal. We'll put you on birth control pills to regulate your cycles." This type of treatment does nothing to correct the underlying disorder creating the problems. It merely places the woman on an artificial cycle, suppressing her ovulation as well as her symptoms, and subjecting her to the side effects of oral contraceptives. With homeopathy, we are able to effect a natural and long-lasting cure.

Menopausal symptoms such as hot flashes, depression, and loss of sexual desire can respond well to homeopathic treatment. As the evidence of negative side effects of estrogen and other hormonal treatments builds up, women may look to homeopathy as a safe alternative to help them through this difficult time of life.

LIMITATIONS OF HOMEOPATHY

Homeopathy cannot cure conditions that stem from structural, long-term, organic changes in the body tissue. It cannot regenerate a cirrhotic liver or cause the diabetic pancreas to start producing insulin. It cannot cure cancer of the breast, ovaries, or uterus. It can, however, palliate the symptoms of these illnesses and enable the patient to be more comfortable and productive.

Most of these organic tissue changes in the body are the result of years of stress, imbalance, and bodily abuse. A person who has been treated homeopathically for many years is generally healthier and less likely to develop a serious disease. Sometimes early stages of a disease can be reversed before more serious symptoms can occur. For example, this author has witnessed the reversal of abnormal Pap results using homeopathy.

Acute infections, such as cystitis, appendicitis, or PID (pelvic inflammatory disease), are situations where there are organic changes in the body that have occurred suddenly. Often we are able to treat these homeopathically by strenthening the body's own defense mechanisms with an appropriate remedy. However, if the person is not treated early enough in the illness or the wrong remedy is used, the illness can progress. Most homeopaths would turn to antibiotics, surgery, or other allopathic treatments in this situation. After the acute episode passes, a homeopathic remedy can be given as an overall constitutional treatment to make the person less susceptible to future recurrences.

A CASE STUDY

A case study can be interesting and illustrative of many of the principles of homeopathy.

Sally B, a 29-year-old unmarried customer-service representative, was seen for the problems of menstrual cramps, sinus congestion, and migraine headache. She has suffered cramps since she was in her early teens, which had been alleviated for a five-year period during which time she took oral contraceptives. With each period, she experiences two days of severe, sharp, throbbing pain, worse in the area of the right ovary and accompanied by nausea, headache, and dizziness. She also notices constipation during the week preceding her period. Her mood gets "vicious" at this time, being short-tempered and often yelling at her coworkers.

Sally also has severe migraine headaches two or three times a year, as well as continual sinus congestion that causes a headache about once every two weeks. Both types of headache are throbbing and are centered over the right eye and forehead. She has a lot of abdominal gas and occasional soreness of the left knee.

When looking at her general symptoms, we find that Sally has a strong craving for sweets, especially before her period. She tends to have cold feet and hands, an average amount of thirst, and finds a problem with low energy, especially in the late afternoon from 4 to 7 P.M. She gets irritable and annoyed when subjected to loud noise.

She describes her personality as shy and reserved, as well as emotionally very sensitive. She states she has a short fuse and can get sarcastic and nasty when angered; she becomes impatient with others. She is extremely neat and well organized and worries a lot about money, her job, and the state of the world.

Based on these factors, Sally was given one dose of the remedy Lycopodium, a type of club moss. Lycopodium fits people who have symptoms more on the right side of the body, as we see with Sally's headaches, as well as her menstrual cramps. The Lycopodium person usually craves sweets and is worse from 4 to 7 P.M. This personality tends to be reserved, sensitive, and well-organized, with definite tendencies toward anger and irritability. As we can see, this remedy fits Sally's picture very well.

One month follow-up with Sally showed several changes. Her menstrual cramps were very severe this month, but they only lasted half a day rather than her usual two days. She reported that her sinuses became fluent and ran continually for the week following the remedy (a healing crisis), but now she has no trouble with them at all. Her constipation and gas are better, and she reports the total absence of any type of headaches.

She has noticed small boils erupting on the right side of her face, which she used to get several years ago. (Symptoms coming to the surface.) Her desire for sweets is drastically less, her energy in general is higher, and her "short fuse" is slightly improved. Significantly, she has decided to leave her job, which she doesn't like, even though it means some loss of security.

As one can see, Sally is vastly improved on many levels, as the remedy takes effect on her underlying constitution.

RESPONSIBILITIES OF THE HOMEOPATHIC PATIENT

As one can see, homeopathic treatment depends greatly on the information provided to the practitioner by the patient. It is therefore important for each person to observe carefully her symptoms and know her own body/person as well as possible. A healthy life style is also important to provide a good foundation for homeopathy. Certain substances, such as coffee and camphor, must be avoided as they tend to serve as an antidote to homeopathic remedies. We also ask that people stay off allopathic medicines, both prescription and over-the-counter types.

We prefer people undergoing homeopathy to postpone any other types of holistic treatments such as acupuncture, polarity, etc., because different modalities tend to interfere with each other. Finally, we ask the homeopathic patient to have perseverance and patience. Lasting cures do not occur overnight and sometimes uncomfortable symptoms must be tolerated as the healing process unfolds itself.

REFERENCES

Panos, M., and J. Heimlich, *Homeopathic Medicine at Home*. Los Angeles: J. P. Tardier, Inc., 1980.

Risse, G. et al., *Medicine without Doctors*. New York: Science History Publications, 1977.

SUGGESTED READINGS

Baker, Wyrth, W. Young, and A. Neiswander, *Introduction to Homeotherapeutics*. Washington, D.C.: American Institute of Homeopathy, 1974.

Blackie, Margery, *The Patient, Not the Cure*. London: MacDonald and Jones, 1976.

Clarke, John, *The Prescriber*, 9th ed. Devon, England: Health Science Press, 1972.

Coulter, Harris L., *Homeopathic Medicine*. St. Louis: Formur, 1973.

Gibson, D. M., *First-Aid Homeopathy in Accidents and Ailments*. London: British Homeopathic Association, 1977.

Grossinger, Richard, *Planet Medicine, From Stone Age Shamanism to Post-Industrial Healing*. New York: Anchor/Doubleday, 1980.

Roberts, H. A., *The Principles and Art of Cure by Homeopathy*. Devon, England: Health Science Press, 1976.

Sharma, C. H., *A Manual of Homeopathy and Natural Medicine*. New York: E. P. Dutton & Co., Inc., 1976.

Shepherd, Dorothy, *Homeopathy for the First Aider*. Devon, England: Health Science Press, 1945.

Vithoulkas, G. *Homeopathy, Medicine of the New Man*. New York: Avon Books, 1972.

———, *The Science of Homeopathy: a Modern Textbook*. New York: Grove Press, Inc., 1979.

LISTING OF ORGANIZATIONS FOR HOMEOPATHY

American Association of Homeopathic
  Pharmacists
6231 Leesburg Pike, Suite 506
Falls Church, VA 22044

American Board of Homeotherapeutics
6231 Leesburg Pike, Suite 506
Falls Church, VA 22044

American Foundation for Homeopathy
6231 Leesburg Pike, Suite 506
Falls Church, VA 22044

American Institute of Homeopathy
7297-H Lee Highway
Falls Church, VA 22042

Homeopathic Educational Services
5916 Chabot Crest
Oakland, CA 94618

Homeopathic Laymen's League of
  New York
c/o Mrs. L. C. Becker
90 La Salle Street, Apt. 18-D
New York, NY 10027

Homeopathic Laymen's League of the
  Northeast
c/o Lorina Cooper
Hawley Road
North Salem, NY 10560

Homeopathic Laymen's League,
  Pittsburgh, Pa.
c/o Steffne Witney
120 Genessee Road
Pittsburgh, PA 15241

Homeopathic Study Group of
  Westchester and Fairfield Counties
c/o Phyllis Freeman
27 Spicer Road
Westport, CT 06880

International Foundation for the
  Promotion of Homeopathy
76 Lee Street
Mill Valley, CA 94941

International Homeopathic League
and the San Francisco Homeopathic
Medical Society
c/o Frederic W. Schmid, MD, D-HT
6200 Geary Boulevard
Medical Building at 26th Avenue
San Francisco, CA 94121

National Center for Homeopathy
7297-H Lee Highway
Falls Church, VA 22042

Standard Homeopathic Company
436 West 8th Street
Los Angeles, CA 90014

Women's National Homeopathic
League, Inc.
1911 Walnut Street
Dover, OH 44622

Chapter Twelve

NUTRITION AS PREVENTION AND THERAPY FOR WOMEN'S DISEASES

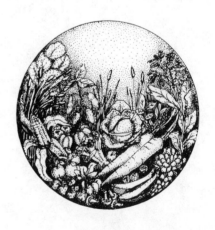

Suza Francina

DIETARY FACTORS IN THE PREVENTION OF DISEASE

Importance of Natural Foods

Observations for centuries have shown that people who live in harmony with natural environmental cycles and eat traditional native foods are not subject to the various diseases of modern civilization. When people adopt modern, fragmented eating habits, they become involved with the symptoms of degenerative disease within a relatively short period (Price 1972).

Perhaps the most outstanding documentation of the effects of denatured, processed foods on health are the studies of Dr. Weston Price, the "Charles Darwin of Nutrition." In the 1920s and 30s, when it was still possible to find areas where modern industrial civilization and its highly refined diet were just beginning to make inroads into traditional food habits, Dr. Price and his wife, Monica Price, R.N., turned from test tubes and microscopes to the unstudied evidence among human beings. They began by comparing various population groups in their native setting, where their natural diet continued unaltered, with the same tribes or ethnic groups where the refined foods brought in by modern civilization had become a major part of their diet. Whole tribes and villages, at varying latitudes, altitudes, and temperatures, provided case studies.

Dr. Price's book *Nutrition and Physical Degeneration* (1972) illustrates that wherever in the world he traveled, those people who remained on their native diet displayed superb health and freedom from "the diseases of civilization." Menstruation and childbirth were also brief and uncomplicated.

Although native foods varied widely as to source and kind, laboratory analysis revealed that they were exceedingly high in proteins, minerals, and other nutrients, all qualities that protect the functions of the organs respon-

209

sible for health—liver, kidneys, heart, brain, etc. On the contrary, analysis of the typical American diet reveals that it not only fails to meet the basic nutritional needs of our vital organs but actually increases the tendency toward menstrual disturbances, cystic mastitis, uterine fibroid tumors, and the current epidemic of breast and uterine cancer.

Distinction between Preventative Diet and Therapeutic Diet

The most important principle of preventative nutrition is that whole foods, nearest to their natural state, are best able to supply the essential nutrients to create a high level of well-being. However, although many different diets can meet the needs of the body so long as the vital organs are in good health, once the functions of the vital organs, especially the liver, become impaired, then another aspect of nutrition—the therapeutic diet—must be considered. A distinction, therefore, must be made between general, preventative nutrition and therapeutic nutrition. *A preventative diet is abundant in all nutrients necessary for the maintenance of high level health and prevention of disease. A therapeutic diet is aimed at correcting past excesses and deficiencies in order to restore balance and health.* This correction may range from simple nutritional changes to high-dose megavitamin (orthommolecular) therapy for inherited or acquired deficiencies.

Common Denominators Found in Natural Diets

The following common denominators are found in natural diets worldwide; these factors ensure health and prevent disease (Price, 1972; Applegate and Connelly 1974):

1. *The food must be grown on highly mineralized soil, with considerable humus content, and without chemical fertilizers or pesticides.* Healthy populations maintain a balance between soil productivity and plant and animal growth.
2. *Whole foods are eaten, not fractionalized or synthesized parts of foods.* The valuable fibers, vitamins, and mineral content are not refined out of the food.
3. *Protein and cholesterol foods are eaten in their unaltered raw form or are cooked lightly.* Fresh or naturally preserved meat, fish, raw milk and milk products, and fertile eggs are used. High heat-altered fat and overcooked protein cause the accumulation of unmetabolized cholesterol in the body and contribute to degenerative disease. Fat-soluble vitamins come from butter, cream, seafoods, and animal organs.
4. *Some iodine-rich sea plants or seafoods are used regularly.*

5. *Sweets are from natural sources and are used in moderation.*

6. *The diet contains some nitrilosides (also known as Vitamin B_{17} or laetrile).* Sources include apricot, peach, and prune pits; apple seeds; bitter almonds; lima beans; and millet. Sprouted grains and seeds are also rich in nitrilosides.

7. *Methods of food preservation and storage that alter the nutrients very little are used: these include earth storage, drying, freezing, culturing, pickling, fermenting, and sprouting.*

8. *Regular periods of fasting, partial abstinence from food, or periods of undereating are observed.* Historically, this came about as a natural result of summer crops being in short supply before the new crops were harvested, or because certain rituals began or ended with days of fasting.

9. *Foods are eaten only when they are in season, according to the cycles of nature.*

10. *Special protective foods are eaten during pregnancy and lactation.*

In general, throughout the following pages, it should be kept in mind that natural sources of vitamins and minerals in food are always preferable to vitamin supplements. However, if whole nutritious food, free of chemicals, cannot be obtained, then supplements may need to be taken. Remember that natural vitamin supplements are superior to artificial synthetic versions, which may be poorly absorbed and metabolized.

MENSTRUAL PROBLEMS AND NUTRITIONAL REMEDIES

One factor in the various contributing causes of menstrual disturbances is excessive estrogen activity, a byproduct of disturbed liver function, which is in turn due to poor eating habits (Fredericks 1977).

The duration and amount of menstrual flow are greatly influenced by diet and life style (Bieler 1974). For example, among primitive women in the Australian bush country who live mainly on fruit and its seeds, the menstrual cycle lasts only about 20 minutes. American pioneering physicians reported that American Indians of the Great Plains had short, uncomplicated menstrual periods, scarcely noticeable. Childbirth and menopause were equally uncomplicated. The same has been reported by anthropologists of other pretechnological peoples.

Misled by the idea that the average represents what is "normal," many women have been persuaded to accept pathological states of menstrual problems simply because they are so prevalent. However, excessive and heavy menstrual flow, cramping, lower back pain, and pelvic congestion may be indications that the liver is failing as a "filter."

Dr. Bieler discusses the problems of menstruation in his book *Food Is Your Best Medicine* (1966):

> When toxic blood seeks an outlet through the womb via the menstrual function, the resulting inflammation and irritation to the delicate mucous membranes throw the organ into spasms which are registered as pain or cramps [or simply congestion if the toxin is more dilute]. . . . Once the flow has started, Nature pours out as much toxic material from the blood as possible. . . . What should be a normal flow develops into a hemorrhage, sometimes lasting for days and reducing the woman to a state of anemia. Nervousness, insomnia, headache, and distressing fatigue may follow. The kidneys may not be able to sufficiently filter certain diffusible poisons so that a mild-to-severe edema occurs, evidenced by an increase in body weight. [P. 172]

The woman who suffers menstrual problems during her menstrual years may also have health problems during menopause, when she can no longer discharge toxins through the menstrual blood. Normal menstruation and menopause in a healthy woman should be virtually symptomless.

General Dietary Rules for Improved Health during the Menstrual Years

Cooked animal proteins should be reduced or eliminated. These include pasteurized and sterilized milk, fried eggs, overcooked meats, etc. The diet should contain adequate amounts of easy-to-digest protein such as sprouts, raw seeds and nuts, whole grains, legumes, cultured raw milk products, fish, poultry, eggs, and green vegetables.

Prior to and during menstruation, a cleansing diet may aid liver function. This can consist of fruits and vegetables and their juices. Nonstarchy green vegetables such as zucchini, celery, parsley, and green beans can be made into soups. These chlorophyl-rich foods are excellent body cleansers/body builders.

A cleansing diet will also prevent constipation, which can increase menstrual cramps. Prunes, prune juice, figs, and herbal laxatives can be used.

Menstrual Problems That Can Be Helped by Diet

Anemia.   Iron-rich foods should be emphasized during menstruation. These include bananas, spinach, prunes, raisins, liver and organ meats, egg yolks, whole grains, green vegetables, grapes, beets, molasses, apricots, kidney beans, and soybeans. Beets are also an excellent liver cleanser, red corpuscle-builder, fibrin dissolver, menstrual regulator, and diuretic. Artificial iron supplements such as ferrous sulfate increase the need for oxygen, pantothenic acid, and other nutrients, as well as inhibiting absorption of vitamins, E, A, and C (Zucker 1958; Davis 1972*b*).

Irregular and abnormal flow.   Irregular and abnormal menstrual flow can be caused by factors other than nutrition, such as increased sexual activity, strenuous exercise, I.U.D., the Pill, and environmental or biorhythm changes. Irregular or profuse bleeding, if caused by thyroid deficiency, can be corrected by a natural source of iodine such as kelp (Davis 1972*a*). Bioflavanoids may also help correct menstrual irregularity, as do vitamins B_{12} and E (Airola 1979). A menstrual flow that continues to be heavy after three or four days has often been corrected by taking 600 units of vitamin E daily (Davis 1972*a*).

Because prolonged, excessive menstruation can be a symptom of uterine cancer, a physician should be consulted if excessive menstruation does not respond to dietary and vitamin/mineral therapy. Vitamin C or citrus should always be taken in the presence of excessive bleeding.

Acne.   Acne is caused by fluctuations in androgen levels at the time of menstruation and can be aggravated by improper diet (refined, greasy, sweet foods). As mentioned earlier, the menstrual period is a time of elimination of toxins, and acne is a sign of elimination of these toxins through the skin. Cleansing diets should be used to speed elimination through normal channels. Recently, vitamin A and zinc have been used therapeutically for acne (Airola 1979; et al.)

Edema.   Salt and foods high in sodium should be restricted to alleviate water retention. Naturally diuretic foods such as cranberry juice, watermelon, cucumber, asparagus, parsley, and strawberries are useful as monodiets (eaten alone). Vitamin B_6 (pyridoxine) alleviates menstrual symptoms in daily dose ranges of 200 mg. daily (Airola 1979; Seaman and Seaman 1979).

Menstrual cramps.   Calcium levels in the blood drop about ten days before menstruation and remain low until menstruation begins (Seaman and Seaman 1979). Low calcium levels are associated with cramping of the uterus and other muscles.

Calcium, phosphorus, magnesium, and other minerals should be present in the diet in proper ratio to one another. For this reason, dietary sources are preferable. Carrot and green vegetable juices are an excellent source of calcium. If calcium intake is more than twice that of magnesium, a magnesium deficiency can occur (ibid). Calcium absorption is also dependent on the simultaneous presence of fat and vitamin D in the intestine. Because sufficient hydrochloric (stomach) acid is necessary for absorption, calcium should be taken on an empty stomach prior to meals.

Refined foods, especially sugar and chocolate, add to mineral deficiencies by leaching calcium out of the system (Stone and Walczak 1974).

Abnormal mineral levels are often found during menstruation. Copper is often high, zinc low. Estrogen medication raises the copper level and lowers the zinc level in the blood. Zinc deficiency can lead to depression and even psychosis, and elevated copper levels contribute to the "blues." Zinc supplements (10–30 mg. daily) may be indicated (Airola 1979; Cheraskin and Ringsdorf 1974).

Note that with most nutritional remedies for menstruation, a trial period of from one to three months may be required to fully assess the effects.

MENOPAUSAL PROBLEMS AND NUTRITIONAL REMEDIES

Vitamin Supplements for Common Symptoms of Menopause

Vitamin E shows promise for relieving common symptoms of menopause (fatigue, leg cramps, hot flashes, vaginal dryness, etc.). Vitamin E is not as dramatic in curing hot flashes as estrogen replacement therapy (ERT), but consistent use of this vitamin is reported to bring marked relief in about one-half to two-thirds of cases (Seaman and Seaman 1979).

Vitamin E as an anticoagulant and antioxidant has many medical uses (Davis 1972a). It has been shown to improve prognosis in heart disease and to lower insulin requirements in diabetes (Shute 1979). However, its use in these conditions should be monitored by a practitioner. It is used therapeutically in the treatment of burns, arthritis, and bursitus (Davis 1972a). Hypertensives should take vitamin E under medical supervision as the vitamin may cause a slight rise in blood pressure in doses over 100 I.U. daily.

Those who are healthy and who are not using any medication with which the vitamin might interact, such as insulin, anticoagulants, digitalis, or other cardiovascular medications may take 400 to 1200 units of vitamin E daily in the form of mixed tocopherols. Start with 100 units daily, and gradually increase until you find the supplementary intake that helps you to feel most fit.

Bone Brittling and Calcium Metabolism

After the hormonal shifts of menopause, women seem to be more susceptible to the action of the parathyroid hormone, which promotes the removal of calcium from the bones. The result is a gradual demineralizing of the bones with increasing age and consequent susceptibility to fractures and collapse of the vertebrae. It has been estimated that such softening of the bones, called *osteoporosis*, is a major orthopedic disorder in about one out of four women who have passed menopause.

Until recently it was assumed that osteoporosis was a natural part of the aging process, a process that could not be prevented, much less reversed. Evidence is accumulating, however, that osteoporosis is more frequent in those with low calcium intake. When a group of women between ages 79–89 were surveyed, it was found that they were getting only about 450 mg. of usable calcium daily from their regular diet—about half the recommended daily allowance of 800 mg. When they took a calcium supplement of 750 mg. each day along with 375 units of vitamin D, the bone density increased over a three-year period. In similar women who were not treated, bone density continued to decrease over that same time period (Ballentine 1978).

Unfortunately, very high intakes of calcium supplements may reduce the absorption of other important minerals such as manganese, zinc, and iron. For this reason, calcium-rich foods are always preferable to mineral supplements. There is also some evidence that osteoporosis is less common and less severe in those who don't eat meat.

One cup of milk (8 oz.) contains about 300 mg. of calcium. Green leafy vegetables are rich in calcium. A cup of mustard greens or collards contains about the same amount as a cup of milk. Broccoli contains about 200 mg. per cup. Probably the richest nondairy source is "lambs quarters" (*Chenopodium album*), usually regarded as a weed in Europe and America. One cup of its cooked green leaves supplies 400 mg. of calcium.

For additional information regarding nutritional therapy during menopause, please refer to books by Barbara and Gideon Seaman and Paavo Airol (see Suggested Readings).

PREGNANCY, CHILDBIRTH, AND LACTATION

Importance of Diet

One of the outstanding changes Dr. Price and other researchers reported after a changeover to the modern refined diet was a decrease in the ease and efficiency of the birth process. For example, a physician reported that during the 36 years he had lived among the Eskimos, he had never been able to arrive on time for a normal birth because labor was so short. However, the first generation of Eskimo women on refined diets had extended labors (Price 1972).

A pregnant woman should eat whatever wholesome natural foods appeal to her, avoiding caffein, alcohol, cigarettes, and drugs (including diuretics) (Brewer and Brewer 1977). If unable to quit smoking, she should be careful not to use cigarettes as a substitute for food, and should take vitamin C and E supplements and aerobic exercise.

The quality of the protein eaten in pregnancy is as important as the quantity. Fertile eggs are superior nutritionally to supermarket eggs from chickens fed with antibiotics, amphetamines, and arsenics. Raw certified milk and milk products contain more vitamins than pasteurized/sterilized milk (Brewer and Brewer 1977; et al.) Avoid yogurt with added sweetners and artificial flavoring and dyes. Good protein sources are nuts, brewers yeast, beans, whole grains, fish, and meat from animals fed without chemical additives (estrogens, testosterones, antibiotics, and arsenics). Organically grown fruits, vegetables, and grains should be used if possible (Ballentine 1978).

Brewers yeast is an excellent source of protein, and is especially recommended for vegetarian mothers. It is among the best food sources of the entire B complex and contains numerous trace minerals needed during pregnancy and nursing—selenium, zinc, iron, and chromium. Brewers yeast is one of the best foods known to stimulate breast milk production.

Yeast also contains the Glucose Tolerance Factor, which is essential for proper sugar metabolism. This will help avoid undue fatigue due to low blood sugar (hypoglycemia). Yeast is a protein food and needs hydrochloric acid to be effectively digested. For this reason it should be taken between meals or at the beginning of a meal when the stomach is empty.

Synthetic vitamins (with the exception of vitamin C) should be avoided during pregnancy and lactation. Natural vitamin supplements, although more expensive, are metabolized more easily. Supplements should be taken just before meals to increase assimilation.

Calcium and vitamin D pills should not be taken to excess as this can result in calcification in the placenta. Another effect could be closure of the fontanelle (normal opening in the top of the infant's skull), which could result in prolonged labor because the infant's head is less able to be moulded and shaped to the birth canal (Price 1972).

Iron supplements, because they inhibit absorption of vitamins E, A, and C, could in some cases contribute to miscarriages or birth defects (Davis 1972b). Adequate iron, plus other nutrients involved in preventing anemia (folic acid, vitamin B_6, vitamins E and C) should be obtained from natural food sources: dark green leafy vegetables, carrots, beets, squash, bananas, apples, grapes, apricots, yeast, egg yolks, and liver.

Pregnancy Health Problems That Can Be Improved by Diet

Nausea. Nausea can occur because of increased hydrochloric (stomach) acid during the first trimester of pregnancy. Some women find if they keep food in their stomachs at all times, they do not become nauseous. Peppermint tea and crackers (which soak up hydrochloric acid) should be helpful.

A cleansing diet emphasizing vegetable soups, broths, and juices (without added meat or fat), fruits, and temporarily eliminating cooked animal proteins, fats, and oils, is recommended. Vitamin B_6 (pyrodoxine) is therapeutic for first-time trimester nausea (Davis 1972*b*).

Edema. Some obstetricians now believe that water retention (edema) is normal during pregnancy and that pregnant women should feel free to salt their food according to taste (Fredericks 1977). This rule may be all right for those women whose taste buds are not addicted to excess salt, but those accustomed to adding salt to everything should be aware that too much salt is a contributing factor in excessive swelling (Bieler 1974). Do not use diuretics to reduce swelling, as this is done at the expense of the sodium/potassium balance. Syptoms of edema are often relieved by reducing salt and adding vitamin B_6 supplements and vitamin B complex (ibid.).

NUTRITIONAL PROBLEMS OF THE ORAL CONTRACEPTIVE

The medical literature contains many reports of metabolic imbalances and nutritional deficiencies caused by the use of the oral contraceptive. Specific vitamin deficiencies in controlled studies of Pill use have been reported by Barbara and Gideon Seaman (1979), along with nutritional corrections.

Nausea, mental and emotional changes, edema, and menstrual disturbances may be due to vitamin B_6 deficiency induced by the Pill (ibid.). Vitamin B_6 will often help correct this problem. Vitamin B_{12} can also relieve Pill-induced anemia.

Vitamin Deficiencies—Symptoms and Remedies

Biotin. Biotin deficiency caused by the Pill contributes to eczema, depression, fatigue, dry hair, and hair loss (Airola 1979). Brewers yeast (2 tbsp. daily) or biotin in tablets (150–300 mg. daily) may be helpful.

Folic Acid. Folic acid is another B vitamin depleted by Pill use (Seaman and Seaman 1979). It is needed to bring about return to fertility in women who fail to ovulate and to ensure normal pregnancies in those who conceive shortly after stopping the Pill. Researchers have demonstrated that several weeks of folic acid therapy can frequently restore Pap smears to normal (ibid.). The abnormal cells found in the Pap smears of many Pill users resemble those observed in patients with folate deficiency anemia. Dosages used (10 mg.) must be obtained by prescription since folic acid supplements in these amounts are not available over the counter. When any B vitamin supplement is taken, it should be taken in the presence of the entire B complex since B vitamins work synergistically, and an excess of one may cause deficiencies of the others.

Vitamin C.   Lowering of ascorbic acid (vitamin C) levels in the blood caused by oral contraceptive use decreases resistance to infections. Bleeding gums, easy bruising, or spider veins can be indications that more vitamin C is needed (ibid.). Since vitamin C only remains in the bloodstream for one hour, it should be taken several times during the day.

Zinc.   Zinc is essential for oral contraceptive users (ibid.). Sources include leafy green vegetables, egg yolks, whole grains, mushrooms, and seafoods. The general dosage is 15–30 mg. daily for Pill users (ibid.). Levels of zinc and other minerals in food depend on adequate zinc in soil, and many soils are deficient (Ballentine 1978).

Selenium and Iodine.   The two trace minerals selenuim and iodine help minimize the carcinogenic effects of the Pill (Airola 1979; Fredericks 1977). The usual dose is 50 mg. of selenium and three or more tablets of kelp daily.

Vitamin E.   Vitamin E helps to dissolve or prevent the formation of fibrin, a material that makes the formation of blood clots possible. An excess of estrogen may contribute to the development of blood clots, and vitamin E can help normalize estrogen levels. Suggested dosage is 200 I.U. daily (Seaman and Seaman 1979).

BREAST DISEASES AND NUTRITION

Various dietary factors are suspected of contributing to benign breast disease—cystic mastitis or fibrocystic disease. Since research links high estrogen levels with increased incidence of gynecological cancers (Fredericks 1977), the relationship between diet and estrogen activity is relevant.

The liver converts estrogen hormones into less active compounds, resulting in the formation of estriol (a less carcinogenic type of estrogen). The estrogen/estriol ratio (as measured in the urine) can make the difference between health and disease. The ability of the liver to effect favorable estrogen conversion is related to diet. Thus any factor that reduces the health and efficiency of the liver (poor nutrition, excessive fat intake, drugs, etc.) can be considered a contributing cause to such diseases (ibid.).

Nutritional Therapy for Fibrocystic Breast Disease

Nonmalignant breast lumps (fibrocystic breast disease) afflect about 50 percent of American women at some time in their lives (McCauley 1979). The lumps can be painful, and they increase the risk of breast cancer eightfold It has been shown that caffein increases the occurrence of breast cysts (Gonzales 1980).

Important in the treatment of breast cysts are elimination of caffein from the diet and the addition of iodine (3 mg. three times daily), magnesium (135 mg. two times daily), and vitamin B_6 (100 mg. three times daily). Vitamin E has been found to be effective in relieving breast cysts and reducing elevated estrogen levels. Dr. Robert London, Director of Reproductive Endocrinology at Mt. Sinai Hospital in Baltimore, studied 26 women with painful breast cysts. Each took vitamin E (600 I.U. daily). Ten women had complete disappearance of the lumps and 12 received moderate relief. Only four were not helped.

FEMALE CANCER, ESTROGEN PRODUCTION, AND DIET

Hormone-Vitamin Interdependence

There is an interaction between vitamins and hormones, and the deficiency of one may lead to the imbalance of another. For example: pituitary dysfunction may lead to nutritional deficiencies, which in turn may impair pituitary function (Airola 1979). Similarly, an underactive thyroid gland can lead to insufficient sex hormone output. Or a malfunctioning parathyroid gland may lead to the derangement of calcium and vitamin D metabolism (Davis 1972*b*). The effectiveness of estrogenic hormones is increased by the simultaneous administration of vitamins B_6, E, and C, PABA and folic acid (ibid.). Taking these vitamins (and acid supplements) at the time of menopause, when the body's estrogen output is decreased, may enhance the effectiveness of the endogenous estrogen without the need to resort to exogenous estrogen replacement therapy (ERT).

The B Vitamins and Estrogen

B vitamin deficiency can raise estrogen levels by interfering with the liver's ability to inactivate excess estrogen. Conversely, high levels of estrogen can cause vitamin B deficiency, often evident in women who take estrogen medications (Bieler 1974).

Experiments with female rats indicate that estrogen production is affected by the presence or absence of B vitamins in the diet (ibid.) Sources of B vitamins include whole grains, wheat germ, seeds, nuts, beans, many vegetables, and yeast. The degradation of estrogen by the liver is inefficient with a diet low in the B's and highly efficient in the presence of an adequate supply of these nutrients. The following statement summarizes the importance of Vitamin B for prevention of female disorders:

> A rise in Vitamin B complex intake . . . will tend to increse the efficiency of hepatic (liver) degradation of estrogen, with frequent and significant improvement in pre-menstrual tension, dysmenorrhea, cystic mastitis, and other disorders which may be related to hyperestrogenism (excessive levels of estrogenic hormone). . . . This nutritional approach may not only lower estrogen activity to a more physiological level, but may tend to raise the output of estriol. Since estriol ratio has been linked with resistance to breast cancer, it may be that early dividends from improvement of a woman's diet may be less significant than the possible long-term reward of increased resistance to estrogen-dependent neoplasms (cancers). . . .
> . . . Any augmentation of estrogen levels—whether endogenous or exogenous origin (given by nature or by prescription)—invites—perhaps demands—the precautionary measure of correction of the patient's dietary habits. [Fredericks 1972, pp. 17–19]

According to Fredericks, epidemiological evidence clearly demonstrates that the estriol/estrogen ratio is a critical factor in determining susceptibility to breast and uterine cancer. Excessive estrogen also contributes to heart and blood vessel disorders (myocardial infarction, strokes, thrombophlebitis, hardening of the arteries). In addition, excessive estrogen impairs carbohydrate tolerance, which can trigger latent diabetes or hypoglycemia, and it can induce water retention (edema) (ibid.).

The relationship between diet and estrogen is even demonstrated in males. In male alcoholics, an early symptom of liver disease is enlargement of the breasts—showing the feminizing effects of elevated estrogen levels (ibid.). Women whose premenstrual rise in estrogen activity increases breast sensitivity or induces temporary breast cysts should explore the diet/liver/estrogen activity relationship.

Dietary Fat

Researchers who correlate high fat intake with breast cancer note that fats overstimulate estrogen production, which in turn is correlated with breast and uterine cancer. Epidemiologists have noted a five to ten times increase in cancer rate in countries with high fat diets (Lauerson 1977).

The geographical distribution of cancer in relation to dietary variables has demonstrated strong associations between the incidence of cancers of the breast and endometrium and the consumption of fat. Furthermore, studies of individuals have shown that the incidence of these cancers is related to estrogen production. The implication is that diet may influence endogenous prolactin and estrogen production: postmenopausal vegetarian women have lower plasma prolactin levels than nonvegetarian women and lower excretion of estrogens in their urine. Estrogen production has thus been associated with total body weight and with dietary fat intake. Therefore it may be possible to relate geographic variation in the incidence of breast and endometrial cancer to diet (Armstrong 1978).

The diet of two groups of women have proved of special interest to researchers of breast cancer rates: These are Northern European women, who have the world's highest breast cancer rate, and Japanese women, whose breast cancer incidence is about one-sixth that of U.S. whites (McCauley 1979). Researchers have found that when Japanese women move to the United States and adopt an American diet, their daughters' and grand-daughters' incidence of the disease rises to meet U.S. rates. It should be noted that the traditional Japanese diet has always been one of fish and vegetables, seafood and kelp, so it is rich in the trace mineral selenium—one component of an enzyme that oxidizes and detoxifies the byproducts of fats taken into the body. This enzyme is deficient in most U.S. diets.

Another example of the correlation of breast cancer with body weight, and fat intake, was demonstrated by Dr. F. de Waard, a Dutch epidemiologist. He reported that when the Nazis invaded the Netherlands, they requisitioned most of the cheese, milk, butter, eggs, and meat, so that the Dutch were forced to live on home-grown vegetables and to decrease their intake of staples like white flour, coffee, and sugar. As a result, from 1942 to 1946, Dutch cancer incidence dropped 35 to 60 percent, depending on the district of the country. After the war, as the food supply returned to normal, so did cancer rates.

When discussing the correlation of cancer incidence and dietary fat, the quality and type of fat consumed are relevant. It is not the *eating* of fat that is harmful, but the *heating* of fat. Few foods are harder on the liver than heated, hydrogenated, refined fats, whether from animal or vegetable sources. Most processed vegetable oils have had their nutrients heated and filtered out of them (vitamins A, E, F). Margarine, shortening, pasteurized (superheated) milk and milk products, heat-altered canned baby formulas, high-heat cooked meats, and eggs all offer an adulterated form of fat difficult for the body to digest and eliminate (ibid.). And any food that interferes with normal liver function contributes to disturbed levels of estrogen and to high blood cholesterol.

Unheated (nonrancid) fats and oils probably do not contribute to cancer risk. However, once liver function is seriously impaired, as is often the case with cancer, all fats should be temporarily eliminated.

In another study of breast cancer differences between Japanese and American women, one researcher found that the breast fluids of cancer-prone American women contained a greater amount of free radicals than did fluids from the fluids from the cancer-resistant breasts of Oriental women (Airola

1979). Free radicals are the chemical byproducts of deteriorated and rancid fats and oils. These may be contained in stale foods (butter, margarine, oil, seeds, nuts, crackers, breads, aged meats, wheat germ). Deep-fat fried foods that have been fried in oil that has been reheated many times are a dangerous source of free radicals. Most grains, nuts, and seeds contain healthful, high-quality natural oils, protected from oxidation by the skins or shells. However, as soon as the germ kernel is broken and oxygen comes in contact with the oil, deterioration begins and toxic products of oxidation begin to form: peroxides, aldehydes, malonaldehydes, and free radicals. If crushed seeds; broken, shelled nuts (nut butters and oils); or grains (whole-wheat flour, wheat germ) are more than ten days old without refrigeration, sufficient peroxidation may have already occurred to cause health damage (ibid.).

This is also true of meat. According to Shamberger (1971), as soon as animals are slaughtered and the fat in the meat (beef contains up to 40 percent fat) is exposed to air, peroxidation begins and carcinogenic malonaldehyde begins to form. Malonaldehyde from aged beef is believed to be one of the contributing causes of cancer of the colon (Airola 1979).

Dietary Iodine

Studies on the relationship between iodine deficiency and breast cancer show that breast cancer reaches its highest incidence in geographical areas where iodine content of the soil is low (Airola 1979). Foods grown in such soil are lacking in iodine.

A deficiency of iodine in the diet interferes with thyroid function and leads to a deficiency in the production of thyroxine, which in turn permits the build-up of excessive amounts of estrogen in the body.

Japan and Iceland both have a low incidence of goiter (disease of the thyroid gland) and an equally low incidence of breast cancer. This is attributed to the presence of iodine in their diet. Conversely, Mexico and Thailand have a high incidence of both goiter and breast cancer. In the United States, the highest death rate from breast cancer is also found in the "goiter belt" in the Great Lakes region where soils are lacking in iodine (Shamberger 1971; Stadel 1976). Poland, Switzerland, the Soviet Union, and Australia showed the same pattern: breast cancer rates are highest in areas where goiter is epidemic.

One researcher confirmed that both thyroxine and vitamin E play important roles in eliminating surplus estrogen, whether natural or synthetic, from a woman's body (Shute 1977). Dietary iodine (as in kelp) may be essential to keep the thyroid glands secreting sufficient thyroxine.

Dietary sources of iodine are seafood and seaweed vegetables (kelp and dulse).

Dietary Selenium

The cancer rate is higher in areas of the United States, Canada, and other nations where the soil is deficient in selenium. Dietary selenium is known to protect against development of breast cancer in animals (Schrauzer, Rhead, and Evans 1973). It is not surprising therefore that the blood of cancer patients also has abnormally low selenium levels. And as noted earlier, selenium is important in the diet for detoxifying fats (Shamberger and Frost 1969). The average American dietary intake of selenium is only 50–150 mg., whereas in Japan, the daily intake averages 200–500 mg. Thus if follows that the cancer rate is lower in Japan.

Many researchers believe that a selenium deficiency can also be a factor in causing hypertension, strokes, and heart attacks (Passwater 1980). Studies show that where selenium in soils and foods is low, the rate for these diseases is higher (USDA Technical Bulletin 1967).

Dietary sources of selenium are kelp and other sea vegetables, mushrooms, whole grains, dairy products, fish and eggs, brewers yeast, and, most notably, garlic. Supplementary selenium should be taken with caution in very small amounts (50–150 mg. daily).

Obesity and Cancer

Recent research verifies the ancient observation that obese women have more breast cancer than those of normal weight (Fredericks 1977; Lauersen 1977). Obesity is also associated with irregular and excessive menstruation. It is also linked with excessive estrogen activity because the adipose tissue manufactures estrogen, elevating the levels of estrogen in the body. A woman who is 20–50 pounds overweight increases her chances of developing a uterine tumor by 300 percent; a woman who is more than 50 pounds overweight increases her chances by 900 percent (Lauersen 1977).

Macrobiotic Diet

Macrobiotic diets are the very basis of Chinese medicine. In macrobiotic eating, the individual, who is seen as the microcosm, assimilates the elements of his/her environment, which is the macrocosm, in every meal eaten. Only foods that grow locally and in season are eaten. Each meal consists of 50 percent whole grains, 30 percent vegetables, 10 percent seafood or animal protein, 5 percent seaweeds, and 5 percent soups containing digestive enzymes (miso/tamari soy sauce). The East-West Foundation in Boston is the major education center for macrobiotic diet in the West and has recorded numerous cases of regressed cancer using this rebalancing method.

THE RELATIONSHIP BETWEEN DIET AND CONSCIOUSNESS

Our belief system, life style, attitudes, emotions, and behavior all affect our nutritional status. Some studies have failed to find any correlation between what is eaten and actual nutrient levels in the bloodstream ("Life Style Correlates" 1980; Ballentine 1978). Rather, they suggest that psychological factors (emotions and attitudes toward food and eating) may be even more important than the type of food eaten.

Western science is recognizing that our emotional/mental makeup affects our digestion, absorption, elimination, and the characteristics of our particular type of metabolism. The unconscious and conscious mind is capable of changing nutrient requirements and even demonstrates the ability to transmute one element into another.

Modern as well as ancient philosophical systems believe that consciousness is able to alter matter, and there have long been reports of spiritual masters who were able to exist with extremely little food. There are also reports of persons able to ingest lethal substances without ill effects. Thus, placing the role of proper nutrition in its broadest perspective would include considering that *both* consciousness *and* food are powerful tools for altering the functioning of the human body.

REFERENCES

Airola, Paavo, *Every Woman's Book*. Phoenix, Ariz.: Health Plus, 1979.

Applegate, William, and Patricia Connelly, eds., *Price-Pottenger Lectures*. San Diego, Calif.: Nutrition Education Research Foundation, 1974.

Armstrong, B., *Proceedings of the Australian Symposium on Nutrition and Cancer*. South Australian Postgraduate Medical Association, Sydney 1978.,

Ballentine, Rudolph, *Diet and Nutrition: A Holistic Approach*. Honesdale, Pa.: Himalayan International Institute, 1978.

Bieler, Henry G., *Food Is Your Best Medicine*. New York: Random House, Inc., 1966.

———, *Natural Way to Sexual Health*. New York: Bantam Books, Inc., 1974.

Brewer, Gail Sforza, with Tom Brewer, *What Every Pregnant Woman Should Know—The Truth about Diet and Drugs in Pregnancy*. New York: Penguin Books, 1977.

Cheraskin, E., and W. Ringsdorf, *Psychodietetics*. New York: Stein & Day Publishers, 1974.

Davis, Adelle, *Let's Get Well*. New York: The New American Library, 1972a.

———, *Let's Have Healthy Children*. New York: The New American Library, 1972b.

Fredericks, C., "Nutritional Management of Estrogen-Dependent Disorders," *Journal of the International Academy of Metabology*, Vol. 4, no. 1 (1972), 17–19.

———, *Breast Cancer: A Nutritional Approach*. New York: Grosset & Dunlap, Inc., 1977.

Gonzales, Elizabeth Rasche, *JAMA*, 244, no. 10 (1980), 1077–79.

Hawaii Performance Medical Group, Inc., *Report*. Kaiser Medical Center, Honolulu, April 1976.

Lauersen, Niels, *Its Your Body: A Woman's Guide to Gynecology*. New York: Playboy Press, 1977.

"Life Style Correlates of Dietary and Biochemical Measures of Nutrition," *Journal of the American Dietetic Association*, March 1980.

McCauley, Carole Spearin, *Surviving Breast Cancer*. New York: E. P. Dutton & Co., Inc., 1979.

Michaelson, Gerd, Lennart Juhlin, and Anders Vahlquist, "Effects of Oral Zinc and Vitamin A in Acne," *Archives of Dermatology*, vol. 113 (1977).

Passwater, R. A., *Selenium as Food and Medicine*. New Canaan, Conn.: Keats Publishing, 1980.

Pottenger, Francis, *Effect of Heat-Processed Foods*. San Diego, Calif.: Price-Pottenger Nutrition Foundation, 1946.

Price, Weston A., *Nutrition and Physical Degeneration*. San Diego, Calif.: Price-Pottenger Nutrition Foundation, 1972.

Schrauzer, G., W. Rhead, and G. Evans. *Bioinorganic Chemistry*, vol. 2 (1973).

Seaman, Barbara, and Gideon Seaman, *Women and the Crisis in Sex Hormones*. New York: Bantam Books, Inc., 1979.

Shamberger, Raymond, an article in *Journal of the National Cancer Institute*, May 1971.

Shamberger, R., and D. Frost, an article in *Canadian Medical Association*, vol. 100 (1969).

Shute, Evan, *The Heart and Vitamin E*, revised Health Science Edition. Evan Shute Foundation for Medical Research. New Canaan, Conn.: Keats Publishing, 1979.

Stadel, B. V., "Dietary Iodine and Risk of Breast, Endometrial and Ovarian Cancer," *Lancet* April 24, 1976, pp. 890–91.

Stone, Harold, and Michael Walczak, eds., *Nutrition Applied Personally*. La Habra, Calif.: International College of Applied Nutrition, 1974.

USDA Technical Bulletin, No. 758, 1967.

Zucker, T.A., an article in *American Journal of Clinical Nutrition*, vol. 6 (1958).

SUGGESTED READINGS

Airola, Paavo, *Every Woman's Book*. Phoenix, Ariz.: Health Plus Publishers, 1979. An excellent self-help nutrition guide covering specific female health problems as well as children's health care.

———, *How to Get Well*. Contains therapeutic diets for 56 of the most common diseases, plus information on how to protect yourself against common poisons in food, water, air, and environment.

———, *Hypoglycemia: A Better Approach*.

Ballentine, Rudolph, *Diet and Nutrition, A Holistic Approach*. Honesdale, Pa.: Himalayan International Institute, 1978. A comprehensive overview of the nutrition field, bringing together the "insight of the East with the science of the West." Excellent section on food and consciousness.

Bieler, Henry, *Food Is Your Best Medicine*. New York: Vintage Books, 1965. A classic discussion on the use of proper food instead of drugs to cure and prevent disease. Menstruation, menopause, case histories of fibroid tumors of the womb eliminated through diet.

———, *Natural Way to Sexual Health*. New York, Bantam Books, Inc., 1974.

Brewer, Gail Sforza, with Tom Brewer. *What Every Pregnant Woman Should Know—The Truth about Diet and Drugs in Pregnancy*. New York: Penguin Books, 1977. In years of clinical experience, obstetrician Tom Brewer came to the conclusion that birth defects are closely associated with weight-control diets, salt-restriction, and drugs—especially diuretics. His advice to pregnant women is simple: Eat all the nourishing foods you want and avoid the use off drugs.

Davidson, Jaquie, *Cancer Winner—How I Purged Myself of Melanoma*. Pierce City, Mo.: Pacific Press, 1977. A very personal account of one woman's victory over malignant melanoma using the Gerson Cancer Therapy.

Fredericks, Carlton, *Breast Cancer: A Nutritional Approach*. New York: Grosset & Dunlap, Inc., 1977. Based on Fredericks's work with 400 women over 20 years, a complete dietary program for breast and uterine problems.

Gerson, Max, *A Cancer Therapy: Results of Fifty Cases*, 3rd ed. Del Mar, Calif.: Totality Books, 1975. Written by an outstanding authority on the treatment of cancer and related diseases. Highly recommended.

Goldbeck, Nikki, and David Goldbeck, *The Supermarket Handbook: Access to Whole Foods*. New York: Signet, 1976.

Hofmann, Lieselotte, ed., *The Great American Nutrition Hassle*. Palo Alto, Calif.: Mayfield, 1978.

Kaslow, Arthur, and Richard Miles. *Freedom from Chronic Disease*. Los Angeles, Calif.: J. P. Tarcher, 1979. Explains that some diseases, written off as incurable, are in many cases the results of the body's long-sustained "rejection response" to certain foods.

Kelley, William Donald, *One Answer to Cancer*. Los Angeles, Calif.: Cancer Book House, 1969.

Kervran, Louis, *Biological Transmutations*. Binghamton, N.Y.: Swan House Publishers, 1972.

Kushi, Nichio, *The Book of Macrobiotics*. Brookline, Mass.: East-West Foundation, 1978.

Lauersen, Niels, and Steven Whitney, *It's Your Body: A Woman's Guide to Gynecology*. New York: Playboy Press, 1977. A comprehensive guide to the female body including research on estrogen and role of diet in women's diseases.

Livingston, Virginia, *Cancer: A New Breakthrough*. San Diego, Calif.: Production House Publishers, 1972.

Mae, Eydie, *How I Conquered Cancer Naturally*. San Diego, Calif.: Production House Publishers, 1975.

McCauley, Carole Spearin, *Surviving Breast Cancer*. New York: E. P. Dutton & Co., 1979. An in-depth report on the latest theories of causation and alternative treatments.

Pottenger, Francis, *Effect of Heat-Processed Foods*. San Diego, Calif.: Price-Pottenger Nutrition Foundation, 1946. Data on raw vs. cooked foods. Fascinating photos of changes in the internal organs of cats caused by various diets.

Price, Weston, *Nutrition and Physical Degeneration*. San Diego, Calif.: Price-Pottenger Nutrition Foundation, 1938. An outstanding collection of nutritional data. Details common nutritional denominators of native diets worldwide. Emphasizes the importance of preconception diet.

Pritikin, Nathan, *The Pritikin Program for Diet and Exercise*. New York: Grosset & Dunlap, Inc., 1979.

Seaman, Barbara, and Gideon Seaman, *Women and the Crisis in Sex Hormones*. New York: Bantam Books, Inc., 1977. Highly recommended reading on all aspects of women's health, including nutrition and the Pill and nutritional remedies for health problems during menstruation and menopause..

Simonton, Carl O., Stephanie Mathews-Simonton, and James Creighton, *Getting Well Again: A Step-by-Step Self-Help Guide to Overcoming Cancer for Patients and Their Families*. Los Angeles, Calif.: J. P. Tarcher, 1978.

Timms, Moira, and Zachariah Zar, *Natural Sources: Vitamin B17/Laetrile*. Mallbrae, Calif.: Celestial Arts, 1978. A well-researched investigation into the causes and treatments of cancer. Clears up common misconceptions about vitamin B_{17} (Laetrile.)

U.S. Senate Select Committee on Nutrition and Human Needs, *Dietary Goals for the U.S.* Washington, D.C.: U.S. Govt. Printing Office, February 1977.

LISTING OF ORGANIZATIONS FOR NUTRITION

American Academy of Medical
   Preventics
11311 Camarillo Street
North Hollywood, CA 91602
(213) 878-1234

Cancer Control Society
2043 N.. Berendo Street
Los Angeles, CA 90027
(213) 663-7801

George Ohsawa Macrobiotic Foundation
1544 Oak Street
Oroville, CA 95965
(916) 533-7702

Hippocrates Health Insitute
25 Exeter Street
Boston, MA 02116
(617) 267-9525

International Academy of
   Biological Medicine, Inc.
P.O. Box 31313
Phoenix, AZ 85046

International Academy of
   Preventive Medicine
10409 Town & Country Way, Suite 200
Houston, TX 77024
(713) 468-7851

International Association of Cancer
   Victims and Friends
7740 West Manchester Avenue
Suite 110
Plaza del Rey, CA 90291
(213) 822-5032

The Kushi Institute
P.O. Box 1100
Brookline, MA 02147

Society for the Protection of the Unborn
   through Nutrition (SPUN)
Suite 603
17 N. Wabash
Chicago, IL 60602
(312) 332-2334
(914) 271-6474

Chapter Thirteen

VITAMIN C AND PREGNANCY

Linus Pauling

The use of very large amounts of vitamins in the control of disease has been called *megavitamin therapy*. Megavitamin therapy is one aspect of orthomolecular medicine. It is this author's opinion that in the course of time, it will be possible to control hundreds of diseases by megavitamin therapy. For example, Drs. A. Hoffer and H. Osmond have reported that many patients with schizophrenia are benefited by megavitamin therapy (Hoffer 1962; Hoffer and Osmond 1966). Their treatment includes the administration of the B vitamin (niacin) or nicotinamide (niacinamide) in amounts of 3 g. to 18 g. per day, together with 3 g. to 18 g. per day of ascorbic acid, and good amounts of other vitamins (Hawkins and Pauling 1973; Pauling 1974).

IMPORTANCE OF EXTRA VITAMIN C FOR GOOD HEALTH

It is usually thought that a drug that is claimed to be a cure for many diseases cannot have any particular value for just one of them. Yet there is evidence that a large intake of vitamin C helps to control a great many diseases: not only the common cold and the flu but also other viral and bacterial diseases, such as hepatitis, and some quite unrelated diseases, including schizophrenia, cardiovascular disease, and cancer. There is a reason for this difference between vitamin C and ordinary drugs. Most drugs are powerful substances that interact in a specific way with one kind of molecule or tissue or agent of disease in the body so as to help to control a particular disease. The substance may, however, interact in a harmful way with other parts of the body, thus producing the side effects that make some drugs dangerous. Vitamin C, on the other hand, is a normal constituent of the body, required for life. It is involved in essentially all of the biochemical reactions that take place in the body and in all of the body's protective mechanisms. With the ordinary intake of vitamin C, these reactions and mechanisms do not operate effeciently; the peson ingesting only the recommended daily amount of 60 mg. is in what might be called "ordinary poor health"—what the physicians and nutritionists call "ordinary good health." However, the optimum intake of vitamin C, together with other health measures, can provide *really* good health, with increased protection against all diseases.

We have been slow to recognize the value of vitamin C and other vitamins. In 1937, Szent-Györgyi wrote that "vitamins, if properly understood and applied, will help us to reduce human suffering to an extent which the most fantastic mind would fail to imagine." Only now, 40 years later, are we beginning to accept this idea.

A large rate of intake of ascorbic acid is required for optimum protection against infectious disease. The use of ascorbic acid to provide protection against the common cold, influenza, rheumatic fever, pneumonia, and other infectious diseases may well be the most important of all methods of orthomolecular medicine.

It has been known for over 30 years that pregnant women need more vitamin C than other women. Part of the reason for this extra need is that the developing fetus needs a good supply of this vitamin, and there is a mechanism in the placenta for pumping vitamin C from the blood of the mother into that of the fetus. In one early study (Javert and Stander 1943), the ascorbate concentration in the blood of the umbilical cord was found to be 14.3 mg. per liter, four times that of the blood of the mother. Depletion of the maternal blood for the benefit of the infant continues even after parturition, as ascorbate is secreted in the mother's milk. Cow's milk is much less rich in vitamin C than human milk; however, the calf does not need extra vitamin C because it manufacturers its own in the cells of its liver.

In normal pregnancy, women with the usual low intake of vitamin C have been reported to show a steady decrease in blood plasma concentration from 11 mg. per liter (average for 246 women), to 5 mg. per liter at four months, and then to 3.5 mg. per liter at full term (ibid.). These low values correspond to poor health, not only for the mother but also for the infant. A low value of the blood concentration of vitamin C has been shown to be correlated with incidence of hemorrhagic disease of the newborn. Javert and Stander concluded that for good health, an intake of 200 mg. per day is needed by the pregnant woman, and it is likely that for most pregnant women, the optimum intake is still greater, that is, 1 g. or more per day (ibid.). Other nutritional needs must, of course, also be satisfied. Brewer (1966) has emphasized that a good intake of protein and other nutrients is essential to prevent puerperal eclampsia and that the diuretics and diet restrictions that are used to control the increase in weight during pregnancy are harmful.

A good intake of vitamin C also has great value in controlling threatened, spontaneous, and habitual abortion. In their study of 79 women with threatened, previous spontaneous, or habitual abortion, Javert and Stander (1943) had 19 percent success with 33 patients who received vitamin C together with bioflavonoids and vitamin K—only three abortions—whereas all of the other 46 patients who did not receive the vitamin aborted. In his analysis of the management of habitual abortion, Greenblatt (1955) concluded that vitamin C with bioflavonoids and vitamin K is the best treatment, the next best being progesterone, vitamin E, and thyroid extract.

During the last seven years, various authorities in the field of nutrition who write newspaper columns have repeatedly stated that a high intake of vitamin C can cause abortions. The basis for this statement seems to be a brief paper by two physicians in the Soviet Union (Samborskaya and Ferdman 1966). They reported that 20 women in the age range 20 to 40 years whose menstruation was delayed by 10 to 15 days were given 6 g. of ascorbic acid by mouth on each of three successive days, and that 16 of them then menstruated. This author wrote to Samborskaya and Ferdman, asking if any test of pregnancy had been carried out. In reply, they only sent another copy of their paper.

Hoffer (1971) has stated that he has used megadoses of ascorbic acid, 3 g. to 30 g. per day, with over a thousand patients since 1953, and has not seen one case of kidney-stone formation, miscarriage, excessive dehydration, or any other serious toxicity.

It seems unlikely that ascorbic acid causes abortions to any great extent, although it may help to control difficulties with menstruation. Lahann (1970) has reviewed the literature, especially that in German and Austrian journals, and he has concluded that noticeable improvement in menstruation has been observed through the oral intake of 200 mg. to 1000 mg. of ascorbic acid per day. Moreover, the utilization of ascorbic acid increases sharply in the course of the menstrual cycle, especially at the time of ovulation, and measurement of this utilization can be used for determining the end of ovulation and accordingly for determining the time of optimum conception in relation to the problem of overcoming sterility (Paeschke and Vasterling 1968).

REFERENCES

Brewer, T. H., *Metabolic Toxemia of Late Pregnancy: A Disease of Malnutrition*. Springfield, Ill. Charles C. Thomas, Publisher, 1966.

Greenblatt, R. B., "Bioflavonoids and the Capillary: Management of Habitual Abortion," *Annals of the New York Academy of Sciences*, 61 (1955), 713–20.

Hoffer, A., "Ascorbic Acid and Toxicity," *New England Journal of Medicine*," 285 (1971), 635–36.

Hawkins, D., and L. Pauling, *Orthomolecular Psychiatry*. San Francisco: W. H. Freeman & Company, Publishers, 1973.

Hoffer, A., *Niacin Therapy in Psychiatry*. Springfield, Ill.: Charles C. Thomas, Publisher, 1962.

Hoffer, A. and H. Osmond. *How to Live With Schizophrenia*. New Hyde Park, N.Y.: University Books, 1966.

Javert, C. T. and H. J. Stander, "Plasma Vitamin C and Prothrombin Concentration in Pregnancy and in Threatened, Spontaneous, and Habitual Abortion," *Surgery, Gynecology, and Obstetrics*, 76: (1943), 115–22.

Lahann, H., *Vitamin C, Forschung un Praxis*. Darmstadt, West Germany: Merck, 1970.

Paeschke, K. D., and H. W. Vasterling, "Photometrischer Ascorbinsäure-Test zur Bestimmung der Ovulation, verglichen mit anderen Methoden der Ovulation-sterminbestimmung," *Zentralblatt für Gynäkologie*, 90 (1968), 817–20.

Pauling, L. "On the Orthomolecular Environment of the Mind: Orthomolecular Theory," *American Journal of Psychiatry*, 131 (1974), 1251–57.

Samborskaya, E. P., and T. D. Ferdman, "The Problem of the Mechanism of Artificial Abortion by Use of Ascorbic Acid," *Bjulletin Eksperimentalnoi Biologii i Meditsinii*, 1966, vol. 635–36.

Szent-Györgi, personal communication, 1937.

LISTING OF ORGANIZATIONS FOR MEGAVITAMIN THERAPY

Academy of Orthomolecular Psychiatry
1691 Northern Boulevard
Manhasset, NY 11030
(516) 627-7260

California Orthomolecular Medical
   Society
2340 Parker Street
Berkeley, California 94704
(415) 848-8595

Chapter Fourteen

HERBAL
TREATMENTS FOR
WOMEN

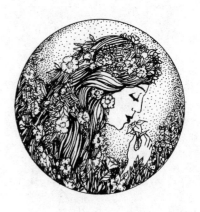

Jeanne Rose

> *And the fruit thereof shall be for meat,*
> *and the leaf thereof for medicine.*
>
> *[Ezekiel 47:12]*

Is there any scientific truth regarding the medicinal value that herbs are reputed to possess? Such questions have been asked of herbalists especially in the last years that herbs/plants have been given recognition as healing agents by the medical establishment and by allopathic physicians.

An herbalist is one who collects, studies, and uses plants; an herb doctor is one who uses plants in a medicinal way, for healing. An herb is "a plant or plant part valued for its medicinal, savory, or aromatic qualities" (*Webster's Third New International Dictionary* 1965). An herb can be any plant part, from leaf to root, or algae to tree.

HERBS—EARLIER FORM OF MEDICINE

The cave woman caring for her mate and children was probably the first herbalist, using different types of vegetation at different times, for healing and well-being. The cave woman was solely responsible for the health of her family, and she administered various plants as curatives. This knowledge was passed down from mother to daughter for millennia, from the time of foraging to the time of agriculture, when people began to plant the medicinal plants they had used in the wild. This knowledge was based on simple observation of what worked and had nothing to do with magic or witchcraft, although the wonder of such simple healing from plants must surely have made these people curious.

Herbalism is the earliest known form of medicine. For humans this knowledge of healing disease using the simple green plants of the fields was probably as instinctive as it was for the animals seeking out appropriate plants for their ills.

It is interesting to speculate as to why this simple herbal healing, as practiced by the early cave woman, became the exclusive domain of the priests/magicians and then of the primarily male doctors of our times. This wonderful simple knowledge of using plants as allies in healing became the esoteric and secret knowledge of the magician priest/physician and later of the studied academics of modern-day medical schools. Early herb doctors in every civilized country, for over 5000 years, have regarded healing as a divine art, a gift from the gods, a natural occurrence. Medicine and magic became linked to herbals in early times when organized medicine took from laywomen the right to practice their age-old craft.

NEW EMPHASIS ON THE USE OF HERBS FOR MEDICINAL PURPOSES

Women must again take charge of the health of their families. Using plants is a simple task; many of the ancient well-known "weeds" have been documented as having medicinal and curative properties. For instance, there are dozens of plants known for their estrogenic activity (Verdeal and Ryan 1979); others are known to relieve premenstrual water retention (Amann 1979) and acne (Amann 1975).

Herbs should be taken along with other health measures, including a wholesome (unprocessed) diet, exercise, moderate living, and nutritional supplements. It is not "normal" to have heavy menstrual discharge or to lack the menses altogether. It is not "normal" to have extremely painful childbirth or to lack milk for one's newborn. We can have menstrual regularity; control our cycle; use herbs as natural abortives; and have relatively painless childbirth—all with only minimal knowledge of plant use. But we cannot expect to take an herb tea for a few days to undo ten years of poor habits, or to take herbal capsules just prior to birth to ensure a normal delivery. Herbal medicine requires that the user live a moderate life, eat a wholesome, fresh, unprocessed diet, and exercise with some regularity.

Each person is a unique creature with different cultural and genetic background. Herbal formulations can be designed individually to account for these differences; if one herbal mixture fails, the competent herbalist can design another that will work. Thus herbalists can design herbal mixtures individually for each case, whereas an allopathic physician with a limited pharmacoepia must use general formulas that may work in the majority of cases, but not all.

Individual herbs have occasionally been "scientifically" studied and their medicinal value qualitatively and quantitatively determined. But in most cases, we must at this time use herbs that have been relied upon for thousands of years—without the "stamp of approval" of investigative scientists. Where possible, scientific references are given in the following pages; more often we recognize that the formulas work because herb doctors have previously used them with success.* The herbs/plants that are mentioned here will always be capitalized, according to the English way to distinguish them for the novice.

HERBAL FORMULAS FOR LATE MENSES AND TO STIMULATE ABORTION

There are various herbal alternatives to surgical intervention when a woman wishes to terminate a pregenancy or to establish regularity in the menstrual cycle. The herbal methods used have not to this author's knowledge been closely studied, but the knowledge gained from many women indicates that these methods can work with success *when used together*. A woman must first know her body and its rhythm, so that she knows when she ovulates and when her menses is due. If the menstrual cycle is late, then several plant products can be used in combination, as described below:

1. Apricot kernals, which are suspected to have anticancer qualities and which might treat the developing fetus as just another foreign body, can be taken eight at a time three times a day, from ovulation until the day 1 of the menstrual cycle (when bleeding first occurs).They must be finely chopped and carefully chewed.

2. Three days before the period is due, a sprig or two of freshly washed and clean whole Parsley (which contains progesterone) is wadded up into the shape of a tampon and is inserted into the vagina. This herbal plug is left for two to three days before it is removed and replaced with a fresh sprig. This can be repeated every two days until the period is well established.

3. In folk medicine, Carrot seeds have been ingested from ovulation to the end of the cycle to inhibit the egg from implanting on the uterine wall, or to ensure that the menses will begin, or even as an abortive after the period has been missed and until the next ovulation is due. Carrot (seed) oil has been investigated and been shown to be a direct cardiac depressant and to have a relaxing effect on the uterus of some mammals (Bhargava, Ali, and Chauhan 1967). This effect may be the reason that it has been effective as an abortive (to inhibit implantation) in women.

*See the "History of Herbs" from *The Herbal* by Jeanne Rose to be published by Bantam Books, Inc., in 1982.

4. High prostaglandins soften and prime the cervix to prepare it for expansion during labor. A lovely flower, the Evening Primrose, is the source of a fluid extract that has been used by women prior to labor or as an abortive. Formerly the fluid extract (infusion) was ingested as well as being used as a vaginal douche. The oil contains gamma linolenic acid, precursers to prostaglandin production in the body. Current usage prescribes oil of Evening Primrose capsules three times per day from ovulation until the period is due, to ensure its arrival if birth-control measures have been lax. The oil is also directly applied to the cervix several times a day just before the period is due.

5. Pennyroyal tea (not to be confused with oil of Pennyroyal which is a deadly poison), is taken a quart a day, for not more than four days beginning on the day before the period is due and until day 4 if the period is late. This tea (infusion) is made by taking ½–1 lb. of the dried herb and adding to it 4–6 quarts of hot water. The herb is allowed to soak in the water for at least 24 hours, then strained. The tea is drunk, one-half cup at a time, every waking hour, for four days.

6. Diet is very important when there is a suspected pregnancy that the person wants to terminate or when a women wishes to establish menstrual regularity. A 70 to 80 percent fresh, raw, or steam vegetable diet is encouraged. This includes vegetables, fruits, potatoes of all kinds, and millet as a grain; but the diet limits other grains, meats, and nuts to 20 to 30 percent. Just before a woman's period, she is encouraged to eat lightly of whole foods and to drink plenty of water, herb teas, and vegetable juices.

7. Finally, exercise is needed—hard vigorous exercise as constantly as possible—until the menses is well established.

These seven steps are done simultaneously to "bring on" a period when it is late for any reason. Steps, 2, 5, 6, and 7 are also used to establish menstrual regularity.

MENSTRUAL REGULATION FORMULATIONS

It has long been known that there are naturally occurring estrogens in plant foodstuffs (Verdeal and Ryan 1979), as well as in certain medicinal herbs. Licorice root and Angelica have been carefully examined and found to be characterized by conbsiderable amounts of estrogens (Goryachev, Pauzner, and Muinova 1970; Tuskaev 1971). In addition, Licorice root when given in large amounts has caused premature sex maturation in young animals (Murav'ev and Kononikhina 1972). Some herbalists use Licorice and Red

Clover* for their plant estrogens in the estrogen phase of the menstrual cycle (Madoyan et al. 1973) and then Sarsaparilla and Blessed Thistle in the progesterone phase, these latter two because of their plant progesterone content. *Agnus Castus* is also taken because it is thought to exert a beneficial effect on the pituitary to create a balancing effect on hormone production. Table 14-1 gives recipes for estrogen and progesterone tea. The tea is made in the standard way: 1 oz. of the dried mixed herbs is steeped (infused) in 1 quart of water, kept just under a boil, for at least 20 minutes. The tea is strained and the liquid drunk, 6 oz. four times per day, during the days indicated in Table 14-1.

TABLE 14-1. Herbal tea recipes

Estrogen Tea—take from Day 1–10	Progesterone Tea—take from Day 10–27
Licorice root—1 part	Sarsaparilla—4 parts
Angelica root—1 part	Blessed Thistle—2 parts
Peony root—1 part	Raspberry leaf—4 parts
Agnus Castus—1 part	Ginseng—1 part
Red Clover—1 part	Agnus Castus—1 part

On days 27, 28, and day 1, or the comparable days when the cycle is normally longer or shorter, the Parsley tampon and the dietary advice are recommended.

FORMULAS FOR PREMENSTRUAL TENSION, ACNE, AND WATER RETENTION

A light diet is encouraged for symptoms of premenstrual tension, acne, and water retention, with the deletion of all refined foods, sugar, alcohol, and stimulants. A tea of Agnus Castus with Rosemary (for its tonic effect) can be taken several times a day for several days just prior to the menses. Some supplements such as calcium in the form of bone meal, vitamin C, and others may also be helpful. Agnus Castus has been shown to have a favorable effect on premenstrual water retention (Amann 1979) as well as to relieve several forms of acne.

Note: Red Clover has been shown to induce sterility when eaten in large amounts by forage animals. It smaller amounts it stimulates reproductive function because of its estrogenic content.

VAGINAL INFECTION

Most forms of vaginal infection, including PID (pelvic inflammatory disease), Gardnerella, fungus, yeast, and bacteria, will respond to the use of two herbal treatments: (1) an herbal bolus inserted into the vagina, and (2) herbal capsules. The herbal capsules include: Echinacea root, which encourages the production of white blood cells to fight infection; Yellow Dock root used as a blood cleanser; Goldenseal, which acts as an antibacterial and antiviral; and Ginseng to encourage the health of the lymphatic system. Equal parts of these dried, powdered herbs are mixed together, stuffed into size 00 gelatin capsules, and the capsules are taken three at a time, three times a day for ten days.

Along with the capsules, the herbs Slippery Elm bark, Comfrey root, and Marshmallow root are added to the basic formula, mixed with just enough melted cocoa butter to hold the mass together. A piece, ½ inch in diameter and 1 inch long, is inserted into the vagina every 36 hours. It can be held in place with a tampon and should be douched out at the end of 36 hours with an herbal mixture. This mixture includes Yellow Dock, Goldenseal, and Comfrey root infusion, simmered, strained, cooled to body temperature, and then applied with a douche bag. The bolus and douche are used for six days, then nothing for one day, then repeated at least twice more for a total of three to six weeks or until or until the infection has completely cleared up. These formulas also require the same dietary, and exercise, recommendations as noted above.

In addition, specific recommendations for various vaginal disorders include yogurt as a douche for yeast infections, or the yogurt can be inserted by using a standard birth-control applicator. Plain vinegar and water are also used as a douche to reestablish the normal acidity of the vagina.

Garlic has been extensively studied as to its medicinal aspects (Ikram 1972) and has been shown to have antiviral, antibacterial (Subrahmanyan 157; Kakelik 1970), antifungal (Lesnikov 1947), and pesticidal properties.

In addition to the general recommendations for vaginal infections, trichomoniasis can be treated with Garlic suppositories. A small piece of Garlic is wrapped in thin cheesecloth and inserted into the vagina. The Garlic is replaced every 12 hours until the infection is cleared up. Garlic (4 chopped cloves per one-half cup yogurt) can also be infused (soaked or steeped) in plain yogurt for several days, then strained out, and this yogurt inserted into the vagina with a vaginal applicator.

Bacterial infections, including Gardnerella (Hemophilus) and PID, are best treated with the herbal capsules and the bolus.

BLADDER AND KIDNEY INFECTIONS

Cystitis (bacterial infection in the bladder) may occur in women due to intercourse or childbirth, or as a result of using standard medicinal drugs prescribed for treating vaginitis. Cystitis can be easily cured at home by using the recommended diet already mentioned and drinking 1 quart of unsweetened Cranberry juice, or taking up to 10 g. of vitamin C per day. These two substances—Cranberry juice and vitamin C—act as antiseptics in the bladder and sterilize the urine. Several herbs can be soaked in the Cranberry juice to increase its effectiveness, and these herbs can also be taken in a standard infusion at intervals throughout the day. In addition, when cystitis is the result of strenuous intercourse, it is wise to check the vulva for external cuts or bruises; these can be treated with sitz baths of Comfrey root. The individual should void both before and after intercourse to flush out whatever bacteria may be lurking in the bladder and should drink plenty of water or herb tea throughout the day.

A good herbal formula for cystitis is:

2 oz. Uva Ursi	1 oz. Buchu leaves
1 oz. Couch grass	1 oz. Parsley root
1 oz. Marshmallow root	1 oz. Comfrey root
½ oz. Juniper berries	½ oz. Goldenseal root
½ oz. Echinacea root	

The dried herbs are mixed together and 1 quart of the infusion is drunk in small quantities at ½-hour intervals throughout the day until the quart is gone. This should be taken for at least five days and preferably for at least three days after the infection has seemingly cleared up.

Folia Uvae Ursi or Uva Ursi is an official drug in the world pharmacopeia. Its medicinal activity is due to arbutin and anthocyanins. There are other species in the *Ericaceae* family that also contain these substances, such as Huckleberry and Blueberry, which actually contain more of these substances than *Uva Ursi* (Mihajlov and Janackovic-Milojevic 1968). But Uva Ursi is more often used. Arbutin passes through the body unchanged, then hydrolizes in the urine if harmful bacteria are present. It is then converted to hydroquinone and becomes a disinfectant (Schavenberg and Paris 1977). *Anthocyanins* also occur in this group, and they possess a great affinity for certain tissues such as the kidneys and skin; they increase capillary resistance and decrease capillary permeability (Lietti and Forni 1976; "Anthrocyanin Glucosides" 1961).

PREGNANCY AND CHILDBIRTH

The *Guelder Rose* cramp bark is used as a uterine sedative (Sloan, Latven, and Munch 1949), especially in cases of threatened miscarriage and for dysmenorrhoea. This plant is particularly interesting to herbalists because it has been closely studied, and the folk remedy of using the crude bark as tea has been shown to be stronger than use of the powdered extract prepared under laboratory conditions (ibid.). This is most interesting because many herbalists feel that the entire plant must be used to be effective, rather than any one of its "active" components, because of inherent factors that occur in the natural product that ultimately affect the outcome of the disease. In this one plant this ancient herbal knowledge has proven to be true.

Raspberry leaf contains fragarine, a uterine relaxant, and is the standard herb to be used throughout pregnancy and lactation.

For morning sickness, antispasmodic herbs such as Peppermint, Catnip, and Chamomile are used as teas. Hops, which has been thought to contain estrogens (Strenkovskaya 1968), but usually does not (Fenselau and Taladay 1973), provides a smoothing antispasmodic action as does Basil and Raspberry leaf as teas.

There are some herbs that it is best to avoid during pregnancy, but that can be used with knowledgeable guidance. These have strong medicinal qualities that may affect the developing fetus: Pennyroyal, Tansy, Black Cohosh, Blue Cohosh, Yarrow, Mistletoe, Wild Celery, Rue, Peyote, Squaw Vine, and Uva Ursi.

Some of the herbs that can be used during pregnancy are Alfalfa and Clover, both of which contain phytoestrogens (Tuskaev 1971); Neetle (iron in an easily assimilable form) for its nutritive value (Obretenova et al. 1973); Plaintain for potash; Raspberry leaf to tone the uterine muscle; Comfrey to help in protein synthesis; and Peach leaf for nausea.

At birthing time, many midwives use Basil, Lavender, and Nutmeg as a tea (Koehler, Solomon, and Hunt 1980). Evening Primrose oil applied to the cervix is helpful to soften and prime the cervix for expansion, and Basil tea is drunk to help expel the placenta. After the birth and to encourage milk production, Comfrey, Fennel, Nettle, and Alfalfa are used as teas.

If the baby has runny eyes, a mixture of Comfrey root and Fennel seed may be used as an eyewash. This infusion should be carefully strained to ensure that all herbal bits and pieces are removed from the herbal liquid.

For mastitis, a hot poultice using Comfrey root, Mullein flowers, or Lobelia works very well. Comfrey root, especially if it can be used freshly grated, is preferable. This poultice should be applied until the breast is red. Occasionally, if the breast is very sore, the herbal poultice can be applied ice cold until the swelling is relieved.

For plentiful breast milk, the following herbs may be used: Marshmallow root to strengthen the milk, Blessed Thistle to increase the flow, and Nettle and Comfrey to build up the blood. Europeans also use Fennel seed and Anise seed to improve the breast milk flow.

MENOPAUSE

The mixtures of herbs that are used specifically for menopause (see formulas below) are various combinations of plants that provide both phytoestrogens and progesterone precursors. The estrogen herbs predominate.

> *Formula #1:* Equal quantities of Licorice root, Angelica (Dong Quai), Black Cohosh, Sarsaparilla, Ginseng, Blessed Thistle, False Unicorn, and Spikenard.

> *Formula #2:* One part each of Wild Yam root, False Unicorn root, Licorice root, Comfrey root, True Unicorn root, Life root or False Valerian, Angelica root, Rosemary leaf; and one-half part each of Spikenard (Grinkevich, Koval'skii, and Gribovskaya 1971), Sarasaparilla, Blessed Thistle, Ginseng, and Red Clover.

The dried herbs are mixed together, bottled in a light-proof container, then labeled and stored in a dark cool place. The general dosage is two cups of tea per day, taken at spaced intervals. The tea is made in the usual way; that is, 1 tablespoon of the mixed herbs is simmered in one cup of water for 1 minute and then removed from the heat, cooled to room temperature, strained, and drunk. Honey can be added, and the residue of herbs can be used again for the second cup of tea.

APPENDIX—DEFINITIONS OF SOME SIMPLE HERBAL TERMS

Bolus: A bolus is a suppository, used either anally or vaginally, and made by adding a mixture of powdered herbs to enough melted cocoa butter to make a consistency like pie dough. This mixture is then rolled into a pencil shape in waxed paper, refrigerated until hard, and then cut into 1-inch sections for later use. The bolus is best applied at night, where the cocoa butter will melt at body temperature, to slowly release the virtues of the herbs. The exact quantity of herbs to cocoa butter is difficult to determine due to the different types of plant materials used, but a reasonable beginning is 2 oz. of mixed herbs to ½ oz. of melted cocoa butter.

Infusion: An infusion is a mixture of herbs that has been soaked or steeped in very hot water, although room-temperature water is sometimes recommended. Bring 16–20 oz. of water to a boil, remove from the heat, and add 1 oz. of herb. Steep for at least 20 minutes, then cool and strain. If the plant parts are roots or seeds, they should be brought to the boil with the water, and then this mixture should be added to the leafy or flower parts for steeping.

Poultice: A poultice is a warm, moist mass of powdered infused herbs that is applied directly to the skin and then covered by a warm, preferably woolen, cloth to retain heat against the skin. It is best to make a very thick infusion first. The liquid is then strained off and used as tea or to soak the cloth. The hot herbs are applied to the skin, and the herbal-soaked cloth is then applied and covered by a piece of plastic or a plastic bag.

Sitz Bath: A sitz bath is a shallow bath that one sits in to sooth aching or sore vaginal or anal parts. An herbal sitz bath is simply an infusion of herbs and water, strained or unstrained.

Tea: A tea is a beverage of herbs and water. It is made using 1 teaspoon to 1 tablespoon of herbs to every cup of water. The best method is to bring the water to a boil, adding the tea to the cup, then pouring on the water. Allow to steep 3–5 minutes, then strain and drink. A "tea" can also mean simply a drink of herbs.

REFERENCES

Amann, W., "Acne Vulgaris and Agnus Castus (Agnolyt)," Z. *Allgemeinmed*, 51, no. 35 (1975), 1645–48.

———, "Premenstrual Water Retention: Favorable Effect of Agnus Castua on Premenstrual Water Retension," *ZFA* (Stuttgart), 10, 55, no. 1 (1979), 48–51.

"Anthrocyanin Glucosides," *Laboratoires Chibret*. April 18, 1961.

Bhargava, A. K., S. M. Ali, and C. S. Chauhan, "Pharmacological Investigation of the Essential Oil of Daucus Carota Var Sativa," *Indian Journal of Pharmacology*, 29, no. 4 (1967), 127–29 (Eng.)

Fenselau, Catherine, and P. Taladay, "Is Estogenic Activity Present in Hops?" *Food and Cosmetics Toxicology*, 11, no. 4 (1973), 567–603.

Goryachev, V. S., L. E. Pauzner, and S. S. Muinova, "Estrogenic Activity of Glycyrrhiza Glabra and Clycyrrhiza Uralensis Hay," *Mater, Biol.* (1970), pp. 11–15. (Russ.)

Ikram, M., "Review of Chemical and Medicinal Aspects of Allium Sativum," *Pak. J. Sci. Ind. Res.*, 15, nos. 1–2 (1972), 81–86.

Kalelik, Jan, "Antimicrobial Properties of Garlic," *Pharmazie*, 25, no. 4 (1970), 266–70. (Ger.)

Koeler, Solomon, and Hunt, handouts for natural childbirth preparation. Sebastopol, Calif. 1980.

Lesnikov, E. P., "Data on the Fungicidal and Fungistatic Action in Vitro of Phytocides of Onion and Garlic on Geotrichoid," *Byull. Eksptl. Biol.* 24, no. 1 (1947), 70–72.

Lietti, A., and G. Forni, "Studies on Vaccinium Myrtillus Anthocyanosides. II. Aspects of Anthocyanins Pharmacokinetics in the Rat," *Arzneim-Forsch,* 26, no. 5 (1976), 832–35 (Eng.)

Madoyan, O. O. et al., "Effects of Plant Estrogens on the Reproductive System of Rabbits," *Izv. Sel'skokhoz Nauk,* 16, no. 2 (1973), 67–72. (Armenian)

Mihajlov, Milena, and B. Janackovic-Milojevic, "Comparative Determination of Arbutoside in Some Species from the Family Ericaeceae from Stara Planina," *Lek. Sirovine,* 6 (1968), 57–64. (Serbian)

Murav'ev, I. A., and N. F. Kononikhina, "Estrogenic Properties of Glycyrrhiza Glabra (Licorice)," *Rast. Resuv.,* 8, no. 4 (1972), 490–97. (Russ.)

Obretenova, N. et al., "Chemical Composition and Nutritive Value of Leafy Vegetables Underutilized in Bulgaria," *Bulg. Akad. Nauk.* Vol. II, 1973, p. 5–20.

Schauenberg, and Paris, *Guide to Medicinal Plants.* New Canaan, Conn.: Keats Publishing Inc., 1977. Original French edition, 1974.

Sloane, Aaron B., Albert R. Latven, and James C. Munch, "Rate of Extraction of Uterine Sedative Potency," *Journal of the American Pharmaceutical Association,* vol. 38 (1949). Viburnum Studies, XVI.

Strenkovskaya, A. G., "Estrogenic Hops Extract for Cosmetics," *Moscow Scientific Research Institute Journal,* vol. 45, no. 18 (1968).

Subrahmanyan, V. et al., "Effect of Garlic in the Diet on the Intestinal Microflora of Rats," *Journal of Scientific Industrial Research,* 16C (1957), 173–74.

Tuskaev, A., "Estrogen Activity of Some Fodder Plants in Northern Ossetis," *Rast. Resur.,* 7, no. 2 (1971), 295–98. (Russ.)

Verdeal, Kathey, and Dale S. Ryan, "Naturally Occurring Estrogens in Plant Foodstuffs—A Review," in *Journal of Food Protection,* 42, no. 7 (1979), 577–83.

Webster's Third New International Dictionary. Springfield, Mass.: G. & C. Merriam Company, 1965.

LIST OF ORGANIZATIONS FOR HERBOLOGY

California School of Herbal Studies
P.O. Box 350
Guerneville, CA 95446

Emerson College of Herbology, Ltd.
11 St. Catherine East
Montreal, Canada H2X 1K3

The Dominion of Herbal College Ltd.
of British Columbia
7527 Kingsway
Burnaby, B.C., Canada V3n3C1

Chapter Fifteen

MASSAGE:
THE ROOTS OF
WOMEN'S HEALING

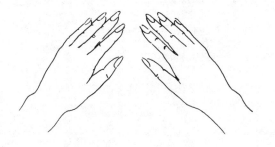

Mirka Knaster

Massage has had a long and checkered history. It has been alternately extolled as a panacea for an extensive list of ailments and rejected as a therapeutic procedure. Despite extravagant claims for and against it, for millennia, massage has been employed successfully. In contemporary times we are witnessing a renaissance in its popularity, possibly the result of a growing public disillusionment with modern depersonalized clinical practices that emphasize surgery and drugs rather than personal contact and self-responsibility or preventative maintenance in health care.

Massage has variously been known as friction, rubbing, kneading, stroking, compression, vibration, and manipulation (Beard and Wood 1964). The word *massage* itself was originated by French physicians early in the nineteenth century (Kamenetz 1980). Massage is a healing art, an act of physical caring, a unique way of communicating without words (Downing 1972). It is also a systematic and scientific manipulation of body tissue producing beneficial effects on the nervous and muscular systems, the local and general circulation of blood and lymph, the skin, viscera, metabolism, etc. Massage is the hub from which other body therapies have radiated.

EARLY HISTORY

The roots of women's massage therapy probably can be traced back to the first woman who massaged herself to relieve menstrual cramps or a sore muscle incurred during her various labors. As likely, it could have been the first woman who ministered to an injured child or other family member or who eased another woman's pain in childbirth. Thus, the very nature of being a woman could have brought on the use of massage as therapy.

Women's biological function has elicited massage in a number of ways: such as to enhance the sexual act (Jex-Blake 1970); to relieve pain associated with the reproductive function (menstruation and other gynecological problems, or birth); to activate that function if it is impeded in some way (infertility); to impede that function if its fruit is not desired (abortion); to facilitate the act of fruition (delivery); and then to soothe, feed, and mold the fruit itself (lactation, baby massage).

Since earliest times, doctors have recommended massage. The ancient Greeks and Romans prescribed massage for everything from a toothache to epilepsy. Soranus of Ephesus, a Greek physician who practiced medicine in Rome (ca. A.D. 100), is best remembered as the author of *Gynaecia,* a treatise on obstetrics, gynecology, and pediatrics. This text represents ancient gynecological and obstetrical practice at its best, and it survived well into the sixteenth century. In it, Soranus prescribes baby massage as well as massage with respect to menstruation, sexual intercourse, abortion, contraception, lactation, and for "hysteria."*

Medical treatment, from ancient times on, included massage, sometimes for several hours a day. Trotula of Salerno, a medical woman of the eleventh century, known for her book *On Curing the Sicknesses of Women, Before, During, and After Parturition,* continued the recommendations of the ancient medical writers before her. She, as well as Avicenna, the famed Arab physician of the early eleventh century, prescribed breast massage to enhance lactation as well as baby massage.

In the Orient, too, massage has long been recognized as a branch of medicine. In China, during the T'ang dynasty (A.D. 618–906), the Imperial Medical Bureau had a Department of Massage, headed by a Professor of Massage who gave lessons in physical exercise and treated cases of fractures, injuries, and wounds (Wong and Lien-teh 1936). In the eighth century in Japan, the Medical College of Nara gave regular courses in massage (Casal 1962). The author Fijukawa also spoke of Japanese medical practice in the eighth century:

> In the second year of the Taiho Era (702 A.D.), the Code of Laws . . . of the Emperor Mommu contained regulations concerning medicine and education analogous to those of the Tang Dynasty from which they were derived . . . The medical high school, which was in the city of the Imperial residence . . . [was comprised of] five divisions, viz: the medical part, acupuncture, exorcism, massage, and pharmacology [1900, pp. 5–6].

Hysteria, from the Greek word for "uterus," was believed as late as the twentieth century to be a female affliction. Eventually, it was proven to be an illness suffered by both sexes and not the result of the "wandering of the uterus" (Rawson 1973).

FACTORS CONTRIBUTING TO THE DECREASE OF MASSAGE

Why then is massage both lauded and scorned? What are the factors that promoted or undermined its popularity? The rise and fall and rise again of massage appear to reflect the cyclical changes in the concepts of physical care and beauty and in medical practice itself.

In ancient Greece, a person achieved and maintained a state of physical well-being and beauty through a combination of bathing, exercise, and massage, all of which could be carried out in one location. The Romans continued this Greek tradition when they took over the existing buildings that housed the facilities for such practices. They also constructed new buildings and further developed Greek medicine. However, when Roman civilization degenerated, therapy declined too, and abuses proliferated in the baths. Massage and bathing became a facile avenue to sexual exploits instead of optimal health. It is this association with sexual activities that has put massage into disrepute. Also contributory has been the practice of therapy by "quacks" and "charlatans," as the medical profession is wont to call those whom they consider untrained or unscientific (Laver 1978; Mackay 1932).

For the most part, the development of massage has, in the West, accompanied that of medicine. While medicine flourished during ancient times, so did massage. And as medicine and its literature declined in the Middle Ages, the use of medical gymnastics and massage fell rapidly too. In the medieval period, "nuns played a conspicuous part in caring for the sick" (Hughes 1943), and secular nurses established their own orders too. Probably their massage was confined to rubbing in medicaments that they had prepared themselves.

In addition to the nuns and nurses, it is likely that the massage techniques that had been used down through the ages as "folk medicine" continued to be employed by other women in the community. However, during this period, such practices were often eyed with suspicion. "Many a poor woman was burned at the stake in northern Europe during the Middle Ages because she knew a little more than other persons and cured suffering men by massage, a magic which was looked upon as a power of Satan" (Nissen 1916, p. 4).* "Witches" were also accused of rubbing themselves with various unguents (Forbes 1966). Touch and nakedness, and concerns with body health and welfare, were deprecated because religious teachings scorned the body as a repository of sin. Under the influence of Christianity, the habit of bathing, long associated with massage and anointing, as during the Greek and Roman times, was minimized in the Latin West.

*This claim is not substantiated by documentation in Nissen's book.

Then, as the various arts and sciences—including medicine—began to reemerge in the Renaissance, massage made its reappearance too. But it was not until the nineteenth century that the spirit of scientific inquiry penetrated the theory and practice of massage, elevating it to a new and higher status.

NINETEENTH AND TWENTIETH CENTURIES—INCREASED RECOGNITION OF THE VALUE OF MASSAGE

During the second half of the nineteenth century, the number of publications on massage and gymnastics increased, especially in Europe (Reibmayer 1889)† Two men in particular did much to broaden the acceptance of massage: Per Henrik Ling, originator of the Swedish movement-cure, a combination of exercise and massage; and Johan Georg Mezger, a Dutch physician whose classification of massage movements (stroking, friction, kneading, tapotement) was adopted by the leading clinicians. During these decades, a growing number of physicians publicly advocated massage,* and numerous research projects were carried out (Kamenetz 1980; Bucholz 1917).

In the late nineteenth century, S. Weir Mitchell, a prominent physician, hailed as one of the founders of American neurophysiology, had a thriving practice of "hysterical" neurotic patients. Both he and Freud, with a similar case load, employed massage as part of their treatment, Freud later giving it up in favor of hypnosis. Dr. William Playfair introduced the Mitchell cure into England, where it became as much the rage as in the United States (1882). One of the major components of the treatment was massage, which expedited the assimilation of greater quantities of food and provided passive exercise for bedridden patients.

At the same time that massage was being advocated for neurasthenia† in women by Mitchell and his followers, it was also resuming its place in gynecology as a result of the efforts of Thure Brandt of Sweden, and of those who furthered his form of gynecological massage. Many works on diseases

†Dr. Reibmayer's tract on massage contains a bibliography from that period listing over 250 items in several languages, many of them dealing with the use of massage for female conditions.

*Drs. Douglas Graham, Benjamin Lee, and S. Weir Mitchell of the United States and Drs. William S. Playfair and James Mennell of England are the best known in the English language. There were many more in Europe, particularly in Germany and the Scandinavian countries.

+Neurasthenia—an atonic condition of the nervous sytem, marked by fatigue, worry, inadequacy, and lack of zest; and often by headache, undue sensitiveness to light and noise, and disturbance of digestion and circulation.

of women were published in the nineteenth century, authored by doctors who recommended massage as part of the treatment. During this century, too, Just Lucas-Championnière popularized the use of massage in the treatment of fractures and other conditions. Doctors in Europe and in the United States wrote about the techniques, benefits, and history of massage. Some administered massage themselves, or they directed trained technicians in the proper use of it. Many foreign treatises, especially in German and Swedish, were translated into English. At the University of Berlin, Dr. J. B. Zabludowski was a full professor of massage.

During this same period, mechanical devices were introduced, obviating the need for personal touch, especially between male technicians and female patients or vice versa, reflecting the shift to industrialization as well as the morality of Victorian society. But increased mechanization had its positive contributions to massage too. Vibratory massage became popular, and a wide variety of machines were manufactured (Hastings and Snow 1912). Along with mechanical apparati, electricity (Despard 1916), heat (thermotherapy), water (hydrotherapy) (Fox 1917), and exercise accompanied the use of massage. Concern with body care also saw the return of many ancient practices.

World War I, and its tremendous requirements for adequate personnel in rehabilitation therapy, further demonstrated the usefulness of massage, particularly in restoring functional activity of injured limbs. Later wars continued this demand for physical therapy (McMillan 1932; "Presidential Messages" 1971).

PLACE OF WOMEN IN THE PROFESSION OF MASSAGE

Not all women are ministered to today by Western-style professionals. In most parts of the world, women continue to turn to their group's traditional healer. In fact, they seek out specialists just as we do in America. Particularly in Asia and the Pacific islands, the general practitioners may incorporate massage as a component in their healing treatment (Hart 1965; Jocano 1973; Nydegger and Nydegger 1966). *Cuanderas* ("witch doctors") and other healers may use massage to extract the evil spirit that is considered the cause of illness in a patient's body. And bone setters may not only set bones to reduce a fracture, but they massage the surrounding and local areas as well.

In the domestic setting, women have been both the receivers and givers of massage with respect to their reproductive function. Throughout the world, midwives have traditionally assisted at home births, which are the rule rather than the exception. They administer massage as part of prenatal and postpartum care. During the birth process, they may massage the shoulders and back to relieve soreness and tension; the abdominal area, as in cephalic version, for better presentation; and the perineum to avoid tearing. A midwife may also be the first person to massage the newborn. Breast massage may be self-administered by the mother or may be provided by the midwife to stimulate the flow of milk and to reduce engorgement. Also among the Maori, "massage of babies was considered highly important and was continued for several years, the mothers using different movements of their hands. Knees and ankles received special attention so that these joints would always be supple" (MacDonald 1973, p. 121).

The nurturing health care that women afford their families through the medium of massage is extended to the public sphere in their role as healing professionals, traditional or modern. For the most part, Western doctors have not massaged a great deal, but ancillary staff—nurses, masseuses, physical therapists—are sometimes employed to perform that function. In the more primitive societies, however, medicine women, *cuanderas*, bone setters, and other folk medical practitioners continue today to administer massage as part of their curing ritual.

RATIONALE FOR THE USE OF MASSAGE

What is the rationale behind employing massage? Whether an evil spirit has invaded and possessed a body or whether lactic acid has accumulated in the muscle, the end sought is a release from some kind of pain—physical, mental, or spiritual. Depending on the belief system of the particular culture, the use of massage may be justified on the basis of its effects on the circulatory and nervous systems. Or, in a society in which people believe in the "evil eye" or "airs," massage may be incorporated in a process aimed at extracting the noxious spirit that is creating disease within the body. In any event, current physiological studies have clearly demonstrated that massage does exert a beneficial effect on the skin, on the circulation of blood and lymph, and on the nervous system, musculature, viscera, etc. As a result of these studies and innumerable clinical cases, massage has earned a rightful reputation today as effective therapy (Beard and Wood 1964, chap. 3; Barr and Taslitz 1970).

NEGLECT BY AMERICAN MEDICAL PROFESSION

Yet, despite its proven efficacy, massage remains largely neglected by the American medical profession, often to the regret of the doctors themselves (Graham 1902). In an address before a state medical society in 1908, Dr.

William Thayer, Professor of Clinical Medicine of Johns Hopkins University, said, "Must we not all on reflection be painfully conscious that not one of us has been properly instructed in massage?" And Dr. J. Madison Taylor voiced a similar sentiment in the *New York Medical Journal* in 1912: "In America, not only is the physician not so instructed, but scarcely one in hundreds has any clear or competent conception of the scope and applicability of these measures" (Jensen 1932, p. 14).

These statements reflect the state of instruction in regard to massage for the medical profession in the United States today. Medical schools give no training in the technique of massage, although some instruction in the theory and art of massage is included in the curriculum of schools of nursing and physical therapy.

Thus, although diverse techniques of massage have been developed in this century, in general the role of massage has diminished. Originally the major component of physical therapy, massage has been dwarfed by other therapeutic agents such as diathermy, ultrasound, and pharmaceutics.

That an adequate massage treatment necessitates considerably more time than highly paid or overloaded medical personnel are willing or able to provide has also led to its decline. Those who do not take time and effort to learn the art of manual treatment cannot know its potentials. Consequently, fewer and fewer therapists believe in its efficacy (Reiter, Garrett, and Erickson 1969). Nevertheless, even as therapists and patients turn to more sophisticated modalities or quicker methods (drugs), massage is still appreciated by some doctors, osteopaths, orthopedists, chiropractors, nurses, physical therapists, psychotherapists, and sports trainers.

Furthermore, although massage does not appear in American medical textbooks, the *Index Medicus* for 1968–1980 lists over 1500 articles from journals around the world referring to the use of massage in medicine and physical therapy, including ocular, gingival, breast, prostatic, lymphatic, and cardiac massage (1981). Massage is also utilized in rheumatism, pneumonia, back conditions, sciatica, joint diseases and injuries, and paralysis, etc. However, this is still a far cry from ancient times when massage was prescribed for almost everything, to promote good health, strength, and beauty as well as to recuperate from illnesses.

REBIRTH OF MASSAGE AS A PRECIOUS AND VITAL TALENT

If massage did not die out at a time when therapeutic arts reached their nadir, it is not likely to fade in the advent of technology either. Massage is more than just physical therapy or mechanical manipulation—it is personal contact. There is communication through the hands, the voice, the energy, or vibration, and the very presence of another breathing human being.

Massage is more than physiology. It is the care and attention afforded by a midwife or masseuse during some trying aspects of pregnancy and birth, by a nurse during an uncomfortable convalescence, by a physical therapist or sports trainer after an accident and injury. Most of all, massage feels good and, in many cases, may immediately relieve distressing symptoms so that an individual can relax enough to allow the healing process to begin.

Combating the decline in personal contact and the increase in technological and pharmaceutical therapy is growing awareness of holistic medicine and the need for touch. People are learning self-responsibility in caring for their body, mind, and spirit. For example, women are taught self-massage of acupressure points to alleviate menstrual pains. Others learn massage to care for their families and friends or to establish themselves professionally. A growing spate of classes and professional schools in a variety of massages is testimony to the need for human touch, for "contact," a human need as basic as the one for food (Montagu 1971; Prescott 1975; Colton 1977). As long as massage ministers to the triune needs of humanity for body/mind/spirit, it will still be relied upon. And it is likely that women will continue to play a central role.

At the same time as the women's movement and the humanistic movement are fostering a growing respect for the feminine side in all of us, recent research on the hemispheres of the brain is pointing in the same direction. Science is demonstrating the importance of the intuitive, nonrational, nonlinear functioning of the right side of the brain. It is the hemisphere that controls the left side of the body, traditionally designated as the female side. It is the side that favors feeling, creativity, and *touch*; it is able to "tune in" and "know" without verbal communication. It is the part that can sense and heal through touch, from a "knowing" that is not based on reason.

In their historical role of ministering to others, women have long been acquainted with and have practiced this "magic medicine." For their own as well as others' survival, it has been a precious and vital talent. It is a natural capacity available to all those who do not eschew its power over that of reason and the kind of medicine that reason produces. It is not a matter of choosing one or the other, but of integrating the two, of creating a balance between nature and reason, female and male, or as in the Orient, between yin and yang.

Women and their ways, long associated with nature and the unconscious, have been the object of derision during the centuries in which nature and human beings have been separated by a belief that consciousness is exclusively rational and human. Women, like natural ways of healing, have been deemed inferior. The mind/body split, developing out of such a philosophy, has had an effect on massage. As "folk medicine," practiced by women, massage was overshadowed by "modern medicine"—until male doctors adapted it scientifically. Women continued to practice massage but as ancillary staff. But in pretechnological cultures, the art of massage has never been lost.

Today, with the resurgence of interest in consciousness and mind/body integration, healing arts from around the world, including different forms of massage, are once again being utilized and respected. Women, who have always been lay healers, are in the forefront of this movement as they express renewed interest in midwifery, natural childbirth, and massage, for themselves, their babies, and others. Women, who have always been intimately involved with the use of touch, will continue to massage effectively and to demonstrate it to others, so that they too may come to understand its magic, whether applied scientifically, intuitively, or both.

REFERENCES

Barr, Jean Scott, and Norman Taslitz, "The Influence of Back Massage on Autonomic Functions," *Physical Therapy*, 50, no. 12 (1970), 1679–91.

Beard, Gertrude, and Elizabeth Wood, *Massage Principles and Techniques*. Philadelphia: W. B. Saunders Company, 1964.

Bucholz, C. Herman, *A Manual of Therapeutic Exercise and Massage. Designed for the Use of Physicians, Students, and Masseurs*. Philadelphia: Lea & Febiger, 1917.

Casal, U. A., "Acupuncture, Cautery and Massage in Japan," *Journal of Asian Folklore Studies*, vol. 21 (1962).

Colton, Helen, *Touch: It's as Vital as Food*. Los Angeles: Forum International Ltd., 1977.

Despard, Louisa L., *Textbook of Massage and Remedial Gymnastics*, 2nd ed., Chapter XV, "Electrical Methods in Conjunction with Massage." London: Oxford University Press, 1916.

Downing, George, *The Massage Book*. New York and Berkeley: Random House—The Bookworks, 1972.

Forbes, Thomas Rogers, *The Midwife and the Witch*. New Haven, Conn.: Yale University Press, 1966.

Fox, R. Fortescue, *Physical Remedies for Disabled Soldiers*, section on Manipulation and Massage Baths. London: Ballière, Tindall & Cox Limited, 1917.

Fujikawa, Y., *Japanese Medicine*, trans. from the German by John Ruhräh, *Clio Medica*, vol. 12. New York: Paul B. Hoeber.

Graham, Douglas, *A Treatise on Massage*, 3rd ed., rev. and enl. Philadelphia and London: J. B. Lippincott Company, 1902.

Hart, Donn V., "From Pregnancy through Birth in a Bisayan Filipino Village," in *Southeast Asian Birth Customs: Three Studies in Human Reproduction*. New Haven, Conn.: HRAF Press, 1965.

Hastings, Mary Lydia, and Arnold Snow, *Mechanical Vibration, Its Physiological Application in Therapeutics*, New York: Scientific Authors' Publishing Company, 1912. Earlier version published in 1904 as *Mechanical Vibration and its Therapeutic Application*.

Hughes, Muriel Joy, *Women Healers in Medieval Life and Literature*. New York: King's Crown, 1943.

Jensen, Kathryn, *Fundamentals in Massage for Students of Nursing*. New York: Macmillan Publishing Co., Inc., 1932.

Jex-Blake, Sophia, *Medical Women: A Thesis and a History*. Edinburgh: Oliphant, Anderson & Ferrier, 1886; republished in New York: Source Book Press, 1970.

Jocano, F. Landa, *Folk Medicine in a Philippine Municipality*, Chapter 6. Manila: The National Museum, 1973.

Kamenetz, Herman L., "History of Massage," in *Manipulation, Traction and Massage*, ed. J. B. Rogoff. Baltimore and London: The Williams & Wilkins Company, 1980.

Laver, Bryan A., "Miracles No Wonder! The Mesmeric Phenomena and Organic Cures of Valentine Great Rakes," *Journal of the History of Medicine and Allied Sciences*, 33 (January 1978), 35–46.

Licht, Sidney, "Mechanical Methods of Massage," in *Manipulation, Traction and Massage*, ed. J. B. Rogoff. Baltimore and London: The Williams & Wilkins Company, 1980.

Macdonald, Christina, *Medicines of the Maori*. Auckland and London: Collins, 1973.

Mackay, Charles. *Extraordinary Popular Delusions and the Madness of Crowds*, chapter on "The Magnetisers." New York: L. C. Page, 1932.

McMillan, Mary, *Massage and Therapeutic Exercise*, 3rd ed. Philadelphia and London: W. B. Saunders Company, 1932.

Montagu, Ashley, *Touching: The Human Significance of the Skin*. New York: Columbia University Press, 1971.

Nissen, Hartvig, *Practical Massage and Corrective Exercises*, rev. and enl. version of *Massage in Twenty Lessons*. Philadelphia: F. A. Davis, 1916.

Nydegger, William F., and Corinne Nydegger, *Tarong: An Ilocos Barrio in the Philippines*. Six Cultures Series, vol. 6. New York: John Wiley & Sons, Inc., 1966.

Playfair, William S., *The Systematic Treatment of Nerve Prostration and Hysteria*. Philadelphia: Henry C. Lea's Son & Co., 1883.

Prescott, James W., "Body Pleasure and the Origins of Violence," *The Futurist*, 9, no. 2 (1975), 64–74.

"Presidential Messages: The First 50 Years," *Physical Therapy*, 51, no. 6 (1971), 619–82. Section on Mary McMillan.

Rawson, Philip, *The Art of Tantra*, illustration 80. Greenwich, Conn.: N.Y. Graphic Society, Ltd., 1973.

Reibmayer, Albert, *Die Massage und ihre Verwerthung in den verschieden disciplinen der praktischen medicin*. Leipzig and Vienna: Franz Deuticke, 1889.

Reiter, Susan, Tom Garrett, and Donald J. Erickson, "Current Trends in the Use of Therapeutic Massage," *Physical Therapy*, 49, no. 2 (1969).

Wong, K. Chimin, and Wu Lien-teh, *History of Chinese Medicine*, 2nd ed. Shanghai: National Quarantine Service, 1936.

SUGGESTED READINGS

Ehrenreich, Barbara, and Deirdre English, *Witches, Midwives, and Nurses*, Glass Mountain Pamphlet No. 1. Old Westbury, N.Y.: Feminist Press, SUNY College at Old Westbury, 1971.

Hughes, Muriel Joy, *Women Healers in Medieval Life and Literature*. New York: King's Crown, 1943.

Szasz, Thomas, *The Manufacture of Madness*, Chapter 6. New York: Harper & Row Publishers, Inc., 1970.

LISTING OF ORGANIZATIONS FOR MASSAGE

The Alliance of Students and
 Practitioners of Medical Massage and
 Related Therapies
c/o The Swedish Institute
875 Avenue of the Americas
New York, NY 10001
(212) 855-1720

American Massage and Therapy
 Association, Inc.
152 West Wisconsin Avenue
Milwaukee, WI 53203
(414) 271-1475

Florida School of Massage
1115 N. Main Street
Gainesville, FLA 32601
904-378-7891

New York State Society of Medical
 Masseurs
P.O. Box 219
Pearl River, NY 10965
(212) 288-6962

Chapter Sixteen

MASSAGE, REFLEXOLOGY, AND WOMEN

Frances M. Tappan

Massage is a healing art.* It is a unique way of communicating without words. Through touching another person, we may communicate the fact that we care, that we want to share our energy with them. Dolores Krieger, Ph.D., R.N., proved in a controlled study that Therapeutic Touch is so beneficial in healing that it can even increase the hemoglobin content of blood (1973).

Krieger's research derives from, but is not the same as, the laying-on of hands. The laying-on of hands is the uniquely human act of concern of one individual for another, which is characterized by touching in a way that aims to heal the person touched. Krieger's ideas concerning the importance of touching to promote healing have a direct relationship to the touching involved in massage.

PHYSIOLOGICAL EFFECTS OF MASSAGE

The effects of massage are psychological, mechanical, physiological, and reflexive in nature. By massage, stimulation is provided to the exteroceptors of the skin and to the proprioceptive receptors of the underlying tissues. Relief of pain is brought about through one of these effects, or by a combination of any of them. Massage functions, not as an isolated healing method, but as part of the total healing plan.

The student of massage should have some understanding of the physiology of the heart and circulation, particularly the peripheral circulation and the return flow of blood and lymph, as taught in basic physiology courses.

*Actual techniques of the massage systems described in this article are presented in detail in the author's book, *Healing Massage Techniques: A Study of Eastern and Western Methods* (1978).

Massage assists the venous flow of blood, encourages lymphatic flow; reduces certain types of edema; provides gentle stretching of tissue; relieves subcutaneous scar tissue; improves nutrition through the skin by the application of special lubricants; increases perspiration, thus removing excretory products; helps to remove dry scaly skin following casting; and assists soft tissue toward normal metabolic balance. In addition, there are reflex effects from the stimulation of sensory receptors of the skin and subcutaneous tissues.

Through mechanical pressure, massage can rid the muscles of toxic products by "milking" these acids into the lymphatic and venous flow toward the heart. As the muscles relax, fresh blood flows into them, bringing necessary nutrition to the area.

Muscular inactivity can bring about poor blood flow, particularly in the limbs where gravity inhibits the normal venous return. Often the results may be varicosity, thrombosis, or pressure on the vessels by edema within the surrounding tissues.

It is obvious that massage should *not* be given if there is a possibility of spreading inflammation; or of disloding a thrombus; thus causing embolism, or if there is such obstruction that the mechanical assistance of massage could not improve the blood flow. However, massage given *first* to the proximal aspects of an injured limb will ensure that these circulatory pathways are open enough to carry the venous flow along toward the heart.

TYPES OF MASSAGE

Effleurage

Any stroke that glides over the skin without attempting to move the deep-muscle masses is called effleurage. Effleurage is used more than any other of the massage techniques. The evaluation the operator can make of the patient's soft tissue with this technique can orient her better than a written or verbal report. During these initial strokes, the operator's sensitive fingers can explore for areas of tenderness or tightness. The hand is molded to the part, stroking with firm and even pressure, usually upward.

Petrissage

Contrary to effleurage, which glides over the skin, petrissage strokes attempt to lift the muscle mass and wring or squeeze it gently. Petrissage consists of kneading manipulations done with hands or fingers, which press and roll the muscles under the hands. This kneading motion of petrissage serves to "milk" the muscle of waste products that collect due to abnormal inactivity. It assists the venous return and will also help to free adhesions.

Friction

Friction is necessary to reach beneath the more superficial tissues. It is performed by small circular movements with the tips of the fingers, the thumb, or the heel of the hand, according to the area to be covered. Small flat ellipsoids are described; these penetrate into the depth of the tissue, not by moving the fingers *on* the skin but by moving the tissues *under* the skin.

Friction is used to massage deep into the joint spaces or around bony prominences such as the patella. It is especially useful around a well-healed scar to break down adhesions between the skin and tissues that are beneath it. However, it cannot affect a deep fibrositis such as might form within a muscle belly.

Vibration

A fine tremulous movement, made by the hand or fingers placed firmly against a part, will cause that part to vibrate. But vibration can usually be better administered with an electrical vibrator, with the exception of the very gentle vibration needed in treating peripheral neuritis and poliomyelitis.

Gentle vibration is used for a soothing effect. The treatment follows the path of the nerve. It has been used in Europe for poliomyelitis patients with such delicacy that the vibrating hand does not even touch the part but merely flutters above it.

MASSAGE OF PREMATURE AND NEWBORN BABIES

Ruth Rice, a nurse, psychologist, and specialist in early child development, researched sensorimotor stimulation of premature infants. She developed a specific stroking and massage technique, which she used in an experimental study of 30 premature babies (1975). The mothers were taught this technique, which includes touching, movement, and the sound of a heartbeat, similar to the conditions the fetus experiences in the womb.

Infant research has shown that this touching, movement, and sound stimulate the nerve pathways and cause the following to occur:

1. An increase in myelination, dendritic processes, and Nissl substance in the brain cells, resulting in a speeding up of neurological growth.
2. A higher output of the growth hormone somatrophin, causing faster weight gain.

3. An increase in the output of the hypothalamus, which serves as a general arousal center, leading to increased cellular activity and endocrine functioning.

The development of Rice's stroking and massaging technique and the success she has had using it have brought national and international recognition from persons in medicine, nursing, psychology, and child development. Rice believes there must be revolutionary changes made in the care of newborn infants and in parent/child interaction if the high incidence of emotional disturbance, learning disabilities, hyperactivity, and many other disorders that have their origins in infancy are to be prevented.

Reflex Massage

Both Eastern and Western medical philosophies agree that isolated pathologies do not exist anywhere in the human body. The entire organism functions as a balanced and coordinated unit if the body is healthy. Thus any disability that disrupts this harmony will affect the autonomic and central nervous systems as well as the hormonal and humoral systems. In other words, the body must be considered as a physiological and psychological whole.

In massage, the hands stimulate the sensory receptors of the skin and subcutaneous tissues, causing a series of reflex effects. The reflex process involves the reception of a stimulus by one organ or tissue and its conduction to another organ, which on receiving the stimulus, produces the effect. The stimuli pass along the afferent fibers of the peripheral nervous system to the spinal cord; from there, it is conceivable that these stimuli may disperse through the central and autonomic nervous systems, producing various effects in any zone supplied from the same segment of the spinal cord. Some of these effects are capillary vasodilation or constriction, relaxation or stimulation of voluntary muscle contraction, and possible sedation or stimulation of pain in an area remote from the area being touched.

The most superficial layer of the tissues forming the body surface is the skin. It is the immediate link with the external environment. It contains the exteroceptors, i.e., specialized nerve endings that react to touch in various intensities and to changes in temperature.

The deepest layer of these tissues is that of the muscles. The muscles contain numerous nerve endings that can alter the tension in the tissue both reflexively and voluntarily. These nerve endings also register alterations in the tension of the tissue by means of proprioceptors, i.e., specialized nerve endings sensitive to alterations in the length of the muscle fiber. Both these tissues—the skin and the muscles—relate to the somatic and the autonomic nervous systems. Therefore, vascular changes occur in both tissues in response to massage. The layer of tissue between the skin and the muscles consists of connective tissue, and this is the layer thought to be of particular importance when applying reflex massage. See Figure 16–1 for the areas on the back that correspond to visceral pathologies.

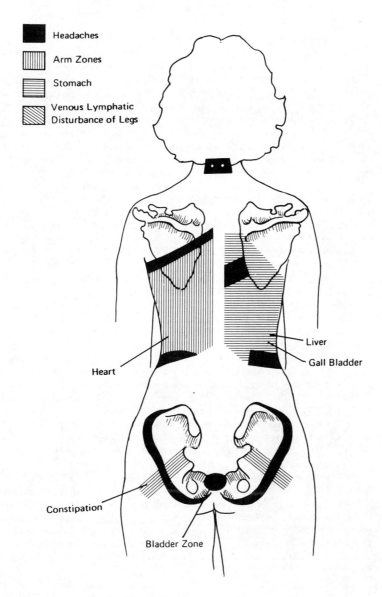

Headaches

Arm Zones

Stomach

Venous Lymphatic
Disturbance of Legs

Liver

Gall Bladder

Heart

Constipation

Bladder Zone

FIGURE 16–1.   Some connective tissue zones and acupuncture points on the back.

Case Study

Elisabeth Dicke was among the first in the Western world to organize the specific routine of reflex massage in her text *Meine Bindegewebsmassage* (1956), and the work of Miriam Jacobs soon followed (1960).

In 1929, Dicke suffered from a severe disturbance in the peripheral circulation of her right leg. As a result of a neglected tooth infection, a general toxemia had developed, which resulted in an endarteritis obliterans of the right leg. The leg was cold and bluish in color, the toes giving the appearance of incipient gangrene. The dorsalis pedis artery was no longer palpable. Dicke was advised to consider amputation of the lower limb.

In addition to the extreme pain in the extremity, she suffered from an almost unbearable backache. While lying on her side she tried to give herself some relief by massaging over the painful areas of her back. She found tht over the sacrum and the right iliac crest, thickenings and infiltrations could be palpated, while toward the left side on the same level, the skin felt tight.

She tried to ease the tension by massage with her fingers across the affected areas, but found that these areas were hypersensitive to the touch. Slight stroking with the fingertips caused great pain. The tension, however, gradually subsided, the pain in the back eased, and an agreeable sensation of warmth took its place. On successive days she persisted with the stroking, which was performed by other people. She gradually felt pins and needles in the affected leg, followed by a sensation of warmth.

In further treatments she incorporated the areas around the greater trochanter and along the iliotibial tract. Gradually the superficial venous circulation reappeared in the thigh and leg. The severe symptoms subsided after three more months of treatment carried out by a colleague under Dicke's direction. Dicke was able to resume her occupation after a year.

Years of investigation followed. During the course of her illness Dicke had experienced pathological function of internal organs in addition to the symptoms in the back and leg. She suffered from a chronic gastritis, the liver showed enlargement, the heart showed symptoms of angina, and she experienced disturbance of kidney function. These visceral complaints cleared up simultaneously with the improvement of peripheral circulation and normalization of tissue changes in the back. Treatment of pathologically affected areas of the body surface apparently helped to clear up pathological changes in affected viscera. Thus she discovered that certain areas on the body surface are definitely related to certain viscera.

Systematic observation of patients in the following years confirmed these findings. Unknown to Dicke at the time, an English neurologist had already described similar findings, showing changes in the same well-defined areas of the body surface, pertaining to specific organs. These alterations appeared when pathological changes took place in affected viscera. Thousands of years previously, the ancient Chinese had already become aware of an increased sensitivity of certain skin areas (called points) when a body organ or function was impaired.*

*A comparison of reflex massage areas and acupuncture points is included in *Healing Massage Techniques: A Study of Eastern and Western Methods*, written by this author (1978).

ZONE THERAPY AND FOOT REFLEXOLOGY

Recently, a great deal of emphasis has been placed on treating disorders of the entire body by treating the bottom of the feet with deep pressure in certain key spots.

According to ancient Chinese medical theory, the total body is reflected in the ear, eye, palm of the hand, and bottom of the foot (see Figure 16–2). Centuries before viscero-cutaneous (organ-skin) and cutaneo-visceral reflex effects were identified in the 1800s, the Chinese had already discovered sensitive areas on the bottom of the feet. Using finger pressure, because needles were too painful, they treated specific areas on the feet to normalize physiological functions in the human body.

This form of massage consists of compression, using the thumbs to apply firm pressure. By doing compression over the entire foot, tender areas will indicate where concentration of treatment should be given. Pressure needs to be firm but not overly painful.

Skilled and experienced thumbs can palpate areas of tightness or swelling on the foot. Medical literature concerning Zone Therapy agrees as to which areas relate to various parts of the body. However, any attempts to explain psychologically why Zone Therapy is effective tend to break down. Thus the term *energy flow* in the human body has been "created" in recent research findings to describe such phenomena.

Other massage systems maintain that the connective tissue and the lymph system throughout the body are the vehicles for energy circuits of a nature not yet analyzed by either Eastern or Western medical science and perhaps cause the release of endorphins, endogenous pain-killing hormones.

By examination of the diagrams (see Figure 16–2), one can readily locate the areas where finger pressure can be applied for at least temporary relief of symptoms. Persistent symptoms should be seen by a doctor.

CREATING POSITIVE ATTITUDES TOWARD HEALING

The art of healing is a two-way street. Massage given by someone who includes the patient as a partner will be remarkably more effective than massage given as a mere technique of body manipulation. The operator who devotes his/her total attention by communicating concern, empathy, and sincere desire to promote the healing process will spur the patient to participate in the effort toward regaining good health.

The purpose is to replace patient dependence with collaborative effort between patient and operator. To establish this relationship, the patient must participate in discussions that include the exchange of ideas, rather

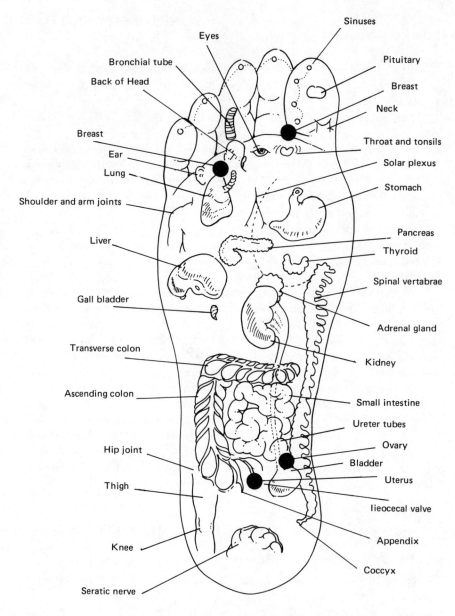

Right foot, bottom view

FIGURE 16–2. Location of major acupuncture points corresponding to organ points on sole of foot. Dots show points important to treatment of female problems. (From *The Massage Book*. George Dowing and Anne K. Rush. New York: Random House, 1974.

266

than simply receiving instructions given by the operator. Such an approach will strengthen positive attitudes and will exclude feelings of despair.

A pleasant atmosphere, the exchange of laughter, a sense of strength and determination, and feelings of love will greatly encourage the human body toward its own constant search for homeostasis. The body itself will then produce more comprehensive chemotherapy (endorphins) than is available at any medical center in the world, be it via Eastern or Western medical approaches.

While giving massage, the operator can encourage the patient to understand the potential source of healing in his/her own consciousness and to be active in his/her own treatment. Skillful encouragement can stimulate the human body's own defense and healing mechanisms.

Current research done with plants, animals, and human beings is proving that positive effects are possible through the "laying-on of hands." For example, in an experiment conducted in 1964, barley seeds that had been soaked in saline to simulate a "sick" condition (1964) were "healed" by the "laying-on of hands." An identical saline-treated flask of barley seeds were not so healed. The seeds treated by the laying-on of hands sprouted more quickly, grew taller, and contained more chlorophyll.

In another experiment, *The Secret Life of Plants* records how Cleve Backster proved that plants respond if touched with affection (Tompkins and Bird 1973). By using lie-detector equipment, Backster confirmed Grad's studies that plants respond to loving care and soft music in a positive way. Conversely, they respond negatively to hard rock music and feelings of hate.

In Eastern cultures, the transference of attitudes between the healer and subject is believed to occur via a state of matter for which the Western culture has neither word nor concept. It is called *prana* in Sanskrit. The nearest translation in the West is "vitality" or "vigor." The Chinese called it *chi*, which translates into "energy." Regardless of what it is called, however, this phenomenon refers to the balanced functioning of the human body and the vital life force of energy that keeps people in good physiological and psychological health. Advocates of this concept believe that the healer can transfer his/her own positive energy to the patient through touch, via any medical approach—pulse reading, acupuncture, or more modern medical methods—to return the patient to normal health. But it is necessary for the patient to have faith in the healer and to possess a strong will to get well.

REFERENCES

Dicke, Elisabeth, *Meine Bindegewebsmassage*. Stuttgart: Hippokrates-Verlag, 1956.

Grad, Bernard et al., "A Telekenetic Effect on Plant Growth, Part 2. Experiments Involving Treatment with Saline in Stoppered Bottles," *International Journal of Parapsychology*, 6 (1964), 473–98.

Jacobs, Miriam, "Massage for the Relief of Pain: Anatomical and Physiological Considerations," *Phys. Therapy Rev.*, 40, no. 2 (1960), 96–97.

Krieger, Dolores, "The Relationship of Touch with Intent to Help or to Heal, Ss In-Vivo Hemoglobin Values: A Study in Personalized Interactions." Paper presented to American Nurses Association, 9th Nursing Research Conference, Kansas City, 1973.

———, "Nursing Research for a New Age," *Nursing Times*, April 1976, pp. 1–7.

Rice, Ruth D., "Premature Infants Respond to Sensory Stimulation," *APA Monitor*, 6, no. 11 (1975), 8–9.

Tappan, Frances M., *Healing Massage Techniques: A Study of Eastern and Western Methods*. Reston: Va.: Reston Publishing Company, Inc., 1978.

Tompkins, Peter, and Christopher Bird, *The Secret Life of Plants*. New York: Avon Books, 1973.

SUGGESTED READINGS

Carter, Mildred, *Helping Yourself with Foot Reflexology*. Englewood Cliffs, N.J.: Prentice-Hall, 1969.

Kaye, Anna, *Mirror of the Body*. San Francisco: Strawberry Hill Press, 1977.

Krieger, Dolores, *The Therapeutic Touch: How to Use Your Hands to Help or to Heal*. Englewood Cliffs, N.J.: Prentice-Hall, Inc., 1979.

Montagu, Ashley, *Touching: The Human Significance of the Skin*. New York: Columbia University Press, 1971.

Chapter Seventeen

ACUPRESSURE FOR WOMEN'S HEALTH

Ann Patterson

Acupressure is a generic word that encompasses any of a number of techniques of applying pressure to stimulate acupuncture points that lie over the entire human body. The three most versatile, well-known acupressure systems are:

Dō-In: Self-massage consisting of tapping, squeezing, stretching, and breathing exercises.

Shiatsu: Rhythmic pressure in a systematic way over the entire body and its acupuncture meridians. It also includes stretching and percussion.

Jin Shin Dō: A meditative technique of holding specific points where muscular tension and energy blockages occur. The points are held gently, two at a time, for 1 to 5 minutes duration.

HISTORY

Acupressure traces its roots back some 5000 to 6000 years as the predecessor of acupunture in China. According to tradition, it grew from the instinctual response of massaging sore muslces by pressing sore points on the body and noticing the immediate relief that followed. Further observation revealed that persons with specific illnesses displayed hypersensitivity in the same skin areas. Other tales relate the correlation between an arrow puncture during battle and the sudden disappearance of a chronic ailment (Chan 1975; Wallnofer and von Rottauscher 1971).

Acupressure was first formalized by Chinese Taoist monks as "Tao-Yinn." *Tao,* "the way," encompasses the philosophy that sees the body and mind of each person as being in harmony with all of nature, with the entire universe. *Yinn,* being the "yin" or gentle approach, described the manner in which this harmony is achieved. The Tao-Yinn techniques had a twofold

271

use: (1) ideally, regular practice maintained a state of supreme health, harmony, and clarity of body and mind; (2) as a therapeutic system, Tao-Yinn was preceded by a week of fasting, deep breathing, visualizations, and meditation to calm the body and the mind and to rid the person of toxic wastes (de Langre 1971). From these ancient beginnings in Taoist philosophy and from centuries of observation and experimentation with points and energy theory, a body of knowledge developed that comprises the present-day Chinese medical theory and practice. It includes acupressure, acupuncture, herbology, and moxibustion (the application of heal to acupressure points).

Tao-Yinn in its present-day form is called *Dō-In*, "the art of rejuvenation through self massage." The instinctive inclination to rub or tap muscles takes on an added purpose when combined with breathing, periods of rest, and knowledge of the electromagnetic energy system that forms the basis of acupuncture (ibid.).

About 1000 years ago, Chinese medicine was brought to Japan and was combined with Japanese massage, which not only expanded the Japanese diagnostic abilities, but added the use of acupuncture points to their manual therapy. More recently, in the last 70–100 years, Western manipulation therapies and physiology were imported and integrated. The resulting form, *Shiatsu* (*shi*—finger, *atsu*—pressure), is very popular in Japan today. In fact, it is authorized by the Japanese Ministry of Health and Welfare, which states:

> Shiatsu therapy is a form of manipulation administered by the thumbs, fingers and palms, without the use of any instrument, mechanical or otherwise, to apply pressure to the human skin, correct internal malfunctioning and promote and maintain health and treat specific diseases. [Masunaga and Ohaski 1977.]

A third form of acupressure, *Jin Shin Dō*, "the way of the compassionate spirit," also had its origins in Japan at the turn of the century and is also based on acupressure theory. This form was originated by Master Jiro Murai as Jin Shin Jystsu and was taught to a small group. One student, Mary Burmeister, brought it to California. Her teachings in California formed the beginnings of Jin Shin Dō as developed by Iona Teeguarden (1978) and of Therap-ease developed by Bonnie Pendleton and Betty Mehling (1980). Unlike Shiatsu's continuous movement along energy pathways, Jin Shin Dō emphasizes a basic 40 points out of the hundreds possible. The points selected are those where the 8 "extraordinary meridians" cross the 12 organ meridians and also coincide with areas of pronounced muscular tension.

HOW IT WORKS

Acupressure is done to release tension and pain, to become healthier, and to learn deep relaxation. It provides an opportunity for individuals to participate actively in their own health care. Acupressure, in Western terms, is a "preventative" health care technique. Based on the Chinese medical tradition of acupuncture, the basic objective of this tradition is to maintain balanced body energy, or life force, and thereby to promote good health, enthusiasm for life, and harmony and peace with oneself and with one's surroundings.

Acupressure points are named for meridians that are invisible continuous energy channels that flow bilaterally up and down the left and right sides of the body, passing six times along the arms and legs. Each body section within the meridians has an internal branch that connects it to an organ—hence the meridian names: lung, heart, gallbladder, kidney, spleen, liver, large intenstine, etc.

Acu means "point." Acupressure involves applying pressure to acupuncture points and meridians. The points are often surrounded by knots or bands of muscle tension and are tender when pressed firmly. They are near the surface of the body, ⅟16- to ½-inch deep.

The electromagnetic energy, the motivating life force common to all living things, has been called by different names—*chi* in China, *ki* in Japan, *prana* in India. Chinese medicine states that the vital force, chi, controls the functioning of the main organs and systems of the body, that it permeates all living cells and tissue, and that it also circulates throughout the body along clearly defined pathways (Giller 1975).

The pathways, called *meridians*, are bilateral, being the same on the left and right sides of the body. There are 12 organ meridians, each taking its name from the organ to which it is connected by internal, secondary branches. Energy is seen to flow continuously in a specific direction through each of the 12, one meridian flowing into another, thereby forming one continuous pathway on each side of the body.

When this energy is flowing freely, undisturbed by subtle blockages in the meridians or by muscular tension around the points, then good health, vitality, and well-being are experienced. In Eastern terms, the body energy is balanced, neither excessive nor deficient in any one meridian. One method of restoring and maintaining this balance is by applying pressure to certain points, in order to loosen the muscular tension, break up the stagnation, and stimulate the circulation of energy.

UNDERLYING PRINCIPLES: EAST MEETS WEST

The techniques of the three forms of acupressure differ, as noted at the beginning of this chapter. The specific power inherent in the points and meridians can be activated by any of these techniques. They are all effective in balancing energy, releasing chronic muscle tension, and promoting health.

The fundamental principle common to all three techniques is the establishment of a deep state of relaxation. This involves (1) a shift of breathing from rapid, shallow, unconscious breaths to slow, deep, inhalations and exhalations—each one fully experienced, and (2) a shift of mental awareness from thinking about things outside oneself and the moment to a concentration on feeling the new body sensations and the flow of the breath.

Each slow exhalation, consciously felt to completion, automatically releases muscular tension throughout the body. When this awareness is accompanied by simultaneous, focused mental awareness of the area being pressed, it brings all the mental energy to this point, dislodging stagnation and increasing relaxation. This is true for both the recipient and the provider. In fact, for acupressure to be most effective, both masseuse and the person being massaged should enjoy full, deeply felt breaths and be very sensitive to the sensations where the fingers meet the tissue around the points. The person applying the pressure will feel a marked relaxation in the muscle as well as a warming sensation in the hands as the blocked energy begins to circulate.

Concentration on body sensation and breathing are major components of the stress and relaxation research and techniques pioneered in the West by Dr. Wolfgang Luthe (autogenic therapy) (1969), Dr. Edmund Jacobson (progresive relaxation) (1962), Dr. Herbert Benson (relaxation response) (1975), Dr. Norman Shealy (biogenics) (1978), Alyce and Elmer Green Menninger Foundation (autogenic biofeedback), and Dr. Hans Selye, (the effects of stress on the body) (1974).

HOW TO DO ACUPRESSURE

Any of the following routines can be done on oneself or for another person. For best results, the recipient lies on his/her back, taking advantage of the body weight to apply the greater sustained pressure needed for the larger, tighter back muscles.

Although massage with movement on the points work well, sustained pressure with attention being given to relaxation through deep breathing and focused attention produces more lasting results.

To Locate the Point

The exact acupuncture point is as precise and minute as the needle used to treat it. However, acupressure involves a much larger muscle area—usually the size of a quarter or silver dollar. Most points are centered in very dense, tight knots or bands of muscle and usually feel tender when pressure is applied. It is the breathing along with attention to feeling the points that bring the changes. Hard pressure only results in soreness.

To Apply Pressure

1. *Press* gently through the soft tissue until you reach the surface of the tighter muscular layers. Apply gentle, steady pressure with one or two fingers. No movement is necessary. The pressure is sustained for 1 to 3 minutes or more.

2. *Breathe* long, slow inhalations and long, very complete exhalations.

3. *Feel* the soreness and tension. Become very aware of what the area feels like and watch for changes in the sensations as the pressure is held over several minutes. The muscles should begin to relax, the tenderness to dissipate, and your fingers to feel warm and tingly.

4. *Be relaxed.* The fingers, hands, and arms should be as relaxed as possible. It is the act of feeling the fingers and the area being held, not hard, painful pressure, that releases both the energy stagnation and muscle tension. If the fingers or hands become too warm or tingly while holding a point, or the arms begin to shake, break contact for a moment and shake out hands, arms, and shoulders while breathing fully.

5. *Be patient, be caring.* It is the repetition of the acupressure technique that will steadily relax the tension that has accumulated over the years.

6. *Afterwards*, notice the events that begin to put tension back or that make changes for decreasing or eliminating the tendency for stress to happen.

TREATMENT TECHNIQUES

There are two possible approaches to the treatment of problems by acupressure: (1) first-aid, and (2) symptomatic and complete energy balancing. The latter gives the more effective, long-lasting results.

As mentioned earlier, acupressure is based on acupuncture theory. To be most effective, it should be administered after a comprehensive history (medical, environmental, and psychological) is made, including pulse diagnosis, physiognomy diagnosis, and tongue diagnosis. With this information, an understanding of the individuals's particular imbalance, its cause, and appropriate treatment can be determined. (See Chapter Ten on acupuncture for a further discussion.)

Acupressure treatment includes two or three steps: (1) general energy balancing, (2) specific attention to the meridians that are the root cause of that imbalance, and (3) (in the Jin Shin Dō form) a neck and shoulder release.

Acupressure can also be used by those who do not have a thorough training in Chinese medical theory. At this level, it is useful as a health maintenance and well-being technique, as an adjunct to professional medical and/or acupuncture care, and as a first-aid technique.

A routine of Dō-In, self-acupressure, or Shiatsu or Jin Shin Dō received on a regular basis from a skilled practitioner will strengthen health and general well-being.

In the following section, the symptomatic approach is taken. The points mentioned are those in the symptomatic area itself or ones that are traditionally associated with the presenting problem. Following the instructions in the preceding section on "How to Do Acupressure" will ensure beneficial results.

ACUPRESSURE FOR SPECIFIC PROBLEMS

Headaches and Arthritis of Arms and Hands

The neck and shoulder area is a catchall for tension in our culture. Releasing this area thoroughly, with patient understanding, promotes relaxation, clear thinking, and the release of emotional tension and muscle stiffness and spasm. It is also an important area to release for hypertension.

The acupressure point, Large Intestine 4 (see Figure 17-1), is traditionally used to relieved headaches and migraines, and to stimulate circulation in the arms and hands. It is located in the muscle webbing between the thumb and index finger and controls the energy of the Large Intestine meridian, which flows through the neck and into the face.

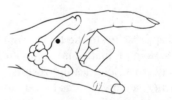

FIGURE 17-1.

Headaches.   All the points in Figure 17-2 are involved with the muscular tension that blocks energy circulation and builds up into headaches. Especially important are the points at the base of the skull and those right on the top of the shoulder, three fingers widths (approximately 1½ inches) out from the base of the neck.

Arthritis.   Arthritic discomfort in the shoulder, arm, and hand is invariably accompanied by extreme muscular tension and blocks in the shoulder area.

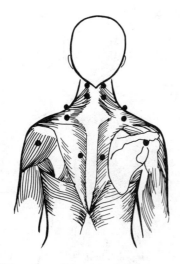

FIGURE 17-2. Neck and Shoulder release.

After acupressure is applied to any of these points that are tense or tender, each hand and every finger should be massaged and gently stretched. It is in the tips of the fingers that one meridian ends and another begins. Massage is important to stimulate the flow of energy up and down the arms.

It should be noted that chronic conditions are best treated with regular weekly or daily acupressure rather than waiting until the pain occurs.

Back Tension and Lower Back Pain

Acupuncture points are spaced approximately 1 inch apart along the muscle bands that parallel both sides of the spinal column. Therefore, any knot of tension you may find on these bands is likely to be a pressure point. There are several of these points that tend to be major areas of tension build-up. These are indicated by the black dots on the diagram (see Figure 17-3). A point in the center of the back of each knee is used to draw pain and tension from the back. In acupressure, this point is pressed gently with one hand, while one or two fingers of the other hand press the back points, one at a time. It is important to finish any work on back points by holding the occipital ridge area. Energy released along the spine could build up in this area were it left unreleased, and could cause a headache.

An optional point, used only in acupressure, is the Center Neck Point, halfway up the neck in the muscles on either side of the vertebrae. It works especially well with the middle and upper back points. For sudden or acute

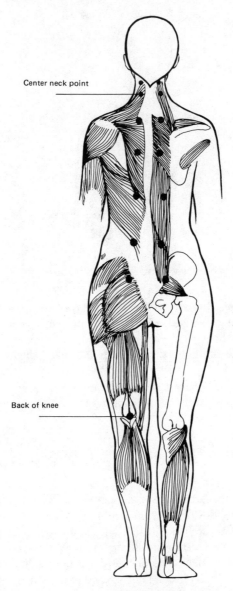

Center neck point

Back of knee

FIGURE 17-3. Important acupressure points in back of body.

pain, that area alone may be held, along with the back of knee or neck point, for immediate relief. Gentle pressure is encouraged, and it may be necessary to begin with points superior and inferior to the pain site. The results are enhanced by imagining the tension and soreness streaming down the leg and out the foot.

Pelvic Disorders

Menstrual discomfort and irregularies involve points in the lower back, sacrum, buttocks, and pelvic region. These areas are massaged, or the specific points indicated are pressed and held bilaterally to loosen the congestion in the pelvic area (see Figure 17-4). Points on the inside of the leg, especially Spleen 10, are held with the pelvic point, Spleen 13, or with the lower back or buttock points, to draw tension out of those areas, helping to relieve the congestion and cramping. Holding Spleen 6 and Spleen 9 together is a quick, though perhaps imcomplete, relief of dysmenorrhea symptoms.

In explaining the relationship between the Spleen meridian and female disorders, Chinese medical theory draws associations between the organ function of modifying blood and the meridian function of effecting menses. There are three yin meridians (i.e., those whose energy most directly affects feminine functions) that travel up the inside of each leg from the foot through

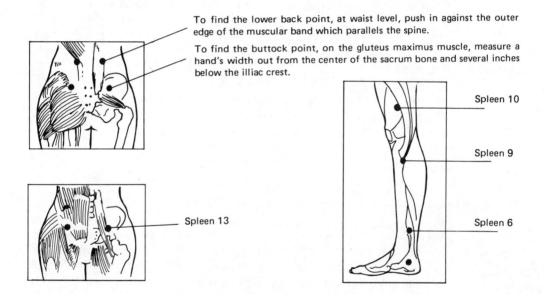

To find the lower back point, at waist level, push in against the outer edge of the muscular band which parallels the spine.

To find the buttock point, on the gluteus maximus muscle, measure a hand's width out from the center of the sacrum bone and several inches below the illiac crest.

Spleen 13

Spleen 10

Spleen 9

Spleen 6

To find *Spleen 13*, on the groin muscle, measure two finger widths in from the top of the pelvic bone and three finger widths down.

To find *Spleen 10*, place palm on your outstretched leg, just above the kneecap, fingers pointing *in*. Spleen 10 is on the inside leg under your index finger.

To find *Spleen 6*, the "three yin meeting point," place your little finger on the top of the inner ankle bone (medial malleolus), and measure up the inside of the leg four fingers. Spleen 6 is at the level of the 4th finger, just behind the tibia.

FIGURE 17-4.

the pelvis into the chest. At one point, four finger widths superior to the medial malleolus, the three meridians converge, forming the "three yin meeting " point, Spleen 6. This point is used in the treatment of virtually all female problems.

Labor and Delivery

Certain points are "forbidden points" for acupunture on pregnant women. These points are often on meridians that have a descending direction of energy flow and are believed to activate descending motion, including that of the fetus. However, very gentle touching over any area can be soothing and relaxing. The so-called forbidden points used during labor to ease pain and encourage contractions should be reserved for that purpose only and should not be used during pregnancy.

A study at the University of Hong Kong found that electrostimulation of Large Intestine 4 and Spleen 6 were useful in inducing labor contractions and as an analgesic (Yip et al. 1976). At the Osaka Medical Center, a similar study of acupuncture anesthesia used these two points in addition to Stomach 36 (Hyodo and Gega 1977). The location of Stomach 36 point is shown in Figure 17-5.

One possible application of these points to acupressure for labor and delivery would be for the expectant mother to hold Large Intestine 4, the muscle webbing, between the thumb and index finger, while her partner holds Spleen 6 and Stomach 36. An alternative combination might be for her partner to hold her hand, pressure Large Intestine 4 with a finger or thumb, and to hold Spleen 6 with the other hand.

Morning Sickness

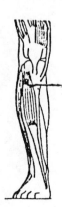

Nausea associated with the first three months of pregnancy, or nausea in general, is treated with Stomach 36, which has the general property of strengthening the stomach, "harmonizing the center," and with Pericardium 6 on the anterior forearm, three finger widths above the crease at the wrist and centered between the ulna and the radius.

According to Chinese medical theory, excess energy blocked or stagnating in the Liver meridian attacks the stomach functioning, causing nausea. The Liver meridian and the Pericardium meridian are connected, forming a channel called *Chueh Yin*. It is the point Pericardium 6 that not only

FIGURE 17-5. Stomach 36, at the top of the tibialis anterior or "shin" muscle, one finger breath outside the tibia or shinbone.

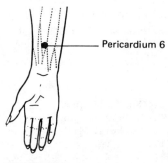

Pericardium 6

FIGURE 17-6.

promotes good blood circulation, but also smooths out the flow of Liver energy, thereby dispersing the attack on the Stomach (see Figure 17-6).

Breasts (Deficient Lactation or Mastitis)

The major points indicated for problems of the breasts are Conception Vessel 17, in the center of the sternum at the level of the nipples, and Stomach 18, directly below the nipple in the depression of the mammillary groove in the 5th intercostal space (Academy of Traditional Chinese Medicine 1975). The Conception Vessel is the meridian that runs along the center of the front of the body from the perineum to the lower lip. It is the most yin of the meridians, and each point along its channel influences surrounding functions. The Stomach meridian begins directly below each eye and travels down, through the nipples, chest, and center of the quadruceps and tibialis anterior muscles, into the toes. The Liver meridian is also associated with the breasts, being a yin or feminine energy channel, and it ends at a point just below the breasts. The Liver meridian's connection to the Pericardium meridian (mentioned above) makes the point Pericardium 6 useful for acupressure treatment of the breast area.

CONCLUSIONS

When used in the gentle, sensitive manner, the acupressure points presented in this chapter can be very helpful. Those interested are encouraged to try the points and technique on themselves and to then share their findings with others. For the serious reader, formal study is strongly suggested to develop skill in the techniques under expert supervision and to gain a greater depth of understanding than can be presented in this brief discussion.

In addition to using the bibliography and reading list that follow, you may contact the author about instruction or to obtain a workbook on this subject.

Ann Patterson
Alternative Therapies Unit
San Francisco General Hospital
2550 23rd Street (Bldg. 9), Rm. 130
San Francisco, California 94110
(415) 821-5139

REFERENCES

Academy of Traditional Chinese Medicine, *An Outline of Chinese Acupuncture.* Peking: Foreign Languages Press, 1975.

Benson, Herbert, *The Relaxation Response.* New York: William Morrow & Co., Inc., 1975.

Chan, Pedro, *Finger Acupressure.* New York: Ballantine Books, Inc., 1975.

de Langre, Jacques, *The First Book of Dō-In.* Magalia, Calif.: Happiness Press, 1971.

———, *The Second Book of Dō-In.* Magalia, Calif.: Happiness Press, 1977.

Forman, Alex, "Acupressure for the Treatment of Dysmenorrhea," *American Journal of Acupuncture,* 6, no. 4 (1978), 139–41.

Giller, Robert M., "Chi Energy and Bioelectric Phenomena," *American Journal of Acupuncture,* 3, no. 4 (1975), 342–46.

Hyodo, Masayoshi, and Osamu Gega, "Use of Acupuncture Anesthesia for Normal Delivery," *American Journal of Chinese Medicine,* 5, no. 1 (1977), 63–69.

Jacobson, Edmund, *You Must Relax: Practical Methods for Reducing the Tension of Modern Living.* New York: McGraw-Hill Book Company, 1962.

Luthe, Wolfgang, ed., *Autogenic Therapy,* vols. 1–6. New York: Grune Stratton, Inc., 1969.

Masunaga, Shizuto, and Watura Ohashi, *Zen Shiatsu: How to Harmonize Yin and Yang.* Elmsford, N.Y.: Japan Publications, Inc., 1977.

Pendleton, Bonnie, and Betty Mehling, *Relax! with Self-Therap/ease.* Calabasas, Calif.: California Publishing, 1980.

Seyle, Hans, *Stress without Distress.* Philadelphia: J. B. Lippincott Company, 1974.

Shealy, Norman, *90 Days to Self-Health.* New York: Bantan Books, Inc., 1978.

Teeguarden, Iona, *Acupressure Way of Health: Jin Shin Dō.* Elmsford, N.Y.: Japan Publications, Inc., 1978.

Wallnofer, Heinrich, and Anna von Rottauscher, *Chinese Folk Medicine.* New York: Mentor Books, 1965.

Yip, S. K. et al., "Induction of Labor by Acupuncture Electro-Stimulation," *American Journal of Chinese Medicine,* 4, no. 3 (1976), 257–65.

SUGGESTED READINGS

Acupressure

Ohashi, Watura, *Do-It-Yourself Shiatsu*. New York: E. P. Dutton & Co., Inc., 1976 (paperback).

Patterson, Ann, *Acupressure Workbook*. Berkeley, Calif., 1980.

Yamamoto, Shizuko, *Barefoot Shiatsu*. Elmsford, N.Y.: Japan Publications, Inc., 1979.

Eastern Health Philosophy and Acupuncture Therapy

Chang, Stephen T., *The Complete Book of Acupuncture*. Millbrae, Calif.: Celestial Arts, 1976.

Connelly, Dianne M., *Traditional Acupuncture: The Law of the Five Elements*. Columbia, Md.: The Centre for Traditional Acupuncture, Inc., 1979.

Manaka, Yoshio, and Ian A. Urquhart, *The Layman's Guide to Acupuncture*. Weatherhill, N.Y.: Weatherhill, 1972.

Mann, Flex, *Acupuncture: the Ancient Chinese Art of Healing and How It Works Scientifically*. New York: Vintage Books, 1973.

Tarthang, Tulku, *Gesture of Balance: A Guide to Awareness, Self-Healing, and Meditation*. Berkeley, Calif.: Dharma Publishing, 1977.

The Yellow Emperor's Classic of Internal Medicine, Ilza Veith, trans. Berkeley, Calif.: University of California Press, 1970.

Self-Health Care, A Western Perspective

Davis, Marth et al., *The Relaxation and Stress Reduction Workbook*. Richmond, Calif.: Harbinger Publications, 1980.

McCamy, John, and James Presley, *Human Life Styling: A Program for Keeping Whole in the Twentieth Century*. Perennial Library, 1975.

Montagu, Ashley, *Touching: The Human Significance of the Skin*, New York: Columbia University Press, 1971.

Chapter Eighteen

ROLFING THE FEMALE BODY

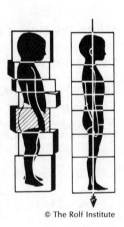

Angwyn St. Just

ADVANTAGES OF ROLFING FOR PREGNANCY— IMPROVED BODY ALIGNMENT

An increasing number of women contemplating pregnancy are choosing to have their bodies "Rolfed" before conception. The advantages this process of structural alignment offers are evident if one considers the predictable strains placed by an enlarging uterus, an altered center of gravity, hormonal changes, and accumulating weight on a "random" or unaligned body. Let us look, for example, at the degree to which the physical changes of pregnancy could stress the improperly aligned body (see Figure 18-1). Given that the center of gravity is located in the pelvis and that the spinal column is best supported by a horizontal pelvic structure, one can see that a body with a tilted pelvis is not in an optimal position for a comfortable pregnancy.

Consider the pattern represented in Figure 18-1. We can see that the forward tilt of the pelvis places heavy strain on the entire spinal column. Since strain at either end of the spine tends to appear in the area of greatest structural weakness (the lower lumbar curve), it is not difficult to see that if this woman were to become pregnant, she would also become a candidate for considerable lower back pain. Looking at her abdominal segment, we find that the pelvic contents are displaced forward and pulled downward. When her abdomen enlarges during pregnancy, the buttocks would need to push even further back in an effort to offset the increasing weight in the front. This, in turn, would cause increasing strain on a weakened lumbar curve as the already short back muscles would need to tighten further in an attempt to compensate for the lengthening of the front.

The potential for a painful situation is even clearer in view of the fact that just 10 pounds of extra weight (half the gain of an average pregnancy)

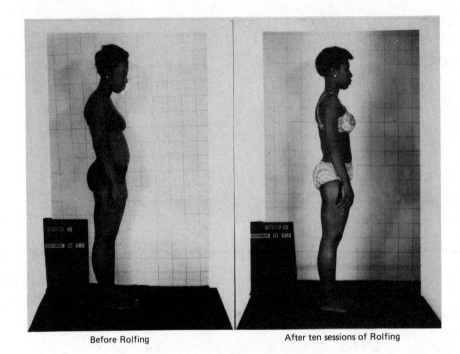

Before Rolfing   After ten sessions of Rolfing

FIGURE 18-1. Before and after Rolfing.

equals 100 pounds of weight in the intervertebral discs (Taylor 1980). The likelihood of discomfort in the lower structure as well, is increased with a torso improperly balanced over the lower limbs so that the abdomen leads the body, and both legs must struggle to fit themselves underneath.

In Figure 18-1, we find a body collapsed through the torso with head bent forward. Although this chronic flexion strains the entire body, we can see that a sagging rib cage has caused specific strain in the region of the seventh cervical vertebra, which gave rise to a "dowager's hump" at the base of the neck. This downward pull on the rib cage has also pushed the lower ribs too close to the brim of the pelvic bone so that the diaphragm is constricted and the breath capacity is diminished. The abdominal segment then suffers the sagging contours of crowded visceral organs, thus offering only minimum space for the uterus to enlarge.

Toneless contours in the abdominal musculature can provide a valuable index to the general health of abdominal and pelvic organs. Poor tone or decreased circulation in this area may indicate equally poor tone in the underlying organs as well as in the ligaments supporting the female organs, bladder, and digestive tract. This is not an ideal situation upon which to place the accumulating weight and hormonal changes of a pregnancy, which will need to stretch muscles, soften ligaments, and loosen joints in order to make room for a growing baby.

After Rolfing, however, it is clear that the body has evolved into a degree of alignment more conducive to a comfortable pregnancy than that offered by the previously random position. It is important to understand that the issue here is the importance of permanently improving structure and not merely correcting faulty posture. Random body patterns cannot be improved by trying to "stand up straight" because the minute the individual ceases to concentrate on posture, the random pattern reasserts itself. The Rolfing process offers women considering motherhood an opportunity for structurally sound, erect carriage, prepared to meet and recover from normal changes of pregnancy without undue strain.

DEFINITION OF ROLFING

What, then is, *Rolfing*? Also known as Structural Integration, Rolfing is a specific form of body work developed by Ida P. Rolf, Ph.D. (1896–1979); see Figure 18-2. Dr. Rolf, who received her doctorate in biochemistry from

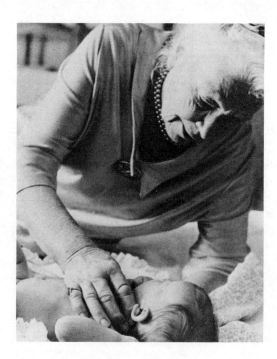

FIGURE 18-2. Ida Rolf.

Barnard in 1920, discoverd that the human body is malleable and therefore changeable. This discovery led her to evolve a system of deep connective tissue manipulation that guides the body toward an anatomical order of increased balance and length centered along its vertical axis. She also found that when the body is aligned, the stress of physical disorder is reduced and less energy reserve is expended, with more energy remaining available for vital functions as well as for emotional and creative expression.*

Dr. Rolf's vision differed from other forms of body work in its emphasis on the relationship between the body and the earth's gravitational field. Basing her work on the belief that only random unbalanced bodies are broken down by gravity, she sought ways of manually aligning the human structure so that its verticality is supported and enhanced by gravity. The result was the Rolfing technique of organizing the body segments along an imaginary plumb line drawn through the ear, shoulder, pelvis, legs, and ankle bone (see Figure 18-3).

CHECKING YOUR OWN ALIGNMENT

If you are contemplating pregnancy and want to check your alignment, you can use the plumb line as a guide. One method would be to have a friend take a full-length photograph of your body. Front and back views are also useful as many of us have never seen our bodies from the back. Or, if you would rather check your alignment yourself, you can stand undressed before a full-length mirror. Beginning with your feet, look to see if they stand parallel with arches slightly raised at the instep. Do your toes point in or out? Do your knees point straightforward? When you walk, do either of your feet turn out or in? If you wear high heels, you may notice that the backs of your legs have become shorter than the front. Elevated shoes shorten the Achilles' tendon above the heel, as well as the calf muscles and entire hamstring group along the backs of the thighs. This shortening may eventually interfere with the function of the knee joints and can cause considerable discomfort in legs and feet. Do your lower limbs feel stable? Stability in the lower structure, offering a reliable base of support, can be a great asset during pregnancy. Competence in the feet and ankle joints will allow for shifting in the center of gravity and for the adjustment of the upper structure during its period of expansion.

*Dr. Rolf's finding was subsequently documented in a study done at the U.C.L.A. Department of Kinesiology by Professor Valery Hunt and Wayne Massey using telemetric electro-myleographic equipment designed to measure muscle response in subjects engaged in activities before and after ten sessions of Rolfing. A status report on the research of Structural Integration can be obtained from the Ida. P. Rolf Foundation for Structural Integration, Box 1868, Boulder, Colo. 80302.

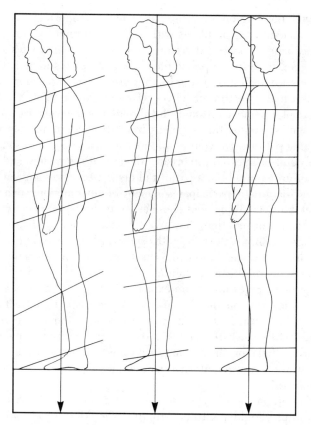

FIGURE 18–3. These illustrations, traced from actual photographs of a woman undergoing structural integration, call attention to the fashion in which vertical and horizontal lines are restored to the body as the body segments become stacked, one above the other.

Next, check the tone of your abdominal segment. Remember that either toneless or overly tight abdominal muscles can lead to backache, and problems with tone can indicate deeper problems within the pelvic organs. Then, look to your iliac crests. Are these bony prominences of your hips horizontal? Is one crest higher, larger, broader, or further from the midline than the other? When you sit on a hard surface, is your weight evenly distributed on the pair of bony prominences at the bottom of your pelvis known as "sitzbones"? The balance of weight on these bones provides an index to the degree of balance in your pelvis. If one bone is higher than the other, your pelvic basin may be rotated as well as tipped. Dr. Rolf believed that imbalance in the pelvic structure is not conducive to good tone in the muscles of the pelvic floor. If muscles of the pelvic floor are prone to sag, they may be especially vulnerable to increased pressure during pregnancy and delivery. The growing uterus, which lies suspended between the bladder and the bowel, depends on this muscular swing for support. If this vulnerable area proves inadequate, problems with urinary continence and sexual dysfunction may arise. It is best, therefore, to begin pregnancy with a balanced pelvis and good tone in the pelvic floor. An added advantage is that when these muscles are healthy and supple, they are able to allow more distention of the vaginal canal at the time of delivery (Deutch; Noble 1976; Rolf 1977).

Now, look to your chest and find the area under your rib cage where the diaphragm separates this segment from the abdominal cavity. Notice your breathing pattern. Do your respiratory muscles allow you to inhale and exhale freely and easily? Can you breathe deeply into your chest and abdomen with ease, or are you held in a pattern of decreased or difficult movement? Although the diaphragm participates in many bodily functions such as crying, singing, coughing, vomiting, and elimination, it also has a special role during pregnancy. Efficient breathing improves circulation for the increased blood volume needed to supply the baby with oxygen and nutrients and to eliminate its carbon dioxide waste. Moreover, the form of deep breathing most frequently taught in childbirth preparation classes is diaphragmatic. This mode of breathing encourages maximum expansion and ventilation in the base of the lungs, which rest on the diaphragm. A preexisting contraction in the diaphragm or collapse in the rib cage can render the entire respiratory function subject to congestive stress as the enlarging uterus expands toward the chest cavity. In labor, the diaphragm is called upon to assist the abdominal muscles with the expulsive uterine contractions during the second stage of labor. (Noble 1976).

Moving up on the body, notice the position of your head and neck in relation to your shoulder girdle. Are your shoulders level and fingertips even? Do your arms hang easily? Finally, see if your head is evenly carried above your torso, and if your neck is forward or pulled to one side. Then have a long look at your overall pattern, weight distribution, and muscle tone.

If you are not entirely pleased with your structure as it is now, you may want to consult with a professional skilled in alignment. Although Rolfing is not the only means of aligning the body, it offers the advantage of a rapid result. The basic ten hourly sessions are usually offered on a weekly basis, although they can be spaced according to individual needs.

POSTPARTUM REALIGNMENT

Although Rolfing is generally not recommended during pregnancy, the process has much to offer after the postpartum period. A series of sessions at this time can assist a woman in giving up her pregnant stance and in restoring her bodily balance, alignment, and comfort. Special attention is given to slackened and overstretched abdominal muscles, rebalancing the pelvis, and stabilizing the sacral bone at the base of the spine.

The sacrum, like all bony members of the spinal-pelvic configuration, is balanced by a myofascial web of muscle and ligaments. During pregnancy, these strong ligaments designed to hold the sacrum in place are greatly taxed by the weight of the growing uterus as well as by softening hormonal changes. The resulting flexibility necessary for the birth process can also allow the increased weight to pull the upper part of the sacrum forward. The lower sacral segments and coccyx of "tail bone" may have to compensate by rotating backward. This can result in disorganizing rotations, displacements, and tensions in the lower half of the body, which do not completely resolve after delivery. The postpartum structure with a weakened or displaced sacrum is left with a lack of adequate "keystone" support for the spinal column above. In order to ensure vertical stability, the body must reenforce this area with extra tissue. The result is a wide-hipped figure. Since this problem is of structural origin, the bottom-heavy body cannot be dieted into proportion. The structural solution offered by Rolfing involves stabilization of the sacrum. Since the sacrum influences the distribution of weight in the lower structure, establishing its strength and alignment is a primary factor in preventing (or if necessary, in removing) the appearance of a "saddle bag" or "riding breeches" configuration where excess tissue gathers on thighs and hips.

In addition to the physical benefits women can obtain from this kind of structural work, the psychological boost of having their bodies fully prepared for and rapidly restored after pregnancy can be very great indeed. Further information about the Rolfing process, a bibliography of material available on the subject, and an international guide to Certified Rolfers can be obtained from: The Rolf Institute, P.O. Box 1868, Boulder, Colo. 80302.

REFERENCES

Deutsch, R. M., *The Key to Feminine Response in Marriage*.

Noble, Elizabeth, *Essential Exercises for the Childbearing Year* Boston: Houghton Mifflin Company, 1976.

Rolf, Ida, *Rolfing: The Integration of Human Structures*. New York: Harper & Row, Publishers, Inc., 1977.

Taylor, Ronald, quoted in "That Aching Back: Latest Word on the Oldest Agony," *Time*, July 14, 1980, p. 33.

SUGGESTED READINGS

Rolf, Ida, *Rolfing: The Integration of Human Structures*. New York: Harper & Row, Publishers, Inc., 1977.

Schutz, W., and Evelyn Turner, *Body Fantasy*. New York: Harper & Row, Publishers, Inc., 1977.

LISTING OF ORGANIZATIONS FOR ROLFING

Aston Patterning Institute
P.O. Box 114
Tiburon, CA 94920
(415) 435-0433

The New York Center for Structural
   Integration and Structural Patterning
165 West 91st Street, #8E
New York, NY 10024
(212) 724-6677

Rolf Institute
P.O. Box 1868
Boulder, CO 80302
(303) 449-5903

Chapter Nineteen

HATHA YOGA FOR WOMEN'S HEALTH

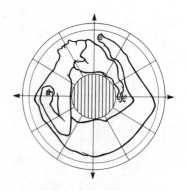

Judith Lasater

In order to understand the relevance of Yoga to the modern woman's health, one must first understand the classic definition of Yoga. Yoga is an Indian philosophical system emphasizing the practice of techniques to obtain the highest degree possible of individual physical, mental, and spiritual integration. The word *Yoga* itself means "to unite or yoke" and implies the discovery of the state of harmony that is existent within each individual. Hatha Yoga is the branch of Yoga that utilizes physical postures (*asanas*) and breathing practices (*pranayama*) to bring a state of relaxed health and harmony to the body and mind.

Many studies have shown Hatha Yoga to be beneficial to overall health, especially to the optimal functioning of the endocrine, circulatory, musculoskeletal, respiratory, and nervous systems (Iyengar 1966). In addition, there is evidence that the practice of Yoga postures and breathing can have salutary psychological effects (Udupa, Singh, and Settiwar 1971). According to a Gallup poll, some five million Americans are presently involved with Yoga, and many of these people report an increased sense of well-being and better health (Gallup 1978). Besides these systemic improvements, Hatha Yoga can have very specific effects on the body and mind, effects that can aid the woman seeking alternatives to the traditional medical approach to the treatment of disease.

Yoga implies that the mind is not separate from the body; rather it is a more refined manifestation of the body. As one's mind becomes clear, better choices are made, choices that affect physical health. And as physical health improves, one has more energy to observe mental patterns that contribute to disease. Many techniques are useful for reducing physical tension, but Yoga allows us to observe the mental attitudes that *create* the tension that leads to disease.

YOGA AS A THERAPEUTIC MODALITY

The physiological changes Yoga can create have only recently begun to be documented by Western science: these include reduced blood pressure, lowered pulse rates, reduction of serum (blood) fats, regulation of menstrual flow and thyroid function, increased range of motion in joints and reduction in joint pain, and a subjectively reported increased feeling of well-being (Copeland 1976).

Although Yoga has been used as a palliative for various physical problems, it is more effective when used to create a basic attitude toward health, namely, that we can control our own health. Yoga restores a state of balance in which the body can heal itself; it is a tool for creating a physical environment in which the body creates its own health.

Because Yoga influences the physical, mental, and spiritual aspects of one's nature, it is difficult to state that a particular pose (asana) is beneficial for any specific health problem. The beauty of the system is that it stimulates the sluggish aspects and quiets the overactive aspects of the organism. The poses (asanas) are homeostatic devices; they help restore the natural physiological balance of the body. This balance is a complex, elusive, and subtle blend of the interrelated functionings of body, mind, and spirit. In order to fit Yoga into a Western model of disease and health, the asanas will be presented here as specific therapeutic tools. However, it is strongly recommended that anyone interested in using Yoga as a therapeutic modality investigate the discipline as a whole.

In all Yoga poses, meticulous attention must be paid to proper structural alignment and to ensure that the body is stressed evenly. This is akin to keeping an automobile in alignment so that the tires wear evenly and energy is expended efficiently. Consultation with an experienced teacher is imperative to learn the precise points of each asana and the proper structural alignment of the body, and to understand the spirit of the practice. As in all health systems, there are contraindications for particular individuals. This article is meant to inspire women to seek guidance from a teacher and then apply Yoga to their own lives.

YOGA POSES FOR FEMALE DISCOMFORTS

Pregnancy

Learning erect posture can prevent the back pain so common in pregnancy. Lower back pain is often related to exaggerated lumbosacral angle commonly found in women (the angle between the lumbar vertebrae and the sacrum). This is an area of potential strain during the latter half of pregnancy when the heavy abdomen increases swayback (Noble, 1976). To help this problem, the Mountain Pose position is used.

The beginning pose of any Yoga practice should be the Mountain Pose (*Tadasana* in Sanskrit) (see Figure 19-1). This pose teaches correct pelvic alignment and encourages the abdominal muscles to support the bulging uterus, preventing fatigue of the uterine ligaments. One study comparing Yoga practitioners with nonpractitioners showed that practice made the performance of the asanas involve less muscular work (Gospal et al. 1975). Continued practice of the Mountain Pose will create a straighter body line during a woman's daily activities, reducing lower back strain.

Many pregnant women find the Cat Stretch (Pelvic Tilt) helpful in alleviating back pain. These poses are especially relieving at the end of the day when the weight of the uterus has been pulling down and forward for hours (see Figures 19-2 and 19-3). Pelvic Tilts bring the uterus into a good

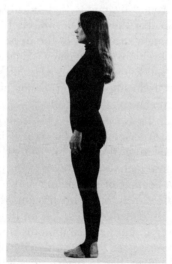

Christopher Wentworth

FIGURE 19-1. Mountain Pose.

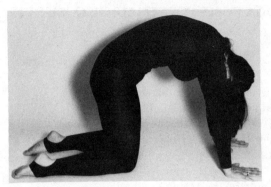

Christopher Wentworth

FIGURE 19-2. Cat Stretch—Step A.

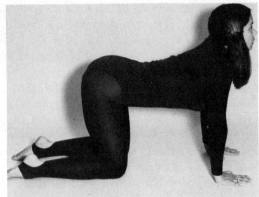

FIGURE 19-3. Cat Stretch—Step B.

Christopher Wentworth

position and work the round ligaments that aid in uterine support. These ligaments are unique in that they contain muscle fibers, which can cramp during pregnancy, causing a sharp pain in the upper groin.

Another common problem of pregnancy is nausea and indigestion. The Hero Pose (*Virasana*) (see Figure 19-6 on page 301) can beneficially affect the digestive system by reducing the compression of the stomach resulting from the enlarging abdomen (Iyengar 1966).

The importance of the Corpse Pose (*Savasana*) (see Figure 19-4) has been demonstrated by experiments in the beneficial effects of relaxation (Benson 1975). This pose brings the body into autonomic balance; physiological parameters of the pose include a decrease of respiratory rate, heart rate, and blood pressure. A feeling of well-being and contentment follows its practice. Long-term effects are to teach conscious relaxation, thus circumventing the deleterious effects that stress has on the body.

The Corpse Pose is an ideal preparation for labor. Maternal relaxation is correlated with a lessened need for pain-relieving drugs during labor. This pose complements all approaches to prepared childbirth. However, when practiced in the second and third trimester, the Corpse Pose should be done while lying on one's side rather than the back, using pillows as necessary to provide comfort. This side-lying position prevents any occurrence of the supine hypotension syndrome, which can result from the heavy weight of

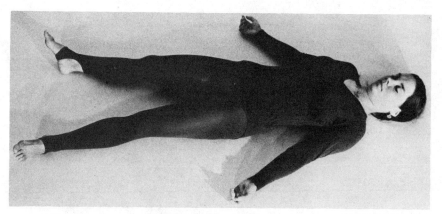

Christopher Wentworth

FIGURE 19–4. Corpse pose.

the uterus pressing on the maternal inferior vena cava artery, causing decreased maternal cardiac return and decreased oxygen to the fetus.

An interesting effect of a partially inverted pose during pregnancy concerns the prevention of breech births (DeSa Souza 1977). Reported at the World Conference of Gynecology and Obstetrics was a study of 744 breech babies, 88.7 percent of whom were maneuvered into a vertex position by having the mother lie on her back for 10 minutes on a hard surface with the pelvis raised by pillows to 9–12 inches above the head. This pose should be practiced twice daily on an empty stomach and should be begun at the 30th week of pregnancy and continued for 4 to 6 weeks. Because the uterus is higher than the head, the pose does not result in supine hypotension. This procedure should be used under the care of a qualified professional.

Postpartum

Yoga is an excellent postpartum approach to regaining strength and muscle tone and can be practiced as vigorously or as gently as the individual desires. Some long-time students of Yoga have begun practicing within 24 hours after a normal delivery and as little as 7 days after a Cesarean birth. Others prefer several months of rest. The major restriction is to avoid inverted (upside down) postures until the postpartum flow of blood is stopped, usually about four to six weeks.

Spinal twisting poses are good postpartum muscle strengtheners because they affect the oblique abdominals that have been stretched during pregnancy (see Figure 19-5). In contrast, the traditional sit-up exercise can strain the abdominals in their weakened postpartum state.

In these poses, the thigh presses against the lower abdomen, stimulating elimination from the intestines and bladder (Iyengar 1966). The direct

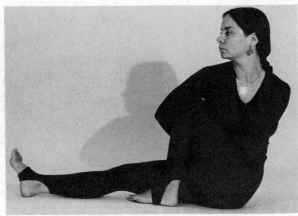

FIGURE 19–5. Spinal Twist.

Christopher Wentworth

pressure against the uterine muscle also aids involution (the return of the uterus to its nonpregnant size).

The problem of prolapsed uterus among older women is best cured by prevention. The best alternative poses are inverted ones in which the uterus is no longer falling down with gravity but moves "up" toward the diaphragm. (See discussion of the Shoulderstand under "Thyroid Problems" on page 303.)

Menstrual Problems

The Hero Pose, mentioned above as a good antidote for morning sickness (see Figure 19-6), can with a slight variation be used to alleviate menstrual cramps (see Figure 19-7). The pressure of the fist just inside the hip bones against the uterus helps the muscle relax, relieving pelvic congestion and inflammation that can contribute to discomfort.

Elevating the legs up the wall, especially with a weight on the abdomen, can also be helpful. (See the discussion under "Fatigue and Depression" below.)

Prevention of Arthritis

Some types of arthritis are caused by mechanical problems at weight-bearing joints, whereas other types like rheumatoid have a systemic component.

The standing poses of Yoga offer a wide variety of movements for the weight-bearing joints (see Figures 19-8 and 19-9). Standing poses include movements with the feet placed approximately three to five feet apart; these poses are beneficial for the maintenance of joint health in the feet, ankles, knees, and hips (Iyengar 1966).

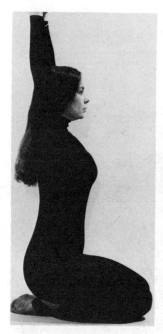
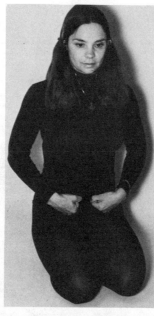
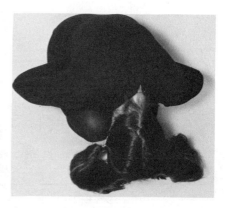

Christopher Wentworth

FIGURE 19–6. (*Left*) Hero pose.

FIGURE 19–7. (*Center and right*)
Hero pose variation.

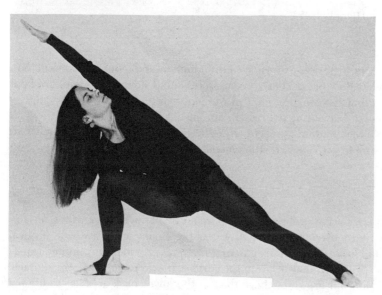

Carol Cavanaugh

FIGURE 19-8. Intensive side angle stretch.

These poses can prevent the development and exacerbation of degenerative arthritic changes often found in the joints. Yoga stresses that movement should be practiced evenly on both sides of the body, so that

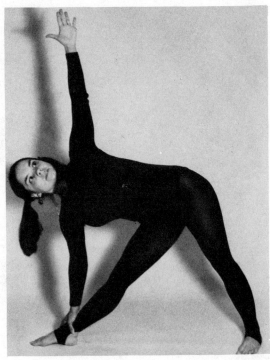

FIGURE 19-9. Triangle pose.

Carol Cavanaugh

complementary flexion-extension and adduction-abduction movements are attempted at the joints. Therefore, muscles on all sides of the joint are kept flexible so that the range of joint movement is free. This allows the joint to be used evenly, avoiding overuse in one plane. Keeping the joint free in all planes, plus maintaining muscle strength and integrity of the ligaments, is the best way to prevent arthritic changes.

Spinal Disc Problems

Disc problems account for about 10 percent of all lower back problems and are difficult to predict and treat. Even the final radical step of surgical removal and fusion of a spinal segment sometimes provides only limited relief.

Disc problems may occur in the cervical (neck) region or in the thoracic (chest) region but are rarer there than in the lower back area. A traditional treatment for lower backs is flexion exercises (forward stretches). These can alleviate symptomatic tightness but may exacerbate the problem because of the design of vertebral anatomy. The disc is the spongy structure between most movable vertebrae; and if there is a rupture of the disc from its normal position, causing pressure on a nearby nerve, that rupture is usually in a

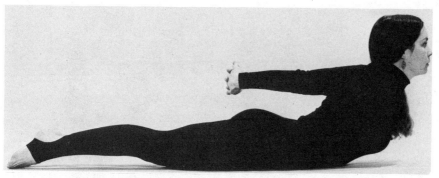

Carol Cavanaugh

FIGURE 19-10. Cobra pose.

posterior or backward direction. Forward flexion of the lumbar spine can overstretch supporting ligaments and muscles of the lower back and can increase pressure on the anterior disc, tending to push it backward. A posterior lateral direction is the most common one for slipped discs.

Backbends are superior to forward bends in preventing pressure on the back portion of the intervertebral disc (see Figure 19-10). By practicing backbends, the pressure is exerted on the disc on its posterior side so that movement is then forced forward, the opposite of the typical position. This may prevent the herniation of disc material backward. In addition, the general health of the disc is improved by movement in all planes, which stimulates fluid circulation in the disc, nourishing it and keeping it from becoming drier and flatter, which would make it more prone to slippage. Sitting in chairs tends to increase pressure on the disc and to flatten it out. To counteract this problem, backbending movements encourage a healthy vertebral column and perhaps can prevent the disk problems that many middle-aged women experience.

Thyroid Problems

Unique to the practice of Yoga is the emphasis on placing the body upside down in the Headstand (*Sirsasana*) and Shoulderstand (*Sarvangasana*).

Benefits attributed to the Shoulderstand are increased flow of venous blood from the lower extremities to the heart, and increased blood flow to the region of the thyroid gland (Funderburk 1977).

The highly vascular thyroid gland is believed to be regulated by the Shoulderstand (see Figure 19-11). This occurs because of the pressure of the chin against the gland during the pose and the sudden release as the student comes down, flooding the area with blood. Metabolism is beneficially effected by enhanced functioning of the thyroid.

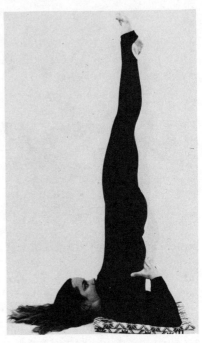

FIGURE 19-11. The shoulder stand.

Carol Cavanaugh

Pelvic Organs

Another possible benefit from inverting the body in the Headstand and Shoulderstand is the effect these poses have on the uterus and other abdominal organs. The effect that gravity, pregnancy, and childbirth have on these organs over the course of a life time perhaps can be ameliorated by allowing these organs to be free of gravity's effects for a few minutes every day during the practice of inverted poses. Perhaps a prolapsed uterus can thus be prevented. The Shoulderstand is also a useful preventative for varicose veins because it accentuates the venous drainage from the legs.

Upside-down poses are not recommended during heavy menstrual flow because the flow could move into the top of the uterus and then, upon standing, flow out the Fallopian tubes into the abdominal cavity. Although no cases of this occurrence have been reported, most women students avoid inverted poses during menstruation.

The Shoulderstand is also contraindicated in cases of high blood pressure; neck problems; infections of the ears, throat, or eyes; or in cases of obesity.

Fatigue and Depression

Backbends are believed to stimulate the adrenal glands, and therefore are antidotes to the fatigue so common among women (Iyengar 1966). Studies have demonstrated a rise in catecholamines after Yoga postures, including backbends (Udupa, Singh, and Settiwar 1971). These hormones increase blood pressure, stimulate the central nervous system, and increase metabolism and blood sugar levels.

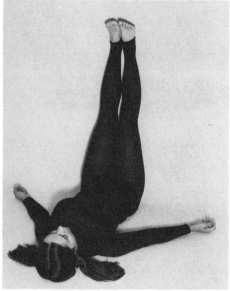

Carol Cavanaugh

FIGURE 19-12. Legs elevated at wall.

Backbends strengthen the long extensor muscles of the back (erector spinae muscles), which are important in maintaining good posture, as was discussed above under "Pregnancy." A slumped posture encourages depression and lethargy. An erect posture is correlated with alertness and energy; it allows the lungs to function more efficiently, ridding the body of excess carbon dioxide, which can depress the central nervous system.

A simple remedy for fatigue at the end of the day is to lie on the floor with the legs elevated up the wall. This enhances venous return from the legs and is excellent after standing for long hours (see Figure 19-12).

Depression and the decreased metabolism that often accompanies it can be alleviated by the daily practice of the Sun Salutation. This vigorous series of movements can be done slowly or quickly, but 10–15 of these has, as the name implies, a warming, stimulating effect on the body and an uplifting effect on the mind. See Figure 19-13.

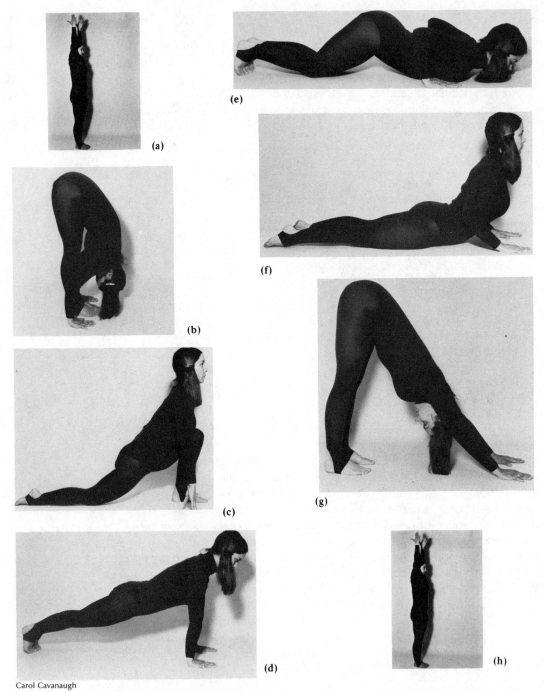

Carol Cavanaugh

FIGURE 19-13 (a–h). The author doing the sun salutation shortly after the birth of her child.

CONCLUSION

It should be remembered that isolated asanas cannot be used like prescriptions to treat specific diseases. If one is interested in improving health through yoga, it is necessary to undertake a well-rounded program of the asanas with the accompanying awareness of diet, relaxation, and breathing. With regular practice, profound changes in the physical and mental functioning can occur. The practice of Yoga results in self-understanding and a clearer view of the choices necessary for maintaining one's health.

See the following appendix to this chapter for a description of the various poses.

CHAPTER NINETEEN—APPENDIX

Pose Descriptions

Figure 19-1. Mountain Pose (*Tadasana*).   Stand tall and evenly on both feet, heels and big toes touching. Tighten knees and point them directly forward. Contract the buttocks, keep stomach in, chest forward, spine stretched up, neck straight, and chin tucked under. Do not bear the weight either on the heels or toes but distribute it evenly on the soles of the feet. Hold, breathing quietly.

Figures 19-2 and 19-3. Cat Stretch.   Kneel so that hands and feet are equidistant. Slowly lift the back up, arching like a cat; then drop the spine to a slight arch. Repeat ten times; inhale when dropping down; exhale when lifting up.

Figure 19-4. Hero Pose (*Virasana*).   Sit on the heels. Try to keep the feet as close together as possible, with toes pointing straight back and spinal column straight. Interlock the fingers and stretch arms straight over head, palms up. Hold, breathing deeply.

Figure 19-5. Corpse Pose (*Savasana*).   Lie on the floor with meticulous attention to the alignment of the body. Legs and arms are equidistant from the spine, hands turned up; the spine is straight, pelvis and shoulder girdles balanced, and chin tucked under. The entire body is profoundly relaxed; eyes are closed and breathing is long and slow, gradually becoming more shallow on its own.

Figure 19-6. Spinal Twist (*Marichyasana III*).   Sit with the left side near the wall, both legs stretched out and the spine straight. Bend the left knee nearer the wall, keeping the sole of the foot flat on the floor. The inner side of the left foot should touch the inner side of the right thigh. Use the right elbow to press against the left knee; place the right hand against the wall for support. The left hand is placed behind the trunk to help keep spine upright. Make sure the twist comes from as low in the spine as possible. There should be no space between the right armpit and the bent left knee. The right leg should remain straight and securely on the floor. Repeat the pose on the other side. Breathe deeply, exhaling on movement.

Figure 19-7. Hero Pose Variation (*Virasana*). Practice Hero Pose described previously, but place the fists just inside the hip bones and bend forward, exhaling, and pressing the fists into the abdomen. The buttocks should remain on the heels and the forehead rests on the floor. Hold, breathing quietly.

Figure 19-8. Intensive Side Angle Stretch (*Utthita Parsvakonasana*). Stand with feet 4 feet apart. Raise the arms sideways in line with the shoulder. Turn the right foot sideways 90 degrees to the right and the left foot in, 30 degrees to the right, keeping the left leg stretched out and tightened at the knee. Bend the right leg at the knee until the thigh and calf form a right angle and the right thigh is parallel to the floor. Place the right palm on the floor by the side of the right foot, the right armpit touching the outer side of the right knee. Stretch the left arm out over the left ear. Keep the head up. Move the chest up and back, bringing the chest, hips, and legs into a line. Hold, breathing deeply. Repeat on other side.

Figure 19-9. Triangle Pose (*Trikonasana*). Place the feet 3 feet apart. Raise the arms sideways in line with the shoulders. Turn right foot sideways 90 degrees to the right and left foot in, 30 degrees to the right, keeping the left leg stretched out and tightened at the knee. Bend the trunk sideways to the right, bringing the right palm near the right ankle. Do not bend the back but keep the spine in a straight line. Keep the right knee pointing directly over the right big toe, and do not let it turn in. Hold, breathe deeply, and repeat on other side.

Figure 19-10. Cobra (*Bhujangasana*). Lie on the floor face downwards; lift the body up from the trunk and throw the head back. Keep the feet together, knees and buttocks tight. Inhale; press the palms on the floor and pull the trunk up until the pubis is in contact with the floor, with the weight on the legs and palms. Exhale, hold.

Figure 19-11. Shoulderstand (*Salamba Sarvangasana*). Place a thick folded blanket on the floor. Lie so that the back is on the blanket but the head and neck are off the blanket. Bring the knees to the forehead. Raise hips from the floor and prop the hands under them by bending the arms at the elbows. Raise the trunk up perpendicularly supported by the hands until the chest touches the chin. Relax the neck. Only the back of the head, neck, shoulders, and backs of arms to the elbows should rest on the floor. Place hand in the middle of the back for support. Hold for 5 minutes with even breathing.

Figure 19-12. Legs Elevated at the Wall. Sit with the left shoulder near the wall and knees drawn to the chest. Simultaneously roll onto the back and swing the legs up the wall. The entire spine should be supported by the floor; this may necessitate moving a few inches away from the wall. Tuck the chin under and place arms comfortably at sides. To come out, bend the knees to the chest, roll onto the side, and sit up slowly.

Figure 19-13(a–g). Sun Salutation (*Surya Namaskar*). Begin by standing in Mountain Pose. Swing the arms up, stretch down, placing the hands even with the feet. Stretch one leg back; then bring the other to match it. Place the chest on the floor, and tightening the buttocks, lift the spine up using the arms as little as possible. Reverse by lifting the buttocks up and pushing with the arms. Bring one leg forward, then the other to match it. Come up with a straight back, arms to the side, and stand in Mountain Pose. Breathing should be normal, with emphasis on exhaling with movement, with the exception of pictures (a) and (f). Repeat as many as ten times.

REFERENCES

Benson, Herbert. *The Relaxation Response*. New York: William Morrow & Co., Inc., 1975.

Copeland, Paul. "The Physiology of Yoga." Unpublished manuscript, 1976.

De Sa Souza, Julet, *Obstetrics and Gynecology News*, January 1, 1977.

Funderburk, James, *Science Studies Yoga: A Review of Physiological Data*. Glenview, Ill.: Himalayan International Institute of Yoga Science and Philosophy, 1977.

Gallup, George. *Gallup Poll*. Princeton, N.J.: American Institute of Public Opinion, February 19, 1978.

Gopal, K. S. et al., "The Effects of Yogasanas on Muscular Tone and Cardio-Respiratory Adjustments," *Yoga Life*, 6, no. 5 (1975), 3–11.

Iyengar, B. K. S., *Light on Yoga*. New York: Schocken Books, Inc., 1966.

Noble, Elizabeth, *Essential Exercises for the Childbearing Year*. Boston: Houghton Mifflin Company, 1976.

Udupa, K. N., R. H. Singh, and R. M. Settiwar, "Studies on Physiological, Endocrine and Metabolic Response to the Practice of Yoga in Young Normal Volunteers," *Journal of Research in Indian Medicine*, 6, no. 3 (1971), 345–53.

Chapter Twenty

AEROBIC EXERCISE AND WOMEN

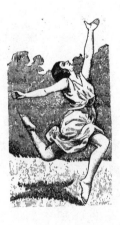

Joan Ullyot

Aerobic, meaning "with oxygen," used to refer to the growth needs of certain microorganisms. Since 1968, however, thanks to the efforts of Dr. Kenneth Cooper, most people who hear the word *aerobic* think immediately of exercise rather than of bacteria. Aerobic exercises, as defined by Cooper, are those that promote the uptake and utilization of oxygen by the working muscles of the body (1978). Regular practice of such exercises automatically improves and conditions the primary oxygen-delivery systems, which include the heart, lungs, and circulation.

Exercises that have the great aerobic training effect are running or jogging, bicycling, swimming, and cross-country skiing. These activities all qualify as full-fledged sports rather than simply *exercise*, a word that carries unpleasant connotations for many readers. One popular and highly successful program of vigorous aerobic exercises set to music calls itself "aerobic dancing" to avoid discouraging recruits. Whatever they are called, all aerobic activities have in common the ability to maintain heart rates and respiration at a high enough level to stimulate adaptation of the oxygen-delivery systems to the increased stress load.

TRAINING PROGRAM

Cooper calls this adaptation the "training effect." Since he first described this effect in his 1968 book, *Aerobics*, much has been learned about the physiological mechanisms involved and the best way to achieve conditioning

311

in various sports. Cooper observed that two factors are involved in training: *time* (duration) and *intensity* (usually speed). In his original system, points were awarded on the basis of these two factors. For example, you could earn the recommended minimum of 30 points per week by running six miles at a pace of 8 minutes per mile, or ten miles at a pace of 10 minutes per mile. The first option would take you 48 minutes per week (preferably divided up into three or four segments of exercise), whereas the second would require 1 hour and 45 minutes of your time, similarly spread out over several days. This system is not for the "weekend athlete"; you must exercise at least every other day or the hard-won training effect is lost.

The original Cooper "point system" had certain drawbacks. The principle concern of some critics was that the emphasis on speed might be detrimental to precisely the type of overworked, compulsive, hard-driving person who most needed the cardiac conditioning. In other words, the aggressive, middle-aged, would-be jock would be tempted to get his point quota as quickly as possible, by running *faster*. At 6 minutes per mile, he could get his 30 points in a scant 30 minutes, or 10 minutes per outing! At this point, however, he would be getting minimal benefit for his efforts, since 10 minutes of exercise, however vigorous, is too short a time to create a good training effect.

In fact, many joggers, especially men, did just that: pushed too hard. The result was injury or pain and boredom. Either way, the tendency to overdo led to early dropouts. Those that persisted, however, including most women, found that regular aerobic exercise led to a host of physiological and psychological benefits that were unsuspected until fitness became a mass movement.

Women learned that maximum speed does not confer maximum benefits. The competitive runner, racing along at top speed, is actually performing less efficiently, in terms of oxygen uptake, than the person who runs only at 70–85 percent of maximal effort. Most runners today use the "talk test" as a guide instead of the pulse rate; if you can converse fairly comfortably while running, rather than gasp for breath, you are within the target zone and are getting maximum conditioning for your efforts.

RESULTS

The primary physiological effects of aerobic exercise are easily observable and generally occur within the first six or eight weeks of workouts. The heart becomes a more efficient pump, increasing its stroke volume; that is, more blood is pumped out per beat. At rest, therefore, the heart pumps less to circulate a given amount of blood, so the *resting pulse* falls to levels that traditional textbooks might characterize as "pathological bradycardia," but which are in fact nothing dangerous at all. The fit individual almost always has a true resting pulse under 60 beats per minute, and not uncommonly as low as 35.

Simultaneously, the amount of blood and oxygen that can be pumped to working muscles increases dramatically. Fit people perform a given work load at a lower heart rate than the unfit.

MEDICAL ASPECTS

The medical profession is primarily interested in aerobic exercise as a possible means to help maintain optimum health, or even to restore good health to victims of heart attacks, emphysema, and other cardiorespiratory diseases. Most medical research has concentrated, therefore, on measuring changes in fitness in various populations participating in different aerobic conditioning programs, or on statistical analysis of cardiovascular "incidents" occurring in groups of subjects with known differences in fitness.

Cardiovascular

Two recent and exciting studies seem to demonstrate that aerobically fit individuals do, indeed, have a certain degree of protection against coronary artery disease and stroke. These two studies are: (1) Dr. Kenneth Cooper's long-term study of participants in his own aerobics program in Dallas (1978), and (2) epidemiologist Dr. Ralph Paffenbarger's study of 10,000 Harvard alumni (1975). Both studies indicate that the protective effects of fitness are not only measurable but also independent of other known "risk factors." It is known that runners, as a group, tend to be lean nonsmokers with low blood pressure; Cooper and Paffenbarger give evidence, however, that fitness reduces the risk of cardiovascular disease independently of these characteristics.

Several pioneering programs of cardiac rehabilitation through aerobic exercise have been developed to emphasize gradual reconditioning of the injured heart, always staying within an individual's "safe" target zone. Many of these patients have astounded conventional medical circles by running full-length marathons (26.2 miles).

Psychological

Participants in aerobic exercise almost unanimously report that their activity confers both energy and peace of mind, an outlet for the stresses and tensions of everyday life. These observations are taken seriously by many doctors.

One running psychiatrist, Dr. Thaddeus Kostrubala, author of *The Joy of Running* (1976), uses running as therapy for patients with both schizophrenia and manic-depressive disorders. This new therapy has proved so successful that Kostrubala now has a unique training program for "running therapists" (ibid.).

Recent neurological research on endogenous (internally produced) chemicals called "endorphins" provides a possible explanation for this exercise-induced calmness and sense of well-being, which is sometimes misleadingly referred to as "Runner's High." The endorphins are hormonelike substances that bind onto and block the brain's receptor sites for morphine and similar narcotics. It is now known that endorphin levels rise dramatically during exercise, and it is suspected that this may be a physiological correlate of the mental effects reported by runners.

Blood Chemistry

Other research has focused on exercise-induced changes in systems other than the cardiovascular one that monopolized early attention. Fit individuals have been found to show a host of deviations from the sedentary "norms." Dr. Peter Wood of Stanford's Heart Disease Prevention Program has documented the high levels of HDL (High Density Lipoprotein) cholesterol that occur in regular runners of all ages and both sexes (1980). HDL, unlike total cholesterol, appears statistically to be a protective factor against coronary artery disease. Male runners over 50 frequently have HDL levels as high as young women in their twenties (a group with very low average risk of heart attack). The HDL levels found in female runners are even higher. The level of exercise necessary to achieve such beneficial levels is not prohibitively high; as little as 30 minutes of running three times a week seems to be almost as effective as intense marathon training (60 miles or more weekly).

Numerous other changes have been reported in the blood chemistry of persons who do regular aerobic exercise. For example, triglycerides and total cholesterol tend to be lower than those of sedentary controls, while certain serum enzymes (SGOT, LDH, and CPK) can be far above the so-called normal range. These latter changes can be deceptively alarming to physicians unfamiliar with the effects of a rigorous training program, so it is wisest for the athlete to seek medical advice only from a sports-oriented doctor!

Long-term study of the blood-chemistry "profiles" of healthy and active people, carried out at San Francisco's Institute of Health Research, shows an intriguing pattern: internal *control* of blood chemistry levels seems to be much tighter in the active. For example, a sedentary but healthy person might have triglyceride levels ranging from 70 to 140 on repeated testing—all in the "normal range." Yet multiple samples from a well-conditioned runner may range only between 56 and 60, a variation entirely ascribable to laboratory procedures. This tight internal control is considered one of the hallmarks of optimum health.

Metabolism

There is considerable general evidence in the medical literature that aerobic activity improves the metabolism of both fats and carbohydrates, even in healthy people. In those with disordered metabolism, such as hypoglycemics and diabetics, the improvement may be clinically observed; many diabetics, for example, can reduce or completely eliminate their insulin dosage by running. Runners with such problems can even complete marathons successfully if they learn to recognize the symptoms of early hypoglycemia and carry a squeeze bottle with juice or some other sweet drink.

Studies on endurance-trained laboratory animals show that metabolic changes occur within the muscle fibers themselves in response to aerobic conditioning. The muscle cells become packed with mitochondria and their associated respiratory enzymes; myoglobin stores increase; and enzymes that oxidize fats replace those that prefer carbohydrate as fuel. Since it established that prolonged muscular contraction such as is required in long-distance swimming, running, and cycling depends on this ability to metabolize fat efficiently, these experiments indicate that training produces the necessary changes at the cellular level.

Other Medical Applications

Much research remains to be done. Although aerobic exercise has been touted as a cure for countless disorders ranging from acne to migraine headaches, there are at present few controlled studies and little scientific basis for guaranteeing any such cures. However, considered and prudent medical judgment can certainly recommend aerobic sports as beneficial, both physically and psychologically. We know of no medical drawbacks to aerobic activity, provided the participant doesn't get carried away by the excitement of the sport and sustain some injury of overenthusiasm! For women in particular, vigorous aerobic exercise appears to be far more effective therapy than the hormones, sleeping pills, tranquilizers, and other nostrums that doctors often overprescribe for assorted "female ills."

Although there are as yet few studies of patients with documented and dramatic improvements, this situation should improve rapidly as increasing numbers of women are drawn to distance running and similar sports. There are already countless testimonials from women who have slimmed down, reshaped their bodies (by losing fat), and eliminated headaches, constipation, and insomnia by exercise. Since exercise is healthy and safe, unlike most other therapeutic modalities, surely it is worth a try!

Menopausal Symptoms

Many women runners of menopausal age report that the classic symptoms such as "hot flashes" bother them far less than they expected from their sedentary friends' experience. A large number of these active women are reluctant to try estrogen replacement therapy because of its dangerous side effects, and opt instead simply to ease their way through menopause by running more.

In this regard, recent studies show that exercise is a very important therapeutic tool in preventing the osteoporosis, or bone thinning, that plagues many postmenopausal women. Runners and other active women develop denser bones, whereas inactivity promotes thinning and consequent stress fractures.

Headaches

"Of course, running cures migrane!" This statement was made to this author by Dr. Otto Appenzeller, a neurologist and editor of the journal *Headache*. Although acknowledging that individual experiences did not constitute proof of the theory, we went on to speculate as to the possible physiological basis for the frequent dramatic "cures" of migraine. Since running seems to alleviate the headaches of hangover and tension as well as migraine, but has no effect on sinus-type headaches and others, perhaps the improved circulation and lowered blood pressure found in regular runners are responsible for this improvement in their health. Again, because the exercise therapy is safe, many doctors prescribe running before resorting to medications for headache. The improvement rate is not 100 percent, but it is high enough to arouse interest in the medical community.

Menstrual Cramps

In the old days, girls used severe cramps as a valid excuse to get out of P.E. class. There was a vague superstition to the effect that exercise could somehow strain or damage the "female organs." In fact, with more women involved in sports and reluctant to miss out on a rewarding activity, the consensus is that aerobic exercise actually alleviates cramps and reduces dependency on drugs for relief.*

*Athletic exercise dramatically reduces the incidence of headache and tension associated with menstruation. (Timonen, Sakari, and Benrdt Procopé, "Premenstrual Syndrome and Physical Exercise," *Aeta Obstet. Gynec. Scandanavia*, vol. 50 (1971).

Similarily, one gynecologist warned that running might cause "pro-lapsed uterus" and was therefore an inappropriate activity for women (or for anyone—men might develop hernias or scotal sag)! In actual fact, athletic women have the tightest pelvic musculature, and hence the best support to their "female organs," of anyone. Their incidence of uterine prolapse (sag) and associated stress incontinence is in fact far lower than is found in sedentary females. This observation has led many gynecologists to prescribe a combination of running and pelvic floor exercises (Kegel exercises) as a successful alternative to surgery for such conditions.

Pregnancy

Pregnant women who are already active in an aerobic sport have been encouraged, in recent years, to continue their exercise program as long as they feel comfortable. All indications so far are that women who do stay active and fit throughout pregnancy have easier pregnancies and much faster postpartum recovery than their sedentary counterparts.

CONCLUSION

In sum, aerobic exercise seems not to be some modern fad indulged in by a handful of "health nuts," but rather a return to a deep-seated evolutionary physiological pattern that is essential to the maintenance of optimal health. We are at lasting returning to the ancient Greek ideal of the sound body as a necessary corollary to a sound mind.

Editor's Note

Recent research conducted by Dr. Joseph Cannon at the University of Michigan indicates that a strenuous workout that raises body temperature can sterilize bacteria and stimulate the body's natural defenses against disease. Heavy exercise is similar to a fever in its ability to reset the internal thermostat upward to create a hostile environment for bacteria. White blood cells are increased and cause an increase in endogenous pyrogen, a protein that kills off bacteria.

REFERENCES

Cooper, Kenneth, *Aerobics*. New York: Bantam Books, Inc., 1968.

———, *The Aerobic Way*. New York: Bantam Books, Inc., 1978.

Kostrubala, Thaddeus, *The Joy of Running*. Philadelphia: J. B. Lippincott Company, 1976.

Paffenbarger, Ralph S., and W. E. Hale, "Work Activity and Coronary Heart Mortality," *New England Journal of Medicine*, 292 (1975), 455–64.

Wood, Peter, *Run to Health*. New York: Charter Books, 1980.

SUGGESTED READINGS

Astrand, Per-Olof, and Kaare Rodahl, *Textbook of Work Physiology*. New York: McGraw-Hill Book Company, 1977. The "Bible" for exercise physiologists and anyone interested in the processes by which the body moves, breathes, and plays. Scholarly and detailed; more technical than Sharkey's or Cooper's books (see below).

Cooper, Kenneth, *Aerobics*. New York: Bantam Books, Inc., 1968. *Aerobics* lucidly describes the physiological effects of training and gives the original testing system and exercise schedules with point values.

———, *The Aerobic Way*. New York: Bantam Books, Inc., 1978. Gives medical data on the health benefits of fitness.

Kostrubala, Thaddeus, *The Joy of Running*. Philadelphia: J. B. Lippincott Company, 1976. Confessions of a psychiatrist who was once a coronary-courting, middle-aged fat boy, but transformed himself into a marathoner who now uses running as therapy for psychosis and depression.

Mango, Richard, Peter Jokl, and O. William Dayton, *The Runner's Complete Medical Guide*. New York: Summit Books, 1979.

Milvy, Paul, ed., *The Long Distance Runner*. New York: Urizen Books, 1978. Subtitled "A Definitive Study," this book lives up to its name. It collects the physiological, medical, epidemiological, and psychological studies presented at the 1977 symposium on "The Marathon."

Paffenbarger, Ralph S., and W. E. Hale. "Work Activity and Coronary Heart Mortality," *New England Journal of Medicine*, 292 (1975), 455–64. Epidemiological evidence for the heart-protective effect of physical conditioning.

Sharkey, Brian, *Physiology of Fitness*. Champaign, Ill.: Human Kinetics Publishers, 1979. A well-referenced overview, detailed, but aimed at the intelligent nonscientist.

Spears, Carola, *The ABC's of Breathing*. New York: Harper & Row, Publishers, Inc.

Ullyot, Joan. *Women's Running*. Mountain View, Calif.: World Publications, 1976. Basic "how-to" about running and racing, aimed specifically at women, with a useful self-help medical section

———, *Running Free*. New York: G. P. Putman's Sons, 1980. This book deals more extensively with physical and psychological questions of concern to athletic women, and with some of the medical controversies concerning fitness and health.

Women's Sports Magazine. Mt. Morris, Ill.

Wood, Peter D., *Run to Health*. New York: Charter Books. A well-written and authoritative guide to running and its health benefits, by the man who discovered several of them.

Chapter Twenty-One

HEAT THERAPY AND WOMEN—SWEAT BATHING

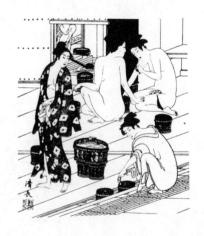

Mikkel Aaland

HISTORICAL SIGNIFICANCE AND WIDESPREAD PRACTICE OF SWEAT BATHING

Sweat bathing is an age-old practice of heating and cleansing the body, still found today among a large part of the earth's population. From Scandinavia to Mexico, many cultures recognize the power of the bath to cleanse and repair the body, mind, and soul.

The sweat bath produces an artificial "fever" and urges every organ of the body into action. Although outwardly relaxed, the inner organs are as active as though one were jogging. The body is being cleansed from the inside out by the skin, the body's largest and most complex organ, and its excretion, sweat.

The oldest known medical document, the *Ayurveda*, appeared in Sanskrit in 568 B.C. and considered sweating so important to health that it prescribed the sweat bath and 13 other methods for inducing sweat. Throughout history, physicians have extolled the medicinal value of the sweat bath in its various forms, such as the Finnish sauna, Russian *bania*, Islamic *hammam*, and the American Indian sweat lodge. (See Figures 21-1 through 21-4.) Today, enthusiasts claim that beyond being relaxing, the sauna gives relief from the common cold, arthritis, headaches, hangovers, and many other ailments. Even if these claims are somewhat exaggerated, medical evidence shows that bathing temperatures of 90° (192°F) has a profoundly beneficial effect on the body. Medical researchers in Finland, Germany, and recently, the United States, have made intensive studies on the phenomenon of sweating and heating the body. Since much of this research is still in progress, many results are still inconclusive.

Among those who believe in the beneficial effects of sweat baths are virtually all North and South American Indian tribes, who have utilized

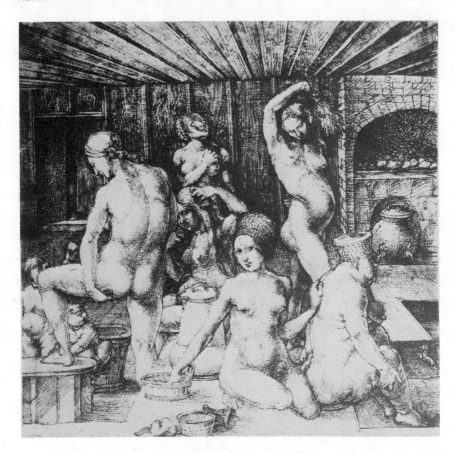

FIGURE 21-1. The woman's bath. (Dürer 1495).

sweats for purification or hygiene purposes. One tribe of American Indians believed that a friendly spirit dwelt inside the sweat lodge rocks and was released through the vapor to penetrate the skins of bathers and to drive out sickness. As a further example, a Finnish proverb says: "If a sick person is not cured by tar, spirits, or sauna, then they will die (Viherjuuri 1952). And an English visitor to Russia a few centuries back, observed:

> In general, the common Russian uses but few medicines; supplying in their place in all cases by the *sweating bath*, a practice universal among them. . . . It is not doubted that the Russians owe their longevity, their robust state of health, their little disposition to certain moral diseases and their happy and cheerful temper, most to the baths. [Tooke 1979]

The largest Mayan dictionary, complied shortly after the Conquest of Mexico, gives the word for sweat bath as *Zumpul-che*, "a bath for women after

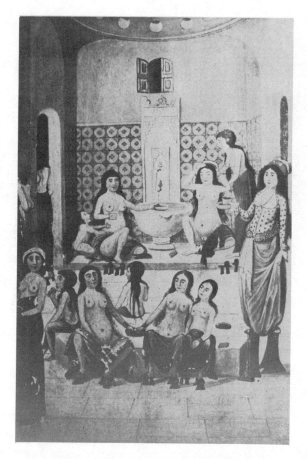

FIGURE 21-2. Rendering of a women's hammam from a folio in the Istanbul
        library, 1791.

childbirth and for sick persons used to cast out disease in their bodies"
(Cresson 1938).

Although modern science has its analytical reasons for the benefits of
sweat bathing, historical explanations were often poetic and imaginative.
Fire is an important element in all sweat baths. Whether shining in heaven
or burning in hell, fire has always commanded reverence. For stealing fire
from the gods and delivering it to humans, Prometheus was credited by the
Greeks with the founding of civilization. The sweat house, by capturing and
controlling the awesome power of flame, became a sacred shrine among
most sweat bath cultures.

When looked on in this spiritual light, the importance of sweat bathing
to many primitive cultures becomes clear. A bather absorbed the heat of a

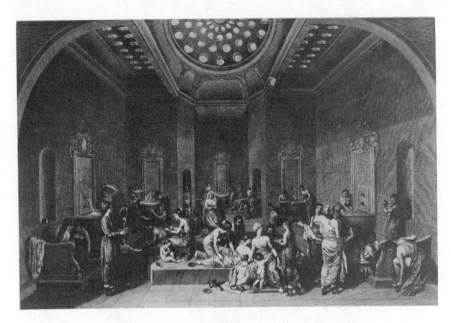

FIGURE 21-3. Eighteenth century women's bath.

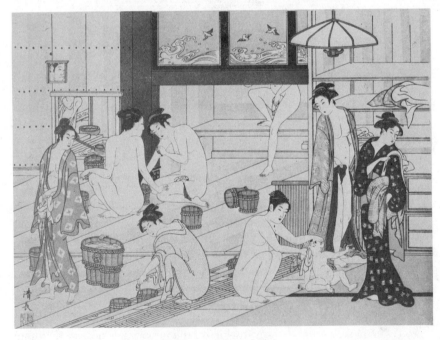

FIGURE 21-4. The power of this kiln bath equals hundreds of medicines.

sweat bath, merging body and fire, and thereby reenacted Creation. In both Russian and American Indian folklore, there are tales of "God" in a sweat bath creating the first man and woman through drops of sweat.

The sweat bath was also often associated with rebirth. The warm, dark moist ambiance inside a sweat bath is easily likened to a womb, even the womb of Mother Earth herself. A tired, dirty bather climbs into the confines of the sweat bath, assumes a fetal position (especially in the small American Indian sweat lodge), sweats out physical and mental impurities, and emerges refreshed and cleansed—reborn.

MEDICAL RESEARCH ON PHYSIOLOGICAL BENEFITS OF SWEAT BATHS

Sources of modern medical information on sweat baths come primarily from West Germany, Finland, and Sweden—perhaps because of a high incidence of sweat bath use in these countries. Unfortunately, because of the relatively low use of sweat bathing in this country, the health potential of the sweat bath is hardly known to the American public. There is a dearth of medical research and professional interest in sweat bathing in America today. At a recent International Sauna Congress attended in West Germany by medical researchers and physicians from around the world, not one American doctor attended.

These researchers have explored almost every aspect of sweat bathing, from careful analysis of the composition of sweat, to the more general effects of heating the body. The sauna or hot-air bath differs sharply from the hot-water bath or hot tub, which has a distinctly different history and physiological effect since hot water baths do not allow the beneficial effects of sweating. As the individual sits in the heat of the sweat bath, the capillaries dilate, permitting increased flow of blood to the skin. Thus the bather's skin becomes red, and the heart is pressed into a faster pace to keep up with the additional demands for blood. Some studies observed lowered blood pressure as the result of relaxed blood vessel walls. Heat-sensitive nerve endings produce acetycholine, a chemical that activates the 2.3 million sweat glands embedded in the skin. Impurities in the liver, kidneys, stomach, muscles, brain, and most other organs are flushed out at a faster rate by the increased flow of body fluids. The skin and kidneys filter these wastes, excreting them in sweat and urine (Hasan, Karvonen, and Püronen 1966).

It is common knowledge that sweating is as essential to our health as eating and breathing. Because the skin eliminates, it is sometimes called the "third kidney." But it is far more complex than the kidney or any other organ except the brain. It is composed of blood vessels, nerve endings, vessels for carrying lymph, pigmentation, oil glands, hair follicles, cells that waterproof and deny entry to bacteria, and, of course, the tubular, coiled sweat glands. It is so important that death by accumulated poisons occur in a matter of hours if the skin, and its sweat packages, are smothered.

Sweat accomplishes three important things: (1) it rids the body of wastes, (2) it regulates the critical temperature of the body at 37°C, and (3) it helps keep the skin clean and pliant. It is significant to note that in this sedentary age, antiperspirants, smog, synthetic clothing, and a physically idle life style all conspire to clog skin pores and inhibit the healthy flow of sweat.

The sweat glands are regulated by the autonomic nervous system. However, this function has ceased to operate smoothly today since modern man surrounds himself with artificial heating and cooling devices. This breakdown has resulted in the skin not being able to perform its backup function for the overworked kidneys. When the skin is not working properly as an organ of elimination, skin discharge occurs. All skin diseases, according to Oriental medicine, can be originally traced back to kidney malfunction (Delavgre 1976).

Ninety-nine percent of what sweat brings to the surface is water. The remaining 1 percent is mostly undesirable wastes. One such waste is salt. Ridding the body of excessive salt carried by sweat is generally believed to be beneficial for cases of mild hypertension. A metabolic byproduct, urea, is also partially excreted through the skin. If not disposed of regularly, urea can accumulate and cause headaches and nausea. In extreme cases, vomiting, coma, and even death can result.

Sweat also drives out lactic acid, another metabolic waste, which causes stiff muscles and contributes to general fatigue.

American researchers have found that sweat bathing flushes out toxic metals such as copper, lead, zinc, and mercury, which the body absorbs in polluted environments. During a 15-minute sauna, sweating can perform the heavy metal excretion that would take the kidneys 24 working hours (Sunderman et al. 1974; Hohnadel et al. 1973). In fact, sweat is such an effective detoxifier that some physicians have recommended home saunas to supplement kidney machines (Synder 1966). And some mental hospitals have used saunas in their rehabilitation programs to pacify patients.

HEAT DESTROYS BACTERIA, VIRUSES, AND CANCER CELLS

Thousands of years ago Hippocrates wrote, "Give me a fever and I can cure any disease." Generations of medical people after Hippocrates have sought this magic "fever." Today, one of the hottest areas of cancer research centers on radical methods of inducing hyperthermia: these include using extracorporeally heated blood, microwaves, ultrasound, or short waves to heat the body to a temperature of 42°C. At this temperature, some types of cancerous cells are found to die sooner than normal healthy cells ("Hyperthermia, Hottest News in Cancer Therapy" 1979).

Research shows that sauna/sweat bathing raises the surface temperature of the skin as much as 10°C and the inner temperature up to 3°C (ibid.). This slight heat increase is enough to kill many bacterial and viral agents that do not survive well at higher body temperatures. It could be also that damaged cells repair themselves quicker in this fever condition due to the increased metabolic rate; recovery from illness then comes easier and quicker.

In men, because of the heat, sperm count slightly decreases during sauna bathing, but "not enough for effective birth control." One hour after sauna, sperm count returns to normal (Procope 1965).

The inner body temperature rise also affects the function of important endocrine glands, the pituitary in particular. The pituitary is known as the master gland because its hormones regulate both metabolism and the activity of other glands such as the thyroid, adrenal, ovaries, and testes. Urged by the heat, the pituitary accelerates the body's metabolism and affects the interplay of several of the body's hormones. An increase in the secretion of the growth hormone is one result. "The growth hormone," suggests one study, "is not only responsible for growth during adolescence but it also stimulates general body repair, perhaps one answer to the question why sauna bathing seems to strengthen the body constitution" (Syvalahti et al. 1974).

As body temperature rises, the oxygen needs of the body increase by about 20 percent, so the lungs, another important eliminator of body wastes, join in the body's quickened pace. Clogged respiratory passages are also opened by heat, giving relief from colds and other minor respiratory problems. However, medical people do *not* recommend sauna/sweat bathing for those suffering from pneumonia or other acute respiratory diseases. In some sweat baths where the humidity is too high, the lungs' rapid exchange of carbon dioxide for oxygen may be hindered. Water condenses on the tiny alveoli where the oxygen-CO_2 exchange takes place, and breathing can be slightly more difficult. On the other hand, there is more danger if the air is too dry, as occurs in many American saunas. Mucous membranes may become dry and damaged in this condition.

When the body is slowly cooled, the effects of heat are reversed—the heart calms, sweat pores close, dilated blood vessels contract, and body temperature returns to normal. The German Sauna Society recommends a warm footbath at this point to reopen constricted blood vessels. The combination of sweating and cooling conditions the body, and a well-tuned body is more resistant to colds, disease, and infection. Abrupt cooling brought on by a plunge into snow or icy water obviously creates a more dramatic effect; for this reason, people with weak constitutions should avoid rapid cooling.

The typical body is 60 percent water by weight, and any kilo loss noticed after sweating will be the result of lost water and thus will be promptly regained. However, sweat baths can have an indirect effect on weight loss. Sitting exposed in the sweat bath, a bather becomes fully aware of the body's condition. It's hard to hide a bulging belly or flabby muscles and self-improvement may be inspired.

POSITIVE EFFECTS OF NEGATIVE IONS

Physiologically, the presence of negative ions in a sweat bath is as important as the heat. The discovery of negative ions in certain types of saunas a few years ago became headline news in Finland. Until then, the healing power of the sauna was attributed to relaxation and increased circulation. Now, the identification of negative ions adds startling new possibilities.

Since the early 1950s, scientists have suspected that ions play an important role in how the body functions and in how we feel. Research has shown that an abundance of negative ions in the air we breathe is highly beneficial, whereas a lack of ions or a higher ratio of positive to negative can cause physical harm. The role played by ions in everyday life has become intensely topical among researchers in the medical profession (Soyka 1977; Teeri 1974).

An ion is simply a molecule with an electric charge, either positive or negative. Ionization, or ion formation, occurs when enough energy acts on a molecule to cause it to discharge an electron. Because electrons carry a negative charge, the molecule stripped off an electron has a greater positive charge and becomes a positive ion. The lost electron scoots around loose until it attaches itself to another molecule, which causes the new molecule to become negatively charged—a negative ion.

Radioactive substances in the earth's crust and cosmic rays cause most ionization, but fire, crashing water (like waterfalls and surf), and plants during photosynthesis can produce negative ions as well. Europeans take ion depletions seriously, and simple negative ion generators have been installed in many businesses, banks, hospitals, passenger cars, and even airliner cockpits. Furthermore, in this country, Europe, and the Soviet Union, negative ion therapy has been used in treatments to help burn victims heal faster, to cure respiratory diseases, to rid the body of general infections, and even to check the spread of some cancers.

Conversely, scientists have found that if the air is charged with too few negative ions and too many positives, we become anxious, fatigued, and tense. This condition is known as "poi-son poisoning" and often occurs as the result of weather disturbances, central air conditioning, smog, and driving too long within the confines of an automobile. Poi-son poisoning has, in fact, been linked to heart attacks, aggravated asthma, migraine headaches, insomnia, rheumatism, arthritis, hay fever, and most allergies.

SIGNIFICANCE OF SWEAT BATHING FOR WOMEN'S HEALTH

For women, sweat bathing has always had special significance, historically and medically. In Islamic countries where women traditionally were home-bound, the *hammam* (sweat bath) was the only sanctioned public meeting place. The hammam became such an important part of a woman's life that if her husband were to deny her visits to the hamman, she had grounds for divorce. In Mexico, Indian women use the *temescal* commonly after childbirth. Oscar Lewis wrote in 1951:

> The *temescal*, which is still widely used even by those women who go to doctors, is usually given eight days after delivery, though some midwives give it after fifteen days. Most women do not take their first *temescal* until after bleeding has stopped.

Finnish women went to the sauna before marriage as a purification ritual. Birthing also took place in the sauna. John Virtanen, a Finnish writer, describes his own birth in a sauna:

> The sauna would provide the warmth, the quiet, the peaceful though primitive environment in which to give birth. The midwife (who accompanyed my mother) washed the baby boy, and there I saw my first candlelight and cried my first sound. [1979]

Sauna and Pregnancy

In today's culture, American women and medical professionals have relatively little experience with sauna and pregnancy. What scientific information that is available is often incomplete or, in some cases, misleading.

An example of misleading information took place a few years ago when researchers from the University of Washington School of Medicine tried to link sauna bathing with anencephaly, a condition where babies are born without brains. In this study, 63 anencephalic pregnancies were restrospec-tively studied. Seven women (11 percent) gave positive histories of hyperther-mia sometime during the first trimester of pregnancy, near the time of fetal anterior neural-groove closure. Most were due to fever, but in two instances, the presumed hyperthermia was thought to be due to sauna bathing (Miller 1978). The restrospective design of this study and lack of follow-up, however, make it impossible to conclude that sauna bathing or even hyperthermia was the cause of the anencephaly. Yet, as a result, many doctors now indiscriminately discourage sauna bathing during all phases of pregnancy, even during normal pregnancies when the sauna could conceivably make the pregnancy easier.

This report from Washington was hotly contested at the 1978 Interna-tional Sauna Congress. In a paper presented to the Congress, Dr. Soiva of the State Maternity Hospital in Helsinki presented statistics that cited Finland as having one of the lowest anencephaly rates in the world—0.32 percent (Rapola, Saxen, and Granroth 1978). "Finnish women bathe regularly in the sauna, even during early pregnancy," the report read, "and if the sauna were dangerous, as the Washington study implies, Finland should have a high rate of anencephaly, which it does not" (ibid.).

Dr. Soiva cited studies that suggest that the sauna may be beneficial for normal pregnancies because of its general conditioning effects and the removal of toxins from the body. He also found that after childbirth, sauna bathing increased lactation. This may be because the milk-producing mammary gland is a modified type of sweat gland.

Dr. Soiva's advice was:

> If the sauna is taken properly, there are no risks for women with normal pregnancies. However, in cases of toxemia, hypertension, anemia, chronic placental insufficiency and the threat of premature birth, sauna should be avoided or taken in moderation. [Ibid.]

Dr. Soiva's advice applies to women who have a history of sauna bathing before pregnancy and who know how to properly use sauna. However, it is believed that sauna can stimulate labor—a large percentage of Finnish women reportedly have given birth on a Sunday or Monday following traditional bathing days (Soiva et al. 1963).

Effect on Menstruation and Menopause

Can the sauna alleviate some of the discomfort associated with menstruation and menopause? No specific research has been done on this subject. However, it is common belief among women familiar with sweat bathing that the heat and subsequent sweating do relieve many of the aches and pains caused by the menstrual cycle. This may result from the removal of excessive water caused by sodium retention, from the discharge of excessive toxins through sweat, aor simply because of a general relaxing effect (Aaland 1978).

In menopause, sweat bathing helps by stimulating the autonomic nervous system, the pituitary gland, the adrenal glands, and the ovaries. Furthermore, some medical people consider menopausal symptoms an elimination crisis that makes sweat bathing even more useful. The theory is that menstruation is more than just an elimination for the uterine linking; it is an eliminative cycle for the entire body. Upon cessation of menstruation, the body must find other ways of ridding itself of toxic accumulations. While the adjustment is going on, uncomfortable menopausal symptoms are felt. Sweat bathing, acting as a general toxic eliminator, reduces some of these distresses.

Editor's Note

Hot flashes (vasomotor fluctuations) might be lessened by the thermal-regulating effect of daily sauna on the body. It is known that both the regulation of estrogen production and the body's heating/cooling mechanisms are controlled by the same gland, the hypothalamus. Heat receptors in the skin transmit information to the hypothalamus, which responds by heating or cooling the body as in hot flashes or chills. (Farmilant 1981). Perhaps the regulation of the heating/cooling mechanism can also help regulate estrogen production.

REFERENCES

Aaland, Mikkel, *Sweat*. Santa Barbara: Capra Press, 1978.

Cresson, Frank M., "Maya and Mexican Sweat Houses," *American Anthropologist*, vol. 40 (1938).

Farmilant, Eunice, "Working Up a Sweat," in *East-West Journal*, August 1981.

Fritzsche, Werner, "Examinations and Observations on Healthy Children during the Sauna Bathing Process." *Sauna Studies*, published by Finnish Sauna Society, 1976.

Hasan, J., M. J. Karvonen, and P. Piironen, "Physiological Effects of Extreme Heat as Studied in the Finnish 'Sauna' Bath," *American Journal of Physical Medicine*, vol. 45, no. 6 (1966).

Hilvers, A. G., "Effects of Hypothalamic Hormones under Normal and Sauna Conditions." Paper read to the Seventh International Sauna Congress, West Germany, 1978.

Hohnadel, David C. et al., "Atomic Absorption Spectrometry of Nickel, Copper, Zinc, and Lead in Sweat Collected from Healthy Subjects during Sauna Bathing," *Clinical Chemistry*, vol. 19, no. 11 (1973).

"Hyperthermia, Hottest News in Cancer Therapy," *Medical World News*, May 14, 1979.

Lewis, Oscar, *Life in a Mexican Village—Tepoztlan Re-Studied*, Urbana, Ill.: University of Illinois Press, 1951.

Miller, Peter et al., "Maternal Hyperthermia as a Possible Cause of Anencephaly," *Lancet*, March 11, 1978.

Procope, Berndt-Johan, "Effect of Repeated Increase of Body Temperature on Human Sperm Cells," *International Journal of Fertility*, vol. 10, no. 4. (1965).

Rapola, J., L. Saxen, and G. Granroth, "Anencephaly and the Sauna," *Lancet*, May 27, 1978.

Synder, Donald, "Sauna Baths Used to Take Kidney's Role." Report read to the 1966 convention of the American Society for Artificial Organs.

Soiva, K., *Sauna und Schwangerschaft* (*Sauna and Pregnancy*). Helsinki: State Maternity Hospital, Institute of Midwifery Sofranlehdowkatu 5,00610 Helsinki 61 Finland.

Soiva, K. et al., "The Effect of Bathing in the Finnish Sauna on the Onset of Labour," *Annals Chirugia Gynaecology*, 52 (1963), 172–77.

Sokya, Fred, *The Ion Effect*. New York: 1977.

Sunderman, F. W. et al, "Excretion of Copper in Sweat of Patients with Wilson's Disease during Sauna Bathing," *Annals of Clinical and Laboratory Science*, vol. 19, no. 11 (1973).

Syvalahti, E. et al., "Effect of the Thermal Stress of the Sauna and the Psychic Stress of Examination on Human Growth Hormone, Immunoreactive Insulin, Aldosterone, Plasma Renin Activity, and Vanilmandelic Acid." *Sauna Studies*. Paper read at the Sixth International Sauna Congress in Helsinki, 1974.

Teeri, N., "The Climatic Conditions of the Sauna." *Sauna Studies*. Paper read at the Sixth International Sauna Congress in Helsinki, 1974.

Tooke, William, *View of the Russian Empire during the Reign of Catharine the Second*. London: Arnold, 1970.

Viherjuuri, H. J., *Sauna, The Finnish Bath* (American edition) Brattleboro, Vt.: Stephen Green Press, 1965.

Virtanen, John, *The Finnish Sauna*. Portland, Continental Publishing: 1974.

Chapter Twenty-Two

BIOFEEDBACK: AN ALTERNATIVE HEALING TECHNIQUE

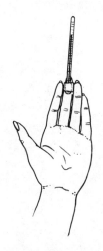

Alyce M. Green

> *So this league of minde and bodie has these two parts. How the one worketh upon the other. For the consideration is double, either how, and how farre, the humours and the affects of the bodie, do alter or worke upon the minde; or again, how and how farre the passions or apprehensions of the minde, do alter or worke upon the bodie. . . .*
>
> *[Francis Bacon 1561–1626]*

Biofeedback is playing an important role in accelerating developments toward more encompassing healing systems. Designated by such terms as "alternative medicine" and "holistic health care," these therapies incorporate a variety of techniques and procedures to achieve the healing, or to maintain the well-being, of the whole person—body, mind, and spirit. Biofeedback is one such technique; biofeedback training is one such procedure.

DEFINITION

What is *biofeedback*? Simply put, it is the feedback of biological information to a person. It is the continuous monitoring, amplifying, and displaying (usually by a needle on a meter, or by a light, or tone) of an on-going internal physiological process, such as heart behavior, blood pressure, muscle tension, temperature, or brain rhythms (brain waves). Biofeedback *training* is using the information in learning to extend voluntary control over normally unconscious autonomic processes and/or neuromuscular processes being monitored (Green and Green 1977a).

The establishing of voluntary control over autonomic "involuntary" nervous system functions, through biofeedback training, rests on the "psychophysiological principle," which postulates:

> Every change in the physiological state is accompanied by an appropriate change in the psychological state, conscious or unconscious; and conversely, every change in the psychological state, conscious or unconscious, is accompanied by an appropriate change in the physiological state. [Green, Green, and Walters 1971]

This principle, when coupled with volition, allows for the self-regulation of a number of autonomic functions and, theoretically at least, for the influencing of every function of the body. Self-regulation of autonomic processes is accomplished through learning to relax and quiet the body, emotions, and mind, imagining and visualizing the change wanted, "feeling" it happen, and, in a detached way, "letting it happen." The biofeedback meter acts as a guide, indicating the degree of success, as when one learns to increase warmth in the hands with the aid of a temperature meter or to control heart rate with the aid of heart-rate feedback.

The aim in biofeedback training is to train various processes of the mind and body to operate in such a way that finally a very brief visualization or self-direction will accomplish the intended change, and the biofeedback instrument will no longer be needed. But how does it work? How is it possible to voluntarily control, to "self-regulate," an autonomic process?

RATIONALE

Figure 22-1, a simplified representation of processes that apparently occur simultaneously in the neurological domain and in the psychological domain, illustrates the mind-body synthesis that makes self-regulation possible (Green and Green 1974 and 1975). Electrophysiologic studies indicate that every perception of outside-the-skin (OUTS) events (upper left box) is associated with electrical activity in both conscious and unconscious structures of the central nervous system (arrow 1), those involved in emotional and mental responses.

The box labeled "Limbic Response" (arrow 2) is placed entirely in the involuntary section of the diagram to indicate its primarily unconscious nature. The limbic structure of the subcortical brain has been intensely studied in animals and humans since Papez's historic paper outlined the possible function of the system in emotional responses (Papez 1937). The limbic system, which has been called the "visceral brain" (MacLean 1949), as well as the emotional brain, is connected by many pathways (arrow 3) to the hypothalamus, the central "control panel" of the brain, which regulates a large part of the body's autonomic and automatic neural machinery. The hypothalamus has an important regulatory effect on the pituitary, the "king gland" of the body, which in turn precipitates changes in the homeostatic balance points of other glandular processes. In this way, alterations in physiologic balance result from changes in limbic processes. To summarize, the perception of OUTS events leads to limbic-hypothalamic-glandular responses. Physiologic change is the inevitable consequence.

The above facts have been known for more than 30 years. What was not known is the fact that if we can become aware of what is going on inside us, we can often modify it voluntarily in a direction we choose. If an internal

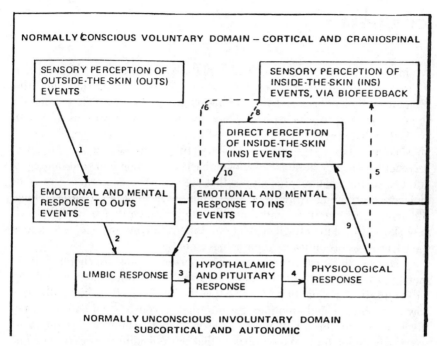

FIGURE 22-1. Simplified operational diagram of "self-regulation" of psycho-physiological events and processes.

physiological change is detected and is displayed on a biofeedback meter, a new mental-emotional response will result (arrow 6), accompanied by an appropriate limbic, hypothalamic and pituitary, and physiologic response (arrows 7, 3 and 4). It is the physiological change that is picked up by the feedback monitor and fed back to the conscious cortex (arrow 5). Thus, a biocybernetic control loop is established as a result of providing the cortex with information about normally unconscious inside-the-skin (INS) processes. Closing the biocybernetic loop bridges the normal gap between conscious and unconscious processes, voluntary and involuntary, between mind and body. We enter the biocybernetic loop at the mental-emotional level and affect the physiological outcome.

Increased sensitivity to internal cues (indicated by arrow 8) is an essential step in closing the internal section of the cybernetic control loop and leads to the development of direct INS perception (arrow 9) and to what might be called, "a self-regulated emotional and mental response" (arrow 10). The use of a feedback device is usually dispensed with as soon as direct awareness and self-regulation are established. Biofeedback thus provides an opportunity not easily available in the past for developing skill in autonomic self-control and for assuming psychosomatic self-responsibility.

PSYCHOPHYSIOLOGIC THERAPY

We in the Voluntary Controls Program of the Menninger Foundation began research in mind-body relationships in 1964, and in 1975 established the Menninger Biofeedback and Psychophysiology Center, in which we conduct clinical work and to which physicians refer patients with various disorders for biofeedback-aided therapy. We call our clinical procedures "psycho-physiologic therapy" (mind-body therapy), and we call ourselves "psychophysiologic therapists." Biofeedback is a major tool, one among a number of therapeutic procedures that we use. We sometimes speak of biofeedback training as awareness training (awareness of physical feelings and sensations, emotions, and thoughts), and through its use, people learn new skills, the skills of self-regulation. Like a mirror, biofeedback guides their learning and indicates their achievement.

During the first session, when a person begins psychophysiologic therapy, the rationale outlined above is carefully explained in terms suitable for that particular client or patient, so that the how and why of biofeedback—how our thoughts and emotions get into the nervous system and how they affect our health (through the limbic system, hypothalamus, and pituitary)—are clearly understood. We emphasize that this is a natural process, happening all the time, with either helpful or harmful results. We emphasize that healing is also a natural process, that it is natural for the body to heal and to be well, and we stress the fact that our minds can play an important part in creating and maintaining our health. Lastly, we emphasize the power of choice, that we can choose to hold one thought rather than another, and can choose to hold one emotion rather than another. By our choice we can move toward disease or well-being. It is the long-held anxiety, anger, frustration, or despair that leads to psychosomatic illness.

When the patient understands the rationale and the process of biofeedback training, we discuss goals. This includes, for example, what is to be achieved in control of temperature, in depth of relaxation, and in the amelioration of the problem for which he/she was referred. Additional goals often include gaining the ability to deal more successfully with interpersonal problems (at home or at work), gaining self-confidence and self-assertiveness, and developing a more adequate sense of self-worth.

During the first session, we also teach the patient the use of the temperature feedback monitor and demonstrate how, by the use of autogenic (self-suggestion) phrases and visualization of warmth in the hands (Schultz and Luthe 1959; Green and Green 1977b), one can increase hand tempera-ture—which means increasing blood flow to the hands. We explain that the blood vessels of the hands are innervated by the sympathetic section of the autonomic nervous system, and the increase in hand warmth signifies relaxa-tion in the autonomic nervous system (the system that controls the functioning of most of our internal biologic processes including blood flow). It signifies the "turn off" of the sympathetic flight-or-fight reaction we inherited from our cavemen ancestors, the "stress response" implicated in much modern disease.

Having learned how to use the temperature feedback instrument and the hand-warming technique, and with the expectation that the patient will, with practice, be able to raise hand temperatures to 94°, 95° or 96°, the patient takes the machine home for twice-daily 15-minute practice sessions. This begins the transfer of self-regulation training to the life situation at the very beginning. (See Figure 22-2.)

The patient comes to the Center once weekly for electromyographic (EMG) training—training in muscle tension control. In most cases, we place the electrodes on the forehead—for relaxation of forehead muscles. The relaxation usually extends to relaxation of the jaw and neck muscles and often generalizes to the whole body. Just as EMG feedback may be used later for relaxation of tense muscles in other parts of the body (e.g., the neck, shoulders, or back), so temperature control, once learned, can be used to bring warmth and increased blood flow to other areas of the body (e.g., the throat, an arthritic knee or back, or the feet) (Green, Green, and Norris 1980).

Other biofeedback modalities may be introduced, depending on the needs of the patient, for example, feedback of brain rhythms, heart rate, or galvanic skin resposne (GSR). Practice of voluntary control of muscle tension and temperature as preliminary learning has proven to be useful in the treatment of many problems—physical, emotional, and mental. It begins to reestablish healthy homeostatic balance and teaches ways of managing stress,

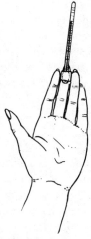

FIGURE 22-2.   An ordinary ambient air temperature thermometer can be taped to the fingertip to measure increase in temperature to the fingers.

which, as mentioned above, plays a major part in modern discomfort and disease.

In addition to biofeedback, we use other techniques when they are appropriate, such as breathing exercises, guided and unguided imagery, internal dialogue with the body, physical exercises (active ones like walking, running, and tennis, or bending and stretching ones as in yoga), and information and suggestions about nutrition. Visualizing what is to be accomplished plays an important part in all our techniques. It helps to make change happen. All of the above are techniques of self-regulation, and as you can see, they combine psychological and physiological procedures.

Of special importance is the transfer of what is learned at the Biofeedback Center to the patient's life situation. For example, we suggest that if a stop light turns red as you approach it, don't clutch the wheel and cuss out the stop light. Instead, say, "Ah, an opportunity." Then relax your hands, take a deep breath—and, if you have time—feel all the tension flow out of your body. You'll be in better shape for driving when the light says "Go," and meanwhile you will have done your body a favor. We also suggest finding reminders, cartoons, or jokes that make you laugh (Cousins 1976 and 1979), a picture or poem that says "untense," or a smiling face that makes you want to smile back, to put under the glass on your desk or on your refrigerator door. We ask patients to develop their own phrases, visualizations, imagery, and other techniques for self-regulation, to free themselves from dependence on the phrases we have given them, from the biofeedback instruments, and from the therapist, thus helping them to realize that both the responsibility and the achievement are theirs.

Beyond the amelioration or healing of a physical disorder, we have found that successful biofeedback therapy usually results in an improved self-image, in a sense of self-direction, self-mastery, and a change in life style. This last, a change in life style, is important if what has been gained is to be maintained. It often seems to happen almost as a "side effect" of the training (Budzynski and Mullaney 1973; Green, Green, and Norris 1980). Successful biofeedback practitioners are often told by clients, "You have changed my life," to which the response is, "No, *you* have changed your life."

HEALTH PROBLEMS SPECIFIC TO WOMEN

Greater understanding is needed of the physical life experiences unique to women. Many important decisions that a woman makes that greatly influence her well-being are related to the health of her reproductive organs. The majority of physicians, gynecologists, and obstetricians are men, and the differences in function of female and male bodies and the physical problems and diseases in women, specific to that difference, have not been given proper consideration. Nor has there been enough understanding of the very real mental and emotional problems engendered by that difference. Many women are dissatisfied with and at times angered by the medical care provided by male doctors, the lack of information sharing and the paternalistic attitude that too often dismisses a problem as "neutrotic," "psychogenic," or even "hysteric," best "treated" by a tranquilizer. In the 1970s, the women's health movement came into being partially as a response to that dissatisfaction.

More and more women all over the world are entering the medical profession; perhaps this will accelerate knowledge and understanding. As one woman physician phrased it:

> Women want basic tools for self-direction and growth; among these tools are knowledge of themselves as psyche and soma, knowledge of their body's rhythms, knowledge of their inner space and how to protect it. [Greenwood 1979]

Menstrual Problems

Menstruation, to which many feminine ills are linked, is a natural process, not a disease, and many women handle it with little discomfort. However, a number of women suffer varying degrees of distress, from mild to disabling, due to one or more of the following disorders (Maddox 1976).

Dysmenorrhea is the term for discomfort in association with the menstrual period.

Premenstrual syndrome (including congestive dysmenorrhea) manifests as one or more physical and psychological distresses that usually occur just before the onset of menstruation but also may occur during menstruation. In some women, premenstrual tension is so severe that it results in feelings of extreme irritability, anxiety, lethargy, and/or depression.

Spasmodic dysmenorrhea, experienced on the first day or two of menses, consists of dull or acute muscle spasms, usually in the lower abdomen and genital area but may include the lower back and the inside of the thighs.

Amenorrhea (absense of menstrual periods) is most often caused by lack of ovulation (anovulation). It may be due to abnormally low hormone release from the hypothalamus. The pituitary is not stimulated, and in turn does not stimulate the ovaries to produce normal estrogen and progesterone. Stress and/or illness may suppress hypothalamic hormones and thus be an underlying cause of amenorrhea.

Although the causes of menstrual distress are not fully understood, studies of the use of biofeedback in the treatment of menstrual problems indicate that biofeedback training for general relaxation and warmth can be helpful in ameliorating spasms and congestion (Tubbs and Carnahan 1976; Dietvorst and Osborne 1978). If necessary, biofeedback can be applied specifically in the areas of discomfort. For example, EMG electrodes (to feed back an indication of muscle tension) can be attached to the lower abdomen as an aid in learning to relax and/or prevent muscle spasms in that area, or they can be attached to the lower back to overcome pain due to muscle tension or spasms there. The thermistor of the temperature meter also can be attached to the lower abdomen as an aid in increasing circulation in that area, or a vaginal-uterine placement of the thermistor may be used (Sedlacek and Heczey 1977). The increase of warmth not only brings sensations of relaxation, calmness, and comfort, but may accelerate expulsion of the menstrual discharge, bringing additional relief from congestion. However, if the skills of relaxation and temperature increase have already been well learned through training, they can often be directed to other areas of the body without further biofeedback.

Since such biofeedback procedures lead to feelings of relaxation and comfort and result in reduction of excessive activity in the sympathetic nervous system, they are helpful in alleviating many of the physical problems associated with dysmenorrhea, such as constipation or diarrhea, headache, nausea, and edema. As they tend to rebalance the limbic-hypothalamic-pituitary system, they may relieve the behavioral or psychological problems of premenstrual syndrome. Further research may also demonstrate the value of biofeedback therapy in the alleviation of amenorrhea. Adler and Adler (1979) make an interesting observation:

> Biofeedback training has many salubrious effects upon hypothalamically mediated visceral functioning, one of which is a reduction of symptoms of dysmenorrhea. [P.74]

They report that in five patients being treated with temperature training for migraine headache, all reported the disappearance of dysmenorrhea. Two of the five also reported the remission of a complete anovulatory state that had accompanied their dysmenorrhea (ibid.).

Hilary Maddox (1976) observes:

> One of the most common causes of both forms of dysmenorrhea is general poor health. Any woman who carried out a regular program of preventive health care will have fewer difficulties with menstruation.

Techniques learned with the aid of biofeedback training clearly contribute to preventive health care.

Instructions that accompany our use of biofeedback and potentiate the healthful effects of the training include breathing exercises, appropriate physical exercises, and relevant suggestions about nutrition.

Control of Ovulation and Spermatogenesis

As discussed above, the most common cause of amenorrehea is anovulation, which may be due to hypothalamic-pituitary malfunction as a limbic response to severe physical or emotional stress. Such considerations have led to speculation as to whether specific biofeedback techniques could be devised by which women might learn to self-control ovulation, not only for the alleviation of amenorrhea but as a method of birth control. To the author's knowledge, no research investigating such a possibility has been reported in the literature.

In the early seventies, research was reported (French et al. 1971) in which a group of male subjects, having been trained to increase blood flow to the hands, transferred the visualization of warmth to the scrotum, making the interal environment hostile to sperm viability and causing temporary infertility. This success intrigued the researchers with the possibility of finding a method by which women might learn self-regulation of ovulation. However, after investigating some of the intricacies involved (e.g., the hypothalamic-pituitary and pH functions), they did not pursue the question (Leeb 1981).

Wolfgang Luthe, at the 1976 Annual Conference of the Biofeedback Society of America, in referring to the above research, urged caution in using biofeedback methods to manipulate the body's normal homeostatic mechanisms—rather than to bring an unbalanced homeostatic process back to normal, as is usually the case. Yet, new areas must be explored, always with caution. It is still too early to say what the limits of self-regulation may be.

Menopausal Problems

Menopause, like menstruation, is a natural process, not a disease. For some women, it is accompanied by relief and a sense of freedom, but for others it too may be accompanied by troublesome symptoms, psychological and physical.

The most commonly experienced physical distress is the menopausal hot flash. A recent study investigated whether biofeedback training in temperature increase and decrease could teach women to control vascular flow in such a way as to reduce the discomfort of hot flashes. The thermistors were placed on "trigger sites," identified by the woman as the place where the hot flash begins. The women in the study were able to increase and decrease both finger and trigger site temperature (i.e., control blood flow to those areas). Six of the seven patients achieved a significant decrease in the frequency of hot flashes, but decreases in intensity and duration did not reach significance. The authors observe that if a replicating study with more patients and more training time proves to be statistically significant in all measures, a new, low-risk therapy may have been found for a prevalent and distressing menopausal problem (Wolf-Willets, Woods, and Betrus 1981).

Psychological problems of menopause—nervous headache, anxiety, depression, loss of self-drive, and memory loss—do not respond to estrogen therapy, and it is not known whether other hormonal changes contribute to these problems. It is clear, however, that hormonal changes during the reproductive years can influence emotional stability. Reacting with stress to problems at home or at work, and to the commonly held values of our youth-oriented culture about ageing (especially ageing in women), definitely affects one's emotional, and therefore physical, well-being. The concept of the "old woman" as valueless, rather than as one to be respected for wisdom gathered through her years (as is true is many other cultures), is damaging.

> A reasonable conclusion is that the emotional problems attributed to hormonal deficiency probably stem from a combination of factors: hormonal, personal, and cultural. [Stewart et al. 1979]

In handling problems arising from personal and cultural factors, biofeedback therapy can help. A change in self-concept toward a better self-image often begins with the first experience of voluntarily controlling an "involuntary" process, such as warmth in the hands. If therapy progresses satisfactorily, and skills of self-regulation increase, the feelings of self-worth and self-mastery continue to grow and radiate out to other areas of one's life, leading to the change of life style that usually accompanies successful psychophysiologic therapy. One learns to be more assertive in fulfilling one's own needs, in finding new interests and satisfactions. One learns to act in new ways in problem situations, rather than to react; and one learns that "if you can't change the stimulus, change the response," i.e., if a stress-producing circumstance in one's life cannot be changed, the reaction to it must be changed.

Feelings of Mourning and Depression

The same self-regulation procedures that lead to feelings of self-direction and self-mastery can be helpful in the periods of mourning and/or depression that often follow hysterectomy, mastectomy, and giving birth (postpartum depression). Such procedures can, in fact, be of value in preparing for any surgery, in undergoing it more calmly, and in recovering more speedily. These procedures have been successfully used in preoperative and postoperative counseling and in the counseling of pregnant women. Dr. Robert Gregg, obstetrician and gynecologist, has written about his use of biofeedback in teaching pregnant women how to control their physiology in different situations. This gives them a greater feeling of independence, confidence, and self-worth, and "skills which they can then apply with assurance and predictability during pregnancy, labor and delivery, post-partum and for years to come" (1979).

Cancer Therapy

Psychophysiologic therapy is being found useful as an adjunctive therapy in the treatment of cancer. Breast cancer and cancers of the reproductive system are the leading causes of death in women. Research has demonstrated that stress impairs the functioning of the immune system, the body's natural defense against disease (Rosch 1979). Research also supports the concept that stress and psychosocial trauma usually precede and are implicated in the incidence of cancer. Thus their alleviation is an important part of the healing process (LeShan 1966 and 1977).

Dr. Carl Simonton, an oncologist, introduced the use of biofeedback and visualization as aids in the treatment of cancer: these include temperature training to demonstrate to a patient that he/she can control an internal physiological process, and meditating while visualizing the white cells of the immune system attacking and destroying the cancer (Simonton and Mathews-Simonton 1978). Each patient develops his/her own visualizations of a strengthened and active immune system destroying the cancerous tissue and of the body returning to health (Norris 1981; Green 1981). A number of biofeedback practitioners have adapted the Simontons' basic concepts to their own procedures (e.g., Pelletier 1977).

To have the ability to call on elements of self-mastery, pain control, and peace of mind in terminal illness is a valuable asset for every human. Patients can be helped to realize that just as it is possible to direct the course of living more intentionally, so is it possible to direct the course of dying more intentionally. If the choice is made by the cancer patient to engage in the struggle to live and be well, as is usually the case, the result may be an extension of life for a few months, or for a few years beyond the time predicted, or it may even be the remission of the cancer. What makes the effort worthwhile is the enriched quality of life as the therapy progresses.

At the Menninger Biofeedback and Psychophysiology Center, we have found stress management techniques—self-regulation skills that encourage feelings of self-mastery and all the psychophysiologic procedures that contribute to emotional and physical well-being—to be of great value. Biofeedback-aided relaxation and specific visualizations pertaining to the medical treatment of cancer have helped patients accept and use chemotherapy and/or radiation in more beneficial ways, and, in varying degrees, to ameliorate adverse effects.

The life stresses that preceded the onset of cancer, as well as the stresses involved in the experience of cancer, are explored and in as far as possible ameliorated. Goals are set and examined and expanded from time to time. New interests are encouraged, and the satisfaction of old interests pursued. Opportunities for laughter and joy are sought. The sense of self-mastery, that one has some power to direct and enhance life even in difficult circumstances, leads to a sense of well-being that gives the mind and body the best environment for self-healing.

A TIME OF CHALLENGE

The present is a time of great opportunity for women, but also a time of great pressure as they strive for equality. Pressure affects the woman who is a homemaker. Her feeling that her role lacks dignity and significance in our society damages her sense of self-worth. Yet what could be more significant than nurturing—physically, mentally, emotionally, spiritually—the members of the coming generation?

Pressure also affects the women striving for equal status in the business, professional, and political worlds in more obvious ways. There is an increase in smoking and in consumption of alcoholic beverages. Women will soon surpass men in the number of deaths due to lung cancer; they already surpass men (in the white poulation) in the number suffering from hypertension.

Obsession with eating to counteract the stress of their self-demand to be successful in a still male-dominated world along with the obsession with being thin in order to be beautiful to achieve that success, has led to an upsurge in the dangerous binge-purge eating syndrome, afflicting thousands of talented young women. Such findings led Kathleen Newland, author of *The Sisterhood of Man* (1979), to say, "It will be a bitter irony indeed if women achieve equality in death before they achieve equality in life."

But a time of pressure is also a time of challenge. The need is for us, as women, individually and together, to find and develop the resources with which to meet the challenge and to apply them in our lives, private and professional. Someone once questioned if we thought biofeedback was a panacea since it is applicable to so many disorders, psychological and physical. Our answer was that biofeedback is a remarkable tool, but only a tool, that if there is a "panacea," it is the potential in human beings to self-regulate their psychological and physical selves, to move toward self-direction, self-mastery, and self-health. The present need is for us to find and choose whatever way—among a number of different methods—is most helpful in recognizing and releasing our potential. Then the challenge will be met, not with self-destructive results but rather with self-developing results, of benefit to ourselves and to our society.

REFERENCES

Acteberg, J. et al., "An Adjunctive Therapy for Persons with Rheumatic Arthritis," *Archives of Physical Medicine Rehabilitation*, vol. 59 (1978).

Adler, Charles S., and Sheila M. Adler, "Biofeedback and Psychosomatic Disorders," in *Principles and Practices for Clinicians*, John V. Basmajian, ed., Baltimore: The Williams & Wilkins Company, 1979.

Budzynski, Thomas H., and Daniel J. Mullaney, "EMG Biofeedback and Tension Headache: A Controlled Outcome Study," *Psychosomatic Medicine*, 35 (1973), 489–96.

Carlson, S. G., and E. N. Gale, "Biofeedback in the Treatment of Long-Term Temperomandibular Joint Pain: An Outcome Study," *Biofeedback and Self-Regulation* (1977), 161–71.

Cousins, Norman, "Anatomy of an Illness (as Perceived by the Patient)," *New England Journal of Medicine*, December 1976.

———, *Anatomy of an Illness*. New York: W. W. Norton & Co., Inc., 1979.

Dietvorst, Thomas F., and David Osborne, "Biofeedback—Assisted Relaxation Training for Primary Dysmenorrhea: A Case Study," *Biofeedback and Self-Regulation*, 3, no. 3 (1978), 301–5.

French, D. J. et al., "Self-Induced Scrotal Hyperthermia in Man Followed by Decrease in Sperm Output. A Preliminary Report," *Andrologie*, 5 (1973), 311–16.

Green, Alyce M., "Psychophysiologic Therapy in the Treatment of Cancer: Review of Two Cases." Paper presented at Advanced Biofeedback Therapy Seminar. Menninger Foundation, Topeka, Kansas, November 1981.

Green, Alyce M., and E. E. Green. "Biofeedback: Research and Therapy," in *New Ways to Health*, Nils Jacobson, ed. Stockholm, 1975.

Green, E. E., and Alyce M. Green, "Biofeedback and Volition." Paper presented at the Conference on New Dimensions of Habilitation for the Handicapped, University of Florida, Gainesville, 1974.

———"Biofeeback: Rationale and Applications," *International Encyclopedia of Neurology, Psychiatry, Psychoanalysis and Psychology*, Benjamin B. Wolman, ed. New York: Van Nostrand Reinhold Company, 1977a.

———*Beyond Biofeedback*. New York: Delacorte Press, 1977b.

Green, E. E., Alyce M. Green, and Patricia A. Norris, "Self-Regulation Training for Control of Hypertension," *Primary Cardiology: Cardiovascular Medicine for Primary Care Physicians* (March 1980), pp. 126–37.

Green, E. E., Alyce E. Green, and E. D. Walters, "Voluntary Control of Internal States: Psychological and Physiological," *Biofeedback and Self-Control*, T. X. Barber et al., eds. Chicago: Aldine Publishing Company, 1971.

Greenwood, Sanja Goldsmith, in "Foreword" to *My Body, My Health: The Concerned Women's Guide to Gynecology*. New York: John Wiley & Sons, Inc., 1979.

Gregg, Robert H., "Biofeedback and Biophysical Monitoring during Pregnancy and Labor," *Biofeedback: Principles and Practice for Clinicians*, John V. Basmajian, ed. Baltimore: The Williams & Wilkins Company, 1979.

Leeb, C. S., personal communication, 1981.

LeShan, Lawrence, "An Emotional Life History Pattern Associated with Neoplastic Disease," *Annals of New York Academy of Science*, 125 (1966), 780–93.

———, *You Can Fight for Your Life: Emotional Factors in the Causation of Cancer*. New York: M. Evans & Company, 1977.

London, Robert H., *JAMA*, 244, no. 10 (1980), 1077–78.

MacLean, P. D., "Psychosomatic Disease and the 'Visceral Brain.' Recent Developments Bearing on Papez Theory of Emotion," *Psychosomatic Medicine* (1949), 338–53.

Maddox, Hilary, "Menstrual Problems," *Woman's Almanac*, Kathryn Paulson, ed. Philadelphia: J. B. Lippincott Company, 1976.

Newland, Kathleen, *The Sisterhood of Man*. New York and London: W. W. Norton & Co., Inc., 1979.

Norris, Patricia A., "The Role of Psychophysiological Self-Regulation in the Treatment of Cancer: A Narrative Case Report. Shifting Paradigms: Awareness, Self-Regulation and Biofeedback," *Proceedings of the Seventh Annual Biofeedback Society of America Advanced Topics Workshop*, October 15–18, New Orleans, 1981.

Papez, J. M., "A Proposed Mechanism of Emotion," *Archieves of Neurological Psychiatry*, 38 (1937), 725–43.

Pelletier, Kenneth, "Adjunctive Biofeedback with Cancer Patients: A Case Presentation." *Biofeedback and Self-Regulation*, vol. 2, no. 3 (1977).

Rosch, Paul J., "Stress and Cancer: A Disease of Adaptation." *Cancer, Stress, and Death*, Jean Tache, Hans Selye, and Stacey B. Day, eds. New York: Plenum Publishing Corporation, 1979.

Schultz, J. H., and W. Luthe, *Autogenic Training: A Physiological Approach in Psychotherapy*. New York: Grune & Stratton, Inc., 1959.

Sedlacek, Keith, and Maria Heczey, "A Specific Biofeedback Treatment for Dysmenorrhea," *Proceedings of the Biofeedback Society of America*, Annual Meeting, 1977.

Simonton, O. Carl, and Stephanie Mathews-Simonton, *Getting Well Again*. Los Angeles: J. P. Tarcher Inc., 1978.

Stewart, Felicia Hans et al., *My Body, My Health: The Concerned Woman's Guide to Gynecology*. New York: John Wiley & Sons, Inc., 1979.

Tubbs, Walter, and Clarence Carnahan, "Clinical Biofeedback for Primary Dysmenorrhea: A Pilot Study," *Biofeedback and Self-Regulation*, vol. 1, no. 3 (1976).

Wolf-Wiletts, Vivian, Nancy Fugate Woods, and Patricia Betrus, "A Pilot Study Comparing the Effectiveness of Skin-Temperature Biofeedback and Relaxation Training for Controlling Menopausal Hot Flashes," *Proceedings of the Biofeedback Society of America*, Twelfth Annual Meeting, March 13–17, 1981.

SUGGESTED READINGS

American Journal of Clinical Biofeedback. New York: Human Sciences Press.

Brown, Barbara, *New Mind, New Body*. New York: Harper & Row, Publishers, Inc., 1974. The history of the development of biofeedback and the formation of the Biofeedback Society of America.

Cook, Stephanie, *Second Life*. New York: Simon & Schuster, 1981. Discusses the dismissing of women's physical diseases as "neurotic."

Jencks, Beata, *Your Body. Biofeedback at Its Best*. Chicago: Nelson-Hall Publishers, 1979.

Pepper, Erik, Sonia Ancoli, and Michelle Quinn, eds., *Mind/Body Integration: Essential Readings in Biofeedback*. New York: Plenum Publishing Corporation, 1979.

LISTING OF ORGANIZATIONS FOR BIOFEEDBACK

Biofeedback Equipment
7186 Glenroy Street
San Diego, CA 92120

Biofeedback Society of America
Psychiatry C268
University of Colorado Medical Center
4200 East Ninth Avenue
Denver, CO 80220
(303) 394-7054

Biofeedback Institute
Headache Pain and Stress Center
3428 Sacramento
Berkeley, CA 94118

Eastern Biofeedback Society
83-91 Woodhaven Boulevard
Queens, NY 11421
(212) 846-2889

Midwest Biofeedback Association
161 East Erie Street
Chicago, IL 60611

Chapter Twenty-Three

MEDITATION AS THERAPY FOR WOMEN

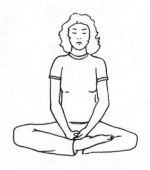

Frances E. Vaughan

Meditation is an ancient practice traditionally undertaken as a spiritual discipline for the purpose of gaining insight into the nature of self and reality. The use of meditation as therapy represents an extension of the traditional purposes of attaining self-mastery, inner peace, and spiritual development. Its current popularity as a method of treatment for various diseases can be attributed partly to research supporting its effectiveness in promoting relaxation and partly to the fact that it is a safe, nonintrusive form of intervention that enables a person to achieve mental states that contribute to his/her well-being.

Although discussing meditation as therapy addresses only a fraction of the potential effects of meditation, data have been accumulating to indicate that meditation can be used effectively in the treatment of both physiological and psychological disorders (Shapiro 1980; Carrington 1978). From a psychological perspective, meditation can be considered not only as an adjunct to psychotherapy but also as a path of sustained personal development. In recent years meditation has become increasingly popular in the West as an effective method of relaxation to counteract stress. It is estimated that over six million people in the United States today have learned some form of meditation.

Meditation as therapy has the additional advantage of not costing anything; and it can be learned by anyone, at any age, who is capable of sustaining a self-administered treatment program. It is a simple, natural process that does not require either technical equipment or medication.

HISTORY

Western medicine was originally informed of the effects of meditation by sporadic reports from British physicians who had served in India during the past two centuries. They had observed that some yogis who practiced meditation were able to regulate such body processes as heart rate, body temperature, and sensitivity to pain. However, it was a woman, French cardiologist Thérèse Brosse, who first attempted to document the value of meditation in medicine when she observed that Indian yogis could actually control activity of the autonomic nervous sytem (1946). More recently, Alyce Green (see Chapter 22) conducted a series of carefully controlled experiments at the Menninger Foundation in Topeka, Kansas, which provided impressive evidence of both the ability of advanced meditators to control autonomic functions, and the ability of untrained subjects to learn such control with the use of biofeedback equipment (1977). Although biofeedback can facilitate learning these strategies, it is not required for the practice of meditation.

Early investigators of meditation as therapy in this country suggested that meditation led to a unique state of low metabolism as measured by oxygen consumption, carbon dioxide production, and blood lactate levels (Wallace 1970). This state has been described as a unique "fourth state of consciousness," as distinguished from waking, dreaming, and sleeping (Bloomfield et al. 1975). Subsequent studies confirmed marked reduction in metabolic rates, and also indicated changes in blood flow and hormone levels. The effects of meditation on consciousness, however, could more accurately be described as offering access to a broad range of states of consciousness, rather than a single state. Nevertheless, the effectiveness of meditation as a tool for self-regulation, which allows the individual to bring various autonomic functions under voluntary control, is well established (Shapiro and Walsh 1982).

HOW TO MEDITATE

See Figure 23-1 for the correct position for meditating. Meditation can be practiced alone or in a group. It can be equally effective either way, but sitting with others can help in the early stages when the necessary self-discipline may be lacking. As familiarity with practice develops, it becomes easier and more pleasant and therefore requires less support from other people. When a doctor recommends meditation, his or her authority and

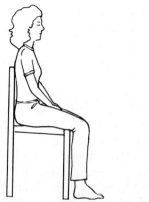 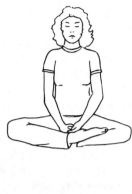

FIGURE 23-1. How to Meditate: The practice of meditation is outwardly very simple. It consists of sitting still, with the spine straight, either cross-legged on the floor on a rug or a cushion, or in a straight-backed chair with feet flat on the floor. Eyes may be closed or slightly open, with a soft gaze directed at the floor or at a specific object of meditation. Breathing is normal and may be used as focus of attention. In every form of meditation the objective is to maintain a wide-awake, alert state of mind, and to develop the ability to focus attention, maintain concentration, and observe subjective experience in a relaxed manner.

encouragement can help sustain continuity of practice in the beginning when it is more difficult to do it alone.

The amount of time allocated to meditation varies. Twenty minutes twice a day, morning and evening, is often recommended for beginners, but shorter periods may also be beneficial (Carrington 1978). Some people prefer longer periods of uninterrupted meditation. The amount of time given to meditation should take into account individual predisposition as well as the effects that are experienced as a result of practice. However, it is a good idea to be consistent in practicing for a certain amount of time each day, preferably at the same time every day, until it becomes an integral part of a daily routine.

TYPES OF MEDITATION

Meditative disciplines may be categorized as either concentrative meditation or open, receptive meditation. Measurable physiological effects may be obtained with either type, and both contribute to developing self-awareness. Attention may be focused on a specific object of concentration, or the meditator may be instructed to maintain an attitude of open, choiceless awareness, wherein all experience is observed and noted without judgment and without trying to hold on to any thoughts in particular.

Meditative practices, developed over many centuries, reflect the cultures from which they derive. However, the wide range and variety of meditative practices share certain common characteristics. They all train attention and attempt to bring the mind under voluntary control. Some practices emphasize sitting and attending to body sensations, feelings, thoughts, and fantasies (Goldstein 1976). Others focus attention on a single object such as the breath, or a specific sound (mantra), or a visual image (Carrington 1978). Still others emphasize the cultivation of specific emotional states, such as calm, equanimity, love, or compassion (Goldstein 1976; LeShan 1974). Personality variables may influence the type of meditation an individual chooses to practice, and the availability of a meditation teacher may also affect the choice of method. But anyone can experiment with meditation independently, with the aid of books of instruction, which are now widely available (Carrington 1978; Goldstein 1976; LeShan 1974; Levine 1978).

People meditate for many different reasons. Needleman considers the heart of psychological discipline in both East and West to be training in self-study (1975). Meditation is essentially such training. Deikman sees meditation as leading to deautomatization of perception and behavior (1966), which implies greater freedom and choice. LeShan suggests that we meditate to find or recover something of ourselves that we have lost (1974). We may begin to meditate in an effort to attain more peace of mind or relaxation. However, the practice can lead to greater self-awareness and psychological development. Wilber suggests that meditation is the means whereby higher states of consciousness begin to unfold (1980). Higher states are defined as those states that possess all the attributes of normal waking consciousness plus additional functions (Tart 1975; Walsh and Vaughan 1980). Higher states are more inclusive, more coherent, and better integrated than what we normally experience, and may therefore be equated with optimal psychological health.

Many research studies have used Transcendental Meditation techniques because of the widespread popularity and adaptability of TM to Western lifestyles (Bloomfield et al. 1975). Studies such as those undertaken by Dr. Benson at Harvard (1975) and Dr. Carrington at Princeton University (1978), using clincially standardized forms of meditation, indicate that meditation need not be affiliated with a formal religious group in order to be effective. Eastern consciousness disciplines traditionally instruct students to practice without being distracted by the contents of consciousness. In the West, however, when meditation is used as therapy, the content that arises in the form of images, feelings, or sensations may be examined for clues to appropriate intervention.

MEDICAL RESEARCH

Meditation has been widely used for health maintenance as a tool for voluntary control of internal states and as self-regulation therapy (Shapiro 1980). Interest among physicians has been supported by the need to find ways to help patients develop more responsibility for their own health care and to offer nondrug alternatives to the treatment of stress-related illness. Increasing sophistication in scientific instrumentation and investigation has also enabled Western scientists to research the validity of some of the claims by Eastern yogis of extraordinary mental and physical control made possible through meditation training (Green and Green 1977).

Meditation research has been focused predominantly on physiological variables since these effects are relatively easy to measure. Marked reductions in metabolic rate have been reported, as shown by reduced oxygen consumption, carbon dioxide production, and blood lactate states (Brosse 1946; Wallace 1970). These physiological measurements indicate a state of deep relaxation that is particularly beneficial in treating stress-related illness. Subsequent studies have confirmed these findings. However, regular practice of meditation is essential to maintaining these good results.

Studies measuring the electrical resistance of the skin (GSR), a measure considered to be an indication of lessening stress, indicate that meditation contributes not only to immediate relaxation but also to a reduction in stress reactivity (Orme-Johnson 1973; Goleman and Schwartz 1976). This implies that meditators are less likely to react adversely to stressful stimuli than nonmeditators. Although reductions in metabolic rate and GSR reactivity may also be induced by other methods, certain patterns of brain-wave activity appear to be unique to meditation (Walsh 1979). Studies of brain physiology during meditation employing the electroencephalograph (EEG) have indicated increased synchronization of brain waves with alpha waves predominating. Such patterns are considered typical of an alert, yet calm and relaxed state of consciousness.

PSYCHOLOGICAL EFFECTS

Subjective reports of how rapidly effects of meditation are experienced vary widely, but almost all meditators report a deepening experience with continued practice. Subjective phenomenological studies commonly report episodes of emotional arousal, relaxation, perceptual clarity, and sensitivity to psychological processes; also reduced defensiveness, nervousness, irritability, restlessness, and boredom; as well as increased self-awareness, insight, empathy, and openness to experience. Occasionally a meditator may also experience self-transcendence and oneness with others and the environment (Shapiro 1980; et al.)

During early stages of meditation, repressed unconscious material may either float to the surface of consciousness or erupt suddenly into awareness. In later stages, creative unconscious potentials tend to unfold and become actualized. Meditation may therefore be considered as a sustained instrumental path for healthy human development (Wilbur 1979 and 1980), as well as a useful adjunct to psychotherapy. Long-term meditators often report profound subjective changes that are also reflected in changes in values and life styles (Elgin 1981). Meditation has been described as a tough discipline that enables one to realize the full human potential. Its practice enables one to feel more able to work effectively, closer to one's fellow human beings, and less anxious and hostile. A good program of meditation may be compared to a good program of physical exercise. Both require consistent effort, and both contribute to overall health and well-being (Levine 1978).

Anxiety

Meditation is particularly effective in the treatment of anxiety. The effects of meditation on anxiety are measurable in metabolic changes and other stress indicators. Physiological indicators of reduced stress support subjective reports of decreased feelings of anxiety as well as indicating faster recovery time after exposure to stressful stimuli (Goleman and Schwartz 1976). Since meditation is a powerful antidote to stress, its value in the prevention of anxiety should not be overlooked. Whether anxiety has reached pathological levels or is simply a source of minor discomfort, meditation can offer immediate relief as well as long-term benefits, and its effectiveness improves with practice.

Patients who meditate tend to worry less and become more relaxed and proficient in their lives. They also gain the confidence that comes from the recognition that they *can* control their own mental and emotional states. The self-discipline required for consistent practice may itself be an indication of increased capacity for self-mastery. The fact that meditation is something the patient can do for himself or herself helps build strength and confidence, and the individual can readily experience the benefits of valuing himself or herself enough to take time to be quiet and tune in to inner experience. It is evident even to a beginner that observing the breath in meditation, for example, can have a calming effect on the mind. Although difficulty in concentration may be frustrating, relaxed deep breathing can provide immediate relief of agitation.

Another advantage of using meditation rather than tranquilizers for the treatment of anxiety is the fact that meditators become more alert rather than sleepy or drowsy as a result of practice. Improved coping ability can therefore be enhanced by improved functioning.

However, although meditation can effectively reduce anxiety, it may be difficult for a person to begin meditating during periods of acute anxiety since beginning practice requires self-discipline and the ability to sit still. Therefore an anxious person may find it easier to begin with short periods of meditation, gradually increasing the length of time as its positive effects are experienced.

Depression

Meditation is not recommended for the treatment of severe depression since severely depressed people tend to resist suggestions that they learn to meditate and are unlikely to sustain practice. However, the use of meditation in the treatment of chronic low-grade depression or transitory depressive moods can have beneficial effects since feelings of well-being are common after beginning practice (Carrington 1978; Bloomfield et al. 1975).

Meditation can also bring underlying emotional factors contributing to depression into conscious awareness. For example, meditation can relieve pressure imposed on someone to engage in what may be perceived as meaningless activity, and instead open a genuine flow of creative inspiration or realignment of purpose. Thus a person who resists participating in normal activities during a period of depression may find therapeutic benefit from turning inward to uncover the source of depression and find a new sense of direction.

Since meditation tends to uncover repressed emotional conflicts, a mildly depressed person who takes up meditation may get in touch with feelings of sadness and anger that were formerly unrecognized. Although this may be considered a problem insofar as the emotional stress may be temporarily increased, effective discharge of repressed emotion can accelerate recovery of subjective feelings of energy and well-being.

Addiction

The use of meditation for combating addiction and drug dependence is indicated by reports that meditators tend to reduce drug usage quite dramatically after commencing practice. In studies of addiction, meditators consistently report a larger decrease in drug usage than nonmeditators (Shapiro 1980; et al.). How much this is the result of group pressure or a predisposition among those who take up meditation is uncertain, and reduced drug usage does not necessarily indicate successful treatment of drug abuse. However, since meditation lowers anxiety, it may reduce the need to take addictive substances and can help patients stay off drugs once they have made the choice to abstain. The use of meditation in alcoholism rehabilitation, for example, has been successful while the patients were in the hospital, but once discharged, they did not sustain practice (Carrington 1978).

It is suggested, therefore, that in combatting addiction, meditation is best used as a preventive measure, and indeed may be a rewarding adjunct to other forms of treatment. Meditation itself is sometimes referred to as a positive addiction, since meditators often report feeling a natural "high" after consistent practice. The relationship between various altered states of consciousness induced by such means as meditation, hypnosis, or drugs has not been clearly established, but evidence suggests that the meditative state may provide an accceptable substitute for some drug users.

EFFECTS ON PREGNANCY AND MENOPAUSE

Meditation may be particularly helpful at times when a woman is undergoing natural changes in hormonal balance. Pregnancy and menopause both involve profound psychological as well as somatic change. At these times, women may be particularly prone to extreme emotional swings between joy and despair. The development of equanimity cultivated in meditation can be a stabilizing factor, and during pregnancy may also benefit the unborn child.

Current research indicates that a harmonious emotional environment is beneficial to the developing fetus. In addition to the fact that the mother's body is producing the hormones that affect the baby's physiological development, there is evident that the baby's emotional development may also be influenced by the emotional tone of the mother's environment during pregnancy. Dr. Schwartz (1981) recommends meditating on the developmental process of the fetus as a way for parents to establish a loving relationship with the baby before birth. The quiet time of meditation can also help the mother more fully appreciate the generative life process taking place in her body and participate more consciously in the reproductive process.

Menopause is a time of hormonal instability that may be accompanied by emotional liability. Meditation can be of benefit to women who feel a loss of meaningful function in connection with the biological changes they are experiencing. By developing sensitivity to the change process and greater voluntary control of internal states, meditation can have a liberating and calming effect during what may be a difficult transitional time of readjustment. By relieving symptoms of anxiety and depression, meditation can help in the process of shifting the focus of life from biological mothering to other forms of satisfying activity or creativity.

DIAGNOSTIC EFFICIENCY

Clinicians who meditate claim that diagnostic efficiency can be enhanced as a result of practice. The enhancement of perceptual sensitivity (Walsh and Vaughan 1980) and greater receptivity to intuitive awareness (Vaughan 1979) evidently contribute to the refinment of diagnostic skills. Diagnostic intuitions developed as a result of meditation are easily amenable to confirmation through standard tests and may be useful in improving accuracy and comprehensiveness (Hastings 1980).

Diagnostic efficiency may also be enhanced by greater acuity in patients' self-reports resulting from meditation. For example, learning to pay close attention to subjective experience may enable a woman to provide more detailed information on her condition. She may also become more sensitive and alert to alterations of condition in response to treatment. In short, by reducing anxiety and unconscious emotional reactions, and encouraging objective, nonjudgmental self-observation meditation can contribute to effective communication between patient and physician.

Developing self-acceptance and learning to maintain alert noninterfering observation of sensations, feelings, thoughts, and images in meditation can enable many people suffering from somatic symptoms to discover contributing factors or even root causes of the problem. It can also be useful in mobilizing inner resources for self-healing and in recognizing and overcoming resistance to getting well.

Moreover, when a patient begins to recognize the power of his/her mind in determining states of physical and emotional well-being, motivation for training in meditation may be increased. The direct experience of the effect of changing states of consciousness on the perception of pain, for example, can provide reinforcement for continuing practice, as well as offering immediate relief in many instances.

CONCLUSIONS

There is substantial evidence that meditation can be used effectively in treating both psychosomatic and stress-related diseases. It has proved effective in the treatment of high blood pressure, peptic ulcers, bronchial asthma, insomnia, tension headaches, chronic fatigue, allergic conditions, and other such problems that are major concerns for both mental health professionals and physicians (Carrington 1978; Bloomfield et al. 1975; Walsh 1979). It also can be prescribed in practical forms for use as an adjunct to other forms of treatment. It has the advantage of not requiring special equipment or a clnical setting. Its validity as a method of self-regulation that enables patients to gain voluntary control of internal states has been affirmed by a number of studies in the past decade and merits further investigation and research (Shapiro 1980; et al.)

Meditation can also be used safely and appropriately as a preventive measure and as an antidote to stressful living conditions. Psychological benefits derived from meditation, e.g., clarity, equanimity, calm, non-judgmental self-acceptance, and inner peace, can help one cope more easily with any problem. It contributes to a holistic approach to maintaining health and preventing illness by sensitizing one to felt needs and tapping inner resources for insight, inspiration, and personal growth. The benefits of meditation may be experienced in spiritual, psychological, emotional, and physical dimensions, and it enables one to maintain a well-balanced integration of all these aspects of well-being. Meditation can be an antidote to both physical and emotional pain, but it is more difficult to begin practice during periods of stress. It is therefore recommended that practice be established before the onset of physical discomfort.

Anyone can practice meditation, but initially it can be difficult. Anyone who undertakes it should be prepared for some periods of restlessness and frustration during initial attempts to bring the mind under conscious control. It does require effort and self-discipline. Furthermore, consistency of practice is essential for effective results. It is therefore best suited to individuals who have sufficient ego strength to maintain practice, and it is especially recommended for those who are willing to assume responsibility for their own treatment program. It is less well suited to those who are severely disturbed.

REFERENCES

Benson, H., and M. Klipper, *The Relaxation Response.* New York: William Morrow & Co., Inc., 1975.

Benson H., and R. K. Wallace, "Decreased Drug Abuse with Transcendental Meditation: A Study of 1862 Subjects," in C. J. D. Zanafonetis, ed., *Drug Abuse Proceedings of the International Conference.* Philadelphia: Lea and Febiger, 1972.

Bloomfield, H. et al., *TM: Discovering Inner Energy and Overcoming Stress.* New York: Delacorte, 1975.

Brosse, T., "A Psychological Study of Yoga," *Main Currents in Modern Thought,* July 1946, pp. 77–84.

Carrington, P., *Freedom in Meditation.* New York: Anchor Books, 1978.

Deikman, A., "Experimental Meditation," *Journal of Nervous and Mental Diseases,* 136 (1966), 329–73.

Elgin, D., *Voluntary Simplicity*. New York: William Morrow & Co., Inc., 1981.

Goldstein, J., *The Experience of Insight*. Santa Cruz, Calif.: Unity Press, 1976.

Goleman, D., and G.Schwartz, "Meditation as an Intervention in Stress Reactivity," *Journal of Consulting and Clinical Psychology*, 44 (1976), 456–66.

Green, E., and A. Green, *Beyond Biofeedback*. New York: Delacorte, 1977.

Hastings, A, "Alternative Forms of Diagnosis," in A. Hastings, J. Fadiman, and J. Gordon, eds., *Health for the Whole Person*. Boulder, Colo.: Westview Press, 1980.

Kornfield, J., "Intensive Insight Meditation: A Phenomenological Study," *Transpersonal Psychology*, 11 (1979), 41–58.

Lesh, T., "Zen Meditation and the Development of Empathy in Counselors," *Journal of Humanistic Psychology*, 10 (1970), 39–74.

LeShan, L., *How to Meditate*. New York: Bantam Books, Inc., 1974.

Levine, S., *A Gradual Awakening*. New York: Anchor Books, 1978.

Maupin, E., "Individual Differences in Response to a Zen Meditation Exercise," *Journal of Consulting Psychology*, 29 (1965), 139–45.

Needleman, J., *A Sense of the Cosmos: The Encounter of Modern Science and Ancient Truth*. New York: Doubleday & Co., Inc., 1975.

Orme-Johnson, D. W., "Autonomic Stability in Transcendental Meditation," *Psychosomatic Medicine*, 35 (1973), 341–49.

Schwartz, L., *The World of the Unborn*. New York: Richard Marek, 1981.

Shafii, M., R. Lavel, and T. Jaffe, "Meditation and the Prevention of Alcohol Abuse," *American Journal of Psychiatry*, 132 (1975), 942–45.

Shapiro, D., *Meditation: Self-Regulation Strategy and Altered State of Consciousness*. Chicago: Aldine Publishing Company, 1980.

Shapiro, D., and R. Walsh, eds., *The Science of Meditation: Theory, Research and Experience*. Chicago: Aldine Publishing Company, 1982.

Tart, C., *Transpersonal Psychologies*. New York: Harper & Row Publishers, Inc., 1975.

Vaughan, F., *Awakening Instution*. New York: Doubleday/Anchor, 1979.

Wallace, R. K., "Physiological Effects of Transcendental Meditation," *Science*, March 27, 1970, pp. 1751–54.

Walsh, R., "Initial Meditative Experiences: I," *Journal of Transpersonal Psychology*, 9, no. 2(1977), 151–92.

———, "Initial Meditative Experiences: II," *Journal of Transpersonal Psychology*, 10, no. 1 (1978), 2–28.

———, "Meditation Research: An Introduction and Review," *Journal of Transpersonal Psychology*, 11, no. 2 (1979), 161–74.

Walsh, R., and F. Vaughan, eds., *Beyond Ego: Transpersonal Dimensions in Psychology*. Los Angeles: J. P. Tarcher, 1980.

Wilber, K., *The Atman Project*. Wheaton, Ill.: Theosophical Publishing House, 1979.

———, "A Developmental Model of Consciousness," in R. Walsh and F. Vaughan, eds., *Beyond Ego: Transpersonal Dimensions in Psychology*. Los Angeles: J. P. Tarcher, 1980.

SUGGESTED READINGS

Benson, H., and M. Klipper, *The Relaxation Response*. New York: Avon Books, 1975.

Bloomfield, H., M. Cains, and D. Jaffe, *TM: Discovering Inner Energy and Overcoming Stress*. New York: Delacorte, 1975. A popular book about transcendental meditation, which provides extensive information on research pertaining to medical effects of meditation prior to the date of publication.

Cade, C. M., and N. Coxhead, *The Awakened Mind: Biofeedback and the Development of Higher States of Awareness*. New York: Delacorte, 1979. An informative account of how Eastern meditative techniques can be combined with biofeedback for increasing effectiveness in personal mind-body control.

Carrington, P., *Freedom in Meditation*. New York: Doubleday/Anchor, 1978. An informative resource book for anyone who is curious about meditation and would like to get started without joining a special group.

Goleman, D., *Varieties of the Meditative Experience*. New York: E. P. Dutton & Co., Inc., 1977. An overview of Buddhist meditation, discussing different approaches to practice, i.e., insight and concentration, and a useful outline of stages of enlightenment on the meditative path.

Goldstein, J., *The Experience of Insight: A Natural Unfolding*. Santa Cruz, Calif.: Unity Press, 1976. An excellent introduction to sitting practice in the Buddhist tradition. This approach is particularly useful in developing self-awareness.

LeShan, L., *How to Meditate*. New York: Bantam Books, Inc., 1974. A good introduction for anyone interested in beginning to meditate. It discusses many types of meditation, the effects of meditation, and its relevance to our Western life style.

Levine, S., *A Gradual Awakening*. New York: Doubleday/Anchor, 1978. A good guidebook for the meditator looking for simplicity, directness, and loving kindness. The author shares personal experiences and insights into how meditation helps us become more aware of ourselves.

Ram Dass, *Journey of Awakening: A Meditator's Guidebook*. New York: Bantam Books, Inc., 1978. A step-by-step introduction that encourages the beginner to investigate meditation practice as a way of finding meaning in being, and provides a number of useful resources for the journey.

Shapiro, D., *Meditation: Self-Regulation Strategy and Altered State of Consciousness*. Chicago: Aldine Publishing Company, 1980. A scientific and personal exploration of the subject that carefully examines the research literature and prescribes indications and contraindications of medical and other therapeutic uses.

Shapiro, D., and R. Walsh, eds., *The Science of Meditation: Theory, Research and Experience*. Chicago: Aldine Publishing Company, 1982. A comprehensive, up-to-date review of the state of the art of meditation. This book will be of interest to serious investigators of the subject.

Sujata, Anagarita, *Beginning to See*. Santa Cruz, Calif.: Unity Press, 1975. A picture book of graphic illustrations on the effects of meditation.

Suzuki, S., *Zen Mind, Beginner's Mind*. New York: Weatherhill, 1970. A classic introduction to the basic teachings of Zen meditation, with wise, poetic, and gentle instructions for the beginner.

Chapter Twenty-Four

SELF-HYPNOSIS WITH APPLICATIONS TO WOMEN'S HEALTH

Freda Morris

Franz Anton Mesmer, the physician who first developed and popularized hypnosis under the name of "animal magnetism," in the late eighteenth century in Vienna and Paris, had almost all women patients. Charcot, the French neurologist who was one of Freud's hypnosis teachers, developed his hypnosis theories through work only with women. And Freud began his monumental work, *The Interpretation of Dreams*, through hypnotic work with a woman patient (1950).

CASE STUDY

For our purpose here we will briefly review a case that Freud published in 1893. It was the case of a mother who was unable to feed her newborn child until hypnotic suggestion intervened. Freud went on to describe the situation.

> I found her lying in bed with flushed cheeks and furious at her inability to feed the baby—an inability which increased at every attempt but against which she struggled with all her strength. I attempted to induce hypnosis by ocular fixation, at the same time making constant suggestions of the symptoms of sleep. After three minutes the patient was lying back with the peaceful expression of a person in profound sleep. I said, "Do not be afraid. You will make an excellent nurse and the baby will thrive." When I came back the next evening she said that she had an excellent appetite and plenty of milk for the baby; there was not the slightest difficulty when it was put to her breast. [1893.]

Freud found it strange that he was given no thanks by either the woman or her husband, nor was hypnotism mentioned. A year later the same problem arose with their next born. After again having striking success, Freud tells the story:

> In face of this renewed success the patient unbent and admitted the motive that had governed her behavior towards me. "I felt ashamed," the woman said to me, "that a thing like hypnosis should be successful where I myself, with all my will-power, was helpless." [1963]

WHO'S IN CHARGE OF ME?

The woman in Freud's story was terribly distressed that "a thing like hypnosis" should be in charge rather than she herself. Think about it. Who *is* in charge of your body? Who decides whether you shall nurse your baby? Who decides whether you will have a pregnancy or not? Who decides whether you shall cramp at the time of your period? Who decides whether you shall have high or low blood pressure? Who decides whether you shall get a cold on weekends or in the middle of the week or at all? Who decides whether you will feel pain or not, even when the dentist is drilling deep with no Novocaine?

You may answer: "My heredity and the stresses under which I work. The ability of the sperm to get to my ovum, naturally. Why, the number of germs in the air, of course. And, certainly, it's natural and unavoidable to hurt when the dentist drills. Some things are outside of the control of willpower."

That's true. But there is another kind of power—an allowing power, a flowing with, a letting it happen. It is a much stronger force than the will and much more broadly applicable. It brings under your control and direction almost every aspect of your self, down even to the very cells and molecules that compose your body. You need only learn how to evoke that special power. It is the purpose of this chapter to give you evidence for its existence, and to tell you how to put it to use to your great betterment.

As children we are taught that diseases and various maladies come upon us from outside. We are responsible for what we do with our striate (ordinary) muscles; that is, we should go to school on time, keep clean, eat well, exercise, and not hit other kids. But if we get sick or hurt, there is nothing to do but stay in bed and take medicine. The functions of our body chemistry, our smooth muscles, glands, and relexes are out of our control, or so we are told.

But when I was 15 years old, I made an amazing discovery that literally demolished at least part of this belief system for me. I was standing before a mirror with a beveled edge such that the edge reflected a focused light, brighter than the rest of the mirror. As I moved my eye into the streak of bright light, I could see my pupil constrict. I knew that it constricted to keep out the excess light. But I said to myself, "There's no one in there except me. I must be constricting it and not knowing it, like I often do things I don't know I can do, or don't intend to do, or don't know that I am doing." So I moved back and forth into and out of the focused light saying, "Dialate" and "Constrict" as appropriate to what my eye was doing. After awhile I simply said the words without changing the light, and my eye responded anyway. Then I just thought the words, and my eye still responded. Finally, I imagined the changes in the light wordlessly, and that worked too. I had been taught that the pupillary reflex was completely involuntary, that the person had absolutely no control over it. Obviously, this was not true. I was in charge of a little bit more of myself than I had thought, and I suspected that there were many more little bits of my self that I was really boss of. I ultimately found that the body chemistry, smooth muscles, and glands are also included.

I came to think of the "boss" as the essence of a person that wants the best for all parts and takes responsibility for the organization of the person as a whole.

This "boss" is "you," the owner and operator of the organization. You send down orders for the outcome, the results you want. Your workers, that is, the various parts of your body, know what to do to create the health, happiness, and success that you request.

COMMUNICATION MODES

You communicate to your blood cells and your bone narrow, to your attitudes, and to your emotions. How this communication takes place is an interesting question, one that has not been satisfactorily answered. Somehow thoughts in your mind are translated into physically expressed information bits that bring messages and produce positive effects.

We don't know how or why some things happen, but we do know some communication modes that are very effective. These are outlined below:

Repetition. Anything that we tell ourselves or are told over and over tends to become a physical reality. For example, "My nose always runs during ragweed season."

Role models. We tend to become like our parents or other admired, feared, or loved persons, especially those we hold in awe. Their communications in word and action influence us strongly and tend to program us to be the way we are.

Authorities. Science says that you should get three colds per year, sleep eight hours per night, and weigh 120 pounds. Therefore you expect and demand these things of yourself.

Strong emotion. During a state of strong emotion we tend to accept what we hear, see, or understand. Gil Boyne, Los Angeles hypnotherapist, tells of a woman who could not shake the feeling that her husband did not love her. With hypnotic regression, it was discovered that on her honeymoon during a highly charged lover's quarrel, she had heard her groom say that he was sorry that he had married her. This no longer meaningful memory was easily replaced by her husband telling her that he was glad he married her while she was in the highly charged state of experiencing orgasm (Tebbetts 1979).

SELF-CONTROL THROUGH PROGRAMMING

In hypnosis we are easily, quickly, and deeply responsive to programming. Hypnosis is a state of consciousness in which we suspend judgment and criticality. We are open and responsive. We tend to clear the deck, or clean the slate, so that new information can come in fresh.

An impressive example of hypnotic suggestion was reported by researcher Black (1969). Although for ten years a patient had had severe attacks of asthma every March, she was able to clean her slate through hypnotic suggestion. She came in for hypnosis for the first time just before the pollen season was to begin, during which she became a "chronic invalid." In the hypnotic treatment, she was simply given suggestions that she would have no difficulty with breathing, running or blocked nose, itching, or sneezing. These suggestions were repeated many times over, during each 30-minute treatment. Her response to this treatment was quite profound: no asthma attacks for the entire pollen season. This case will be referred to again in a later section to demonstrate the effect of the mind on the body chemistry.

In this case, the woman was responding to the suggestions of the doctor; but if in the hypnotic state we maintain a part of our minds to do the programming, to give ourselves the information, we are using *self-hypnosis*. With self-hypnosis we need to have no concern about the suggestions wearing off. We simply give them again as often as need be. We are independent, in charge. We can unprogram those programs that we do not like and plug in new ones.

Salter (1963) gave an example of self-programming: "A woman stutterer would speak impeccably for about two days after a session, and then relapse to her old level. With self-hypnosis she had no occasion to revisit me."

FEMALE HEALTH PROBLEMS HELPED BY HYPNOSIS

Painful Intercourse (Vaginismus)

Fear of sexual aggressiveness from men in a group of 71 women was studied by Fuchs and Hoch (1978). Exactly how the fear was programmed in, they did not say, but we can speculate that it was with repetition, role modeling, and no doubt, with strong emotion. All 71 women suffered from vaginismus, a condition described as "a psycho-physiological syndrome affecting women's freedom of sexual response by severely or totally impeding coital function" (ibid.). Out of fear, a woman may simply clamp her vagina shut, and the man cannot penetrate. It is described as a "spastic contraction of the vaginal outlet which is a completely involuntary reflex, stimulated by imagined, anticipated or real attempts at vaginal penetration (ibid.).

All these women were married and had been suffering from the condition for more than two years. They had also all been treated by gynecologists and psychiatrists for long periods without results.

The hypnotic treatment used was first to teach each woman self-hypnosis. Then all the women were told to vividly imagine erotic situations with their husbands. They moved at their own pace, gradually inserting a finger and than a dilator into the vagina until they gained confidence in their ability to open to their husbands. When they actually began intercourse, they remained on top of their husbands until they became completely confident and were able to experiment.

This is a terrible malady that prevents normal marriage and childbirth, yet it can be treated simply with understanding that a conditioned reflex can come under voluntary control through reprogramming. With regard to the importance of the active role for the woman, the article states:

> Being active, the wife automatically prevents the previously dreaded image of an "attacking husband." The self-esteem and self-confidence gained during therapy will be thus further reinforced by successful intercourse. [Ibid.]

Infertility

General problems of infertility may arise from a similar fearful attitude associated with passivity. Rather than using gross musculature, a woman might prevent penetration of the ovum by the sperm through creating chemical barriers. Although there has been nothing in the literature to support such a contention, there have been two cases (that this author has found through exploration in deep hypnosis) that revealed the feeling that the women were holding the sperm away from the ovum through creating impenetrable walls around it. This realization, together with direct suggestions of opening the barriers, plus images of creating ideal conditions for the sperm, allowed the women to become pregnant (Morris 1979).

Urinary Incontinence

Whatever happens repeatedly begins to be expected, and the internal dialogue reflects this expectancy. A fairly common malady among women is the inability to hold urine firmly during sudden bursts of activity such as coughing, hard laughter, certain movements in sports, and during orgasm. The problem often starts after a urinary infection or after pregnancy. Once it begins, the internal dialogue or expectancy inclines it to continue, even though the physiological reason is absent. Godec reported what he believed to be the first case successfully treated with hypnosis (1980). All he did was teach the young woman to hypnotize herself. While she was in the hypnotic state, he demonstrated to her that her bladder could hold three times as much as she had been able to retain in ordinary consciousness. Although she had to void every 30 minutes and twice at night prior to hypnosis, within one week after learning to hypnotize herself, she was normal.

Obesity

Although American's number one health problem—obesity—is terribly recalcitrant, remarkable changes come about if expectancy is changed. Stanton (1975) reported 100 percent maintenance of weight loss in a two-year follow-up with ten cases. Among the simple direct suggestions for eating changes, he also included suggestions for a change in self-image. "And this is the way you will look, and this is the weight you will be. As you believe this, so it will happen."

Attitude Change

With the internal dialogue changes, the person redefines herself, and a new and healthy expectancy set is developed. Since thoughts control our lives, improved health is inevitable.

We can easily see how attitude change helps in improving general health, but the mystery becomes profound when we begin to probe how the more microscopic changes come about; that is, How do thoughts alone change blood chemistry? The purpose of the next section is to explore some of the more dramatic cases and to attempt to accept the reality without understanding the mechanism.

THE MIND AFFECTS BODY CHEMISTRY

Asthma, Cancer, and Rheumatoid Arthritis

There are three distinct immunological errors on the part of the body that lead to the three different conditions of bronchial asthma, cancer, and rheumatoid arthritis. With asthma the immune system is *over*reactive in fighting off the pollen or other foreign invader. In cancer, it is *under*reactive, thus allowing the undesirable cells to grow rather than killing them. In rheumatoid arthritis, the immune system is *misguided* in its attempts to defend the body, and the immune system responds to its own body's tissue as if it were a foreign invader, a case of mistaken identity.

The power of the mind to profoundly affect the chemistry of the body was clearly shown by skin tests of the woman presented earlier as having no asthma attacks after hypnotic suggestion. Recall that she was hypnotized and told that she would have no sneezing or other symptoms during the pollen season. Her doctors tested her and found that her immediate-type hypersensitivity skin reaction to injected antigens was also eliminated, even though that had not been suggested. One of the researchers inject the patient's serum into his own arm, and then exposed himself to the allergen. Amazingly, he displayed the characteristic hypersensitive skin response. In other words, the woman was somehow inhibiting an allergic reaction to pollen despite the presence of the antibodies in her serum that should have brought about the allergic reaction (Black 1969).

Further research with hypersensitive individuals led other researchers (reviewed by Bowers and Kelly 1979) to conclude that *individuals who responded well to hypnotic suggestions* could reduce or eliminate allergic reactions through hypnotic suggestion even at a blood chemistry level, i.e., through immunological factors.

Of 121 cases of asthma patients treated with hypnosis, another reasearcher, Collison (1975), reported that the 19 who were completely cured were highly hypnotizable. Almost all the rest, the nonhypnotizable, were unaffected by positive suggestions.

Stephanie Mathews-Simonton and co-workers (1978) reported the effects of "meditative visualization" as a supplement to medical treatment of 159 patients who were diagnosed as having incurable cancer. The instructions given to the patients were to visualize the cancerous cells being destroyed in a naturally healthy way, and to visualize the diseased body part as healthy. Twenty-seven percent of this sample were significantly helped, and about 9 percent completely recovered. However, it is important to note that this sample of patients was selected from the much larger group of the Simontons' practice, and made up about 5 percent of it. Bowers and Kelly (1979) speculate that these 159 people were more likely to be *talented in the ability to achieve hypnotic states* than the larger population.

A man who later became a colleague of this author had fairly advanced rheumatoid arthritis, and was scheduled for retirement into a wheelchair. Through his contact with medical doctors during his conventional treatment, he gained some knowledge of the relationship between the disease, stress, and personality factors, but knew nothing about the immunological variables. For the purpose of improving his sleep, which was impaired due to chronic pain, he learned to hypnotize himself. Discovering himself to have *exceptional hypnotic ability*, he treated himself through visualization and suggestion, and reversed the disease process. He now has virtually no symptoms of arthritis (McDowell 1978).

Vaginal Viral Conditions

Conditions caused by viruses have well-documented responses to hypnotic suggestion. Warts, including vaginal warts, are a common and sometimes seriously limiting malady. They have been removed through hypnotic suggestion in odd patterns such as on one side of the body only, so that spontaneous recovery could not be used to explain away the results. Many studies show that the success rate is much higher among persons known to be easily hypnotized (Johnson and Barber 1978).

Menstrual Cramps

A woman who had learned to *achieve deep hypnotic states* in order to enhance her creative writing ability casually mentioned to this author that she suffered agonizing menstrual cramps each month. The cramps were worst just before her period started. Her period was due at the time of my interview with her. I talked to her for less than five minutes, suggesting that she go into a deep hypnotic state and activate the proper hormones from her pituitary gland so as to start her period and carry it out pain-free. I suggested that she would continue to do so indefinitely at just the right times. Her period started within a few hours and was perfectly comfortable. This was several months ago, and her periods have been relatively pain-free since.

In order for the hypnotic suggestions to be effective, the person must become uncritically and imaginatively absorbed in the information or idea received. The ability to do this seems to be almost by definition *a function of the hypnotic ability of the person*. In other words, the ability to translate the message of health into immunological or biochemical action lies in the person, not in the words or images. With such powerful evidence that words and images can be translated into the langauge of the body and acted upon to bring about health-giving changes involving immunological processes, it seems that almost any condition can be prevented and often successfully be treated by hypnosis in people who are capable of receiving hypnotic suggestion. The crucial factor seems to be the capability of the person to get the message of health through to the "workers" at the cellular levels.

In the next section, we discuss how to develop the skill to get the desired messages through both to the body and to those aspects of mind that control habits and attitudes. We also elaborate a plan for maintaining health and well-being through the use of these methods.

SELF-HYPNOSIS AND HYPNOTIC SUGGESTION

Hypnosis can be used to further any human endeavor. By looking at some of the characteristics of a hypnotized person, you will see that the potential benefits of hypnosis are unlimited. When compared with people in ordinary consciousness, people in hypnotic states can:

More readily recall visual memories, feelings, sounds, and ideas from the recent or distant past.

More easily, quickly, and creatively construct mental images (either realistic or fanciful).

More fully remove old attitudes and develop new ones—maintaining the new attitudes after returning to ordinary consciousness.

In addition, they have the ability to:

Change the way they experience the "realities" of life.

Heighten the intensity of sensations, feelings, and emotions.

Block painful sensations.

Gain increased control of physiological functions.

A wonderful quality of hypnosis is that, with proper training, you can use it alone, at will, in minutes, and without complicated procedures. These facts make the benefits readily available throughout life.

The hypnotic state is a naturally occurring state of consciousness that everyone experiences to greater or lesser degrees at times. Following is a description so you'll know the next time you have the good fortune or take the initiative to experience this state.

Hypnotic state: Here are some of the sensations you may experience while in hypnosis: Your arms or legs may seem to float a few inches above the floor, or they may feel heavy, as though they were sinking into the floor. They may seem to be in a different position than they actually are. You may lose conscious awareness of parts of your body, or all of it, and be conscious only of your mind. You may see strange visions or beautifully colored patterns of light. [Tebbetts 1977, used with permission.]

Children achieve hypnotic states easily. This author firmly believes that anyone can relearn this marvelous skill. Certainly people vary widely in hypnotic talent, but skill in achieving the state grows with practice. You have experienced it spontaneously, perhaps without recognizing it, when you are just coming from or going to sleep and often when absorbed in music, a play, a sunset, etc. To get into a hypnotic state deliberately, ask a friend to talk you into sleep. Depending on your personal hypnotic talent (the ease with which you move through various states of consciousness), it may be very easy for you to achieve assisted self-hypnosis simply by sitting or lying still with your eyes closed while your friend counts slowly, or describes in vivid detail some interesting object. My book, *Hypnosis with Friends and Lovers* (1979) is the only one I know of on assisted self-hypnosis.

If you want to work alone, the use of self-made tapes is recommended (Morris 1975; Tebbetts 1977), or commercially made tapes (Boyne 1981). If you have deeply forgotten the skill you had as a child, I recommend that you take a self-hypnosis seminar or see an amateur or professional hypnotist for individual instruction.

In the meantime, begin giving yourself positive helpful suggestions using the methods given below. This list comes from Boyne 1979. As you learn to achieve deeper and deeper hypnotic states, the suggestions will become more and more effective.

Rules for Structuring Successful Suggestions

1. *Use present tense*. A suggestion phrased in the future is not a suggestion but an annoyance. It sounds burdensome and antagonistic. Stated in the present, it's "the truth told in advance," as the great sales trainer Zigler says (1979).

2. *Be positive*. Eliminate every possible unpleasant word or negative phrasing. Do not mention what you are moving away from. For example, say, "I am perfectly comfortable during my menstrual flow," rather than, "I don't have cramps anymore."

3. *Be specific*. Don't make vague statements. Pin yourself down to exactly what you want, knowing that you can correct any errors later.

4. *Be detailed*. By adding details to your suggestions you bring them alive and are able to create the experience now.

5. *Be simple*. Simple words and sentences that make a single point are better than complex sentences that require logical processes to follow.

6. *Use exciting, emotional words.* Use words that are vibrant, sparkling, thrilling, wonderful, powerful, radiant, loving, etc.

7. *Use the active voice.* Don't say that you have the ability to do such and such. Say that you do it.

8. *Be realistic*, but don't limit yourself unnecessarily.

9. *Use repetition.* Keep repeating your suggestion until it comes about, or you replace it with something better.

I recommend that you write out a set of suggestions, and read them onto cassette tape. Listen to the tape regularly while deeply relaxing and occupying your conscious mind with pleasant fantasy. Include in your tape suggestions for a pleasant healthful program of rest, recreation, exercise, food, and positive attitudes toward work and family.

MUTUAL HYPNOSIS

In addition to the beneficial effects of a self-suggestion program, self-hypnosis can be used to explore your deeper personality. It is helpful to have a supportive friend with you when you use self-hypnosis for self-exploration, although this is not essential. Methods and techniques are detailed in my book *Hypnosis with Friends and Lovers* (Morris 1979). The purpose of self-exploration is to gain deep self-understanding by clarifying your feelings, your goals, and your relationships.

WOMEN AS NATURAL HYPNOTISTS

We began this chapter by pointing to women's early experience with the value of hypnosis. In the 1890s, Dr. Freud, a male authority, was the dominating hypnotist, and a woman was embarrassed that she could not do what she wanted to do with her willpower. Yet, using the "mere words" of the doctor, she was able to translate her desire to nurse her baby into a language that her mammary glands understood and thus create milk for her baby. All the hypnotist did was speak; the hypnotee made the dramatic changes within herself. She simply did not have the concept of taking credit for the positive actions of her volitional self.

Women intuitively know the value of deep inner-connectedness. They know the value of deep exploration, and I believe that they are naturals for mutual hypnosis.

Major stresses, both in business and personal life, come primarily from interpersonal relations. Stress and conflict dissolve, however, through the process of mutual hypnosis for assisting each other into hypnotic states and exploring true feelings. Such open relating is much more familiar and natural for women than for men. I believe that as women move more and more into top management in business, industry, and government, these tools of self-discovery and conflict resolution will come more and more into use through the influence of women. As women gain more power, I believe that they will channel more funds into research on the value of hypnosis in the prevention and treatment of disease as well as in the maintenance of health.

In conclusion, I predict that within the next twenty years the increased uses of hypnosis will bring enhanced health and happiness for both women and men.

REFERENCES

Black, S., *Mind and Body*. London: William Kimber, 1969.

Bowers, K., and P. Kelly, "Stress, Disease, Psychotherapy, and Hypnosis," *Journal of Abnormal Psychology*, 88 (1979), 490–505.

Boyne, G., "Rules for Structuring Successful Auto-Suggestion." From a seminar, Los Angeles, 1979.

———, *Catalog of Hypnosis Tapes and Books*. 312 Riverdale, Glendale, Calif.: 1981.

Collison, D., "Which Asthmatic Patients Should Be Treated by Hypnotherapy?" *Medical Journal of Australia*, 1 (1975), 776–81.

Freud, S., *The Interpretation of Dreams*. Basic, 1950.

———, "A Case of Successful Treatment by Hypnotism (1893), in P. Rieff, ed., *Therapy and Techniques*. New York: P. F. Collier, Inc., 1963.

Fuchs, D., and Z. Hoch. Hypno-Desensitization Therapy of Vaginismus," in F. Frankel and H. Zamansky, eds., *Hypnosis at Its Bicentennial*. New York: Plenum Publishing Corporation, 1978.

Godec, C., "Inhibition of Hyperreflexic Bladder during Hypnosis," *American Journal of Clinical Hypnosis*, 22 (1980), 170–72.

Johnson, R., and T. Barber, "Hypnosis, Suggestion, and Warts: An Experimental Investigation Implicating the Importance of 'Believed-in Efficacy,' *American Journal of Clinical Hypnosis*, 20 (1978), 165–74.

McDowell, K., personal communication, 1978.

Morris, Freda, *Self-Hypnosis in Two Days*. New York: E. P. Dutton & Co., Inc., 1975.

———, *Hypnosis with Friends and Lovers*. New York: Harper & Row, Publishers, Inc., 1979.

Salter, A., *What Is Hypnosis?* New York: Citadel Press, 1944.

Simonton, C., Stephanie Matthews-Simonton, and N. Creighton, *Getting Well Again*. Los Angeles: Tarcher/St. Martin's, 1978.

Stanton, H., "Weight Loss Through Hypnosis," *American Journal of Clinical Hypnosis*, 18 (1975), 34–38.

Tebbetts, C., *Self-Hypnosis: The Creative Use of Your Mind for Successful Living*. Los Angeles: Westwood Publishing Company, 1979.

Wall Street Journal. Sperry advertisement, December 23, 1980, p. 17. West Coast edition.

Zigler, Z., sales seminar, Palo Alto, Calif., 1979.

SUGGESTED READINGS

August, Ralph, *Hypnosis in Obstetrics*. New York: McGraw-Hill Book Company, 1968.

Chapman, L. F., Helen Goodell, and H. G. Wolff, "Changes in Tissue Vulnerability Induced During Hypnotic Suggestion," *Journal of Psychosomatic Research*, 4 (1959), 99–105.

Cheek, David, and Leslie M. LeCron, *Clinical Hypnotherapy*. New York: Grune & Stratton, Inc., 1968.

Crasilneck, Harold B., and James A. Hall, *Clinical Hypnosis: Principles and Applications*. New York: Grune & Stratton, Inc., 1975.

Esdaile, James, *Hypnosis in Medicine and Surgery*. New York: Julian Press, 1957.

Frank, Jerome, *Persuasion and Healing*. Baltimore: John Hopkins University Press, 1973.

Haley, Jay, ed. *Advanced Techniques of Hypnosis and Therapy: Selected Papers of Milton H. Erickson*. New York: Grune & Stratton, Inc., 1967.

Hilgard, Ernest, and Josephine Hilgard, *Hypnosis in the Relief of Pain*. Los Altos, Calif.: William Kaufmann, 1975.

Simonton, Carl, and Stephanie Matthews-Simonton, and N. Creighton, *Getting Well Again*. Los Angeles: Tarcher/St. Martin's, 1978.

LISTING OF ORGANIZATIONS FOR HYPNOSIS

The American Society of Clinical
Hypnosis
2400 East Devon Avenue, Suite 218
Des Plaines, IL 60018
(312) 297-3317

International Journal of Clinical and
Expermental Hypnosis
111 North 49th Street
Philadelphia, PA 19139

Psyche Research Institute
10701 Lomas Northeast, Suite 210
Albuquerque, NM 87112
(505) 292-0370

The Society for Clinical and
Experimental Hypnosis
129A Kings Park Drive
Liverpool, NY 13088
(315) 652-7299

Chapter Twenty-Five

SELF-HEALING IN THE TWENTIETH CENTURY: SELF-HELP AND VAGINAL DISEASES

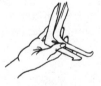

Plastic vaginal speculuum

Carol Downer

At present, there are over one hundred women's health projects around the country. They have many differences in their history, their organizational structure, and their day-to-day activities; but they share a common philosophy of self-help or self-health, which means that self-examination of the breast and genitals and sharing of information form the basis of their health education programs (Federation of Feminist Women's Health, 1981).

In early 1970, women began to learn to do vaginal self-examination and to feel for the size and position of each other's uterus. This first group of women found that it was easy to learn self-examination with the plastic speculum. The walls of the instrument are stretched apart by the two bills of the speculum and are locked into an open position. With a mirror and a light, a woman can see the cervix (the knoblike protuberance that extends into the vagina), the vaginal walls, and any secretions that are coming from the cervical os (the opening of the cervical canal that leads to the uterus). She can also see the color, the shape, and the texture of the face of the cervix. (See Figure 25-1).

The radical possibilities of this health education activity soon became evident. As women shared their health experiences, they found that much of what they had considered the province of the physician, such as fitting diaphagms or cervical caps, and health concerns such as vaginal infections, urinary tract infections, detection of pregnancy, menstrual difficulties, and a myriad of minor problems, were well within their control. Some "problems" turned out not to be problems at all. For example, a tipped uterus or an irregular menstrual cycle is merely a normal and healthy variation of the angle and flexion of the uterus or of the menstrual cycle.

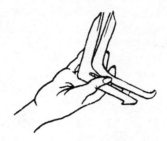

FIGURE 25-1. Plastic vaginal speculuum.

Women also discovered that early detection and quick treatment of such illnesses as a urinary tract infection were not only feasible but far preferable to letting the disease reach crisis proportions before seeking out and obtaining medical treatment, which in many cases consisted of strong and dangerous drugs. The first Self-Help Clinic, The Feminist Women's Health Center in Los Angeles, developed the 'technique of "menstrual extraction," in 1971, a method used to extract the contents of the uterus on or about the day of the expected period. Based on the same technology as vacuum aspiration for early abortion, using a device invented by Lorraine Rothman, this technique promises to give women direct control of the termination of very early pregnancy.

EARLY OPPOSITION BY MEDICAL PROFESSION

The basic political aim of the self-help movement, which rapidly spread across the United States and Europe, in the 1970s is to assert women's rights to control their sexuality and reproduction, to directly deal with a variety of everyday health concerns, and to enable women to become informed and assertive consumers of medical care when it becomes necessary. Obviously, this movement poses a direct threat to the sway of the male-dominated medical profession.

In September 1972, the medical profession moved to counter the threat of Self-Help Clinics. The Feminist Women's Health Center in Los Angeles was raided by police, and two women, the author and Colleen Wilson, were arrested for practicing medicine without a license. Wilson was charged with 11 counts, including demonstrating a menstrual extraction and pulling out a lost tampon. She pled guilty to one count of fitting a diaphragm and was given summary probation and fined $250.00. The author contested the one charge against her based on having helped a woman to insert yogurt into her vagina for the treatment of a yeast condition. Because the police confiscated the yogurt in the Center's refrigerator, this case was dubbed "The Yogurt Conspiracy." The author's trial and acquittal were highly publicized, and the way was opened for women to learn directly about their own bodies.

MAJOR ACCOMPLISHMENT OF WOMEN'S HEALTH MOVEMENT— THE TREATMENT OF VAGINAL INFECTION

One of the major accomplishments of the women's health movement has been the discovery of various ways to effectively prevent, treat, and sometimes permanently cure a vaginal infection. How have medically untrained women been able to solve a problem of epidemic proportions, one that gynecologists have only been able to offer temporary, risky treatments for? The answer is through Self-Help Clinics. Women found that many of them were creating their own infections by trying to get rid of certain secretions from the cervix and vagina, secretions that they felt were abnormal but were really healthy. They were soon able to learn through observation that these secretions vary in amount and consistency throughout the menstrual cycle. Around the time of ovulation, these vaginal secretions are generally clear, slippery, and may be quite profuse. This type of healthy secretion is "fertile mucus" produced by glands in the cervical canal, and it is vital to reproduction. The Catholic Church, because it needed to provide its members with a method of birth control based on abstinence during the fertile period, developed the Billings Method, which demonstrated that fertile mucus literally pulls the sperm into the canal and into the uterus and nurtures them. At other times of the month, the secretions are more creamy and white, sometimes resembling library paste. This "non-fertile" mucus is inhospitable to sperm, blocking their entrance to the cervical canal (Billings 1975). The medical profession has erroneously labeled this whitish secretion, "leukorrhea," a fearsome term to describe what is in fact healthy cervical secretions mixed with cast-off vaginal wall cells.

Because women have not understood the role of these secretions in their healthy functioning, and because huge advertising campaigns have been based on the supposed offensiveness of female odors, many women have been persuaded to use a variety of means to eliminate the odors or to disguise them, such as douching and spraying with deodorant. These efforts have resulted in drying the vagina, changing the vaginal flora, and in the case of deodorant sprays, of causing drying up, irritation, and even injury to the mucous membranes (Hopkins 1975; Fisher 1973). Many a woman has been delighted to find that her "vaginitis" cleared up when she stopped douching or spraying.

Another factor that has increased the incidence of vaginal infections is the current styles of tight pants and nylon pantyhose. If the air cannot circulate, the build-up of heat favors the growth of undesirable organisms. In hot weather, a vaginal infection, usually a yeast condition, may result. Cotton panties and nylon pantyhose with cotton crotches may help prevent such problems.

It may be said that women have brought vaginal infections on themselves through ignorance or through vanity, but certainly the medical profession bears the greater responsibility for causing vaginal infections by prescribing antibiotics and birth-control pills. Antibiotics not only kill the bacteria that are causing an illness but they also destroy the friendly, beneficial bacteria that inhabit the vagina as well. Many women find that they have gotten rid of one problem only to have a raging yeast infection. Birth-control pills, among their many undesirable effects on the body, cause the cells of the vagina to have a higher sugar content, the food of yeast.

TYPES OF VAGINAL INFECTIONS AND RECOMMENDED TREATMENT

There are three basic types of vaginal infections: (1) a yeast condition, (2) trichomoniasis, and (3) bacterial infection. Women have learned that they can distiguish these from one another through observing the odor, color, amount, and consistency of the discharge and other signs.

Yeast Condition

A yeast condition can be recognized by the white, clumpy discharge and its characteristic yeasty odor. Sometimes, the clitoral lips and opening to the vagina will be red and irritated, causing severe itching. At other times, a woman will notice a yeast condition only if she does self-examination. Since the problem arises because the one-celled yeast plants (that are typically found in the vagina) have overgrown, the principle of home treatment is to restore the natural dominance of lactobacilli, the type of bacteria normally present. Thus the application of plain, preferably unpasteurized, yogurt or one or two lactobacillus tablets into the vagina alleviates this condition by reintroducing these bacteria. This treatment is also very soothing to the tissues.

Trichomoniasis

A trichomoniasis infection is caused by the proliferation of one-celled animals called *trichomonads*. These bothersome parasites are passed from person to person by sexual contact. They can live in the male reproductive tract without causing symptoms, but they quickly multiply in the woman's vagina or urethra and within days can begin to cause irritation and discharge. As the infection reaches its height, the discharge has a disagreeable fishy smell. When a woman uses her speculum she can see the discharge, which usually forms a yellowish and frothy pool in the vagina. A greenish discharge, especially direct from the cervix, will alert her that the infection is accompanied by gonorrhea, a not unusual combination. This discharge will keep the inner lips uncomfortably moist, but the vagina will feel dry. The cervix is often covered with red blotches, and the individual generally will have tenderness and pain.

The drug most often prescribed for trichomoniasis, Flagyl, is a classic example of drug abuse. Flagyl (metronidazole) *is* effective in killing trichomonads, but it *also* causes nausea, headache, diarrhea, or a metallic taste in the mouth in many people. Drinking alcohol while taking Flagyl can intensify any of these effects. Furthermore, the white blood cell count is lowered, making the body less resistant to infection. And, to top off the list, the *Medical Letter*, a newsletter published by a nonprofit group of Physicians has printed reports that Flagyl has caused cancer in rats (*Physician's Desk Reference* 1980).

If trichomoniasis were a life-threatening disease, or even if Flagyl were the only effective remedy, the risks of taking Flagyl might be justified. But, on the contrary, there are fortunately several inexpensive, safe, and effective self-treatments available to women. The treatment works on the principle of flushing out the infestation, diluting the number of organisms, or even better, killing them off completely. Some of those remedies are also soothing to the inflamed tissues.

Two types of treatments that directly attack the trichomonads are a garlic suppository and a Betadine douche. The suppository is prepared by peeling a clove, and either inserting it as is, or wrapping it in a strip of gauze and dipping it in vegetable oil before inserting into the vagina. The clove is changed every 12 hours for three-to-five days.

Another treatment, douching daily with a Betadine solution (an over-the-counter iodine-based antibacterial soap) through the menstrual period and for a week following, is generally effective. The need to continue treatment after the menstrual period arises from the fact that the trichomoniasis often reappears after the period is over. If remedies are not reaching all the surfaces of the vagina, any trichomonads left in the creases can multiply, until within a few days or weeks they once again cause inflammation and irritation.

To administer the Betadine douche, one should roll back on the shoulders, raising the hips so that the vagina is upside down. This is best done in the tub. Rest the legs against the wall or the sides of the tub. This ways the vagina balloons out, so there are no creases or crevices. The vaginal opening is gently spread apart either with the fingers or with a speculum.

The Betadine, warmed to body temperature, is then slowly poured into the vagina and is left there for several minutes. Sitting up will force the fluid out of the vagina. A variation on this method is to put one-half cup of Betadine into the vagina and swab another one-half cup onto the vagina walls and the entrance to the vagina, using cotton gauze pads or cotton balls held with a pair of kitchen tongs. The pain of trichomoniasis results from the millions of trichomonads biting the flesh. After this Betadine blitz, the pain immediately ceases, and within hours the cervix becomes clear and the inflammation goes down.

Herbal douches used once or twice a day for a week or more will also clear up this type of infection. Teas that have antiseptic properties and that can relieve inflammation are: Bayberry, Goldenseal, and Slippery Elm. Brews from these plants can be prepared by steeping one oz. of cut or powdered herb in a pint of boiling water for 15 to 20 minutes. Cool and strain.

Bacterial Infections

Bacterial infections can be caused by many types of organisms and are often the most difficult type of vaginal condition to clear up. Potentially harmful bacteria are present in the healthy vagina without causing problems, but when they multiply greatly or are introduced in great numbers from the nearby rectum where they live, they can cause itching, pain, and a runny (or sometimes thick and profuse), foul-smelling, grayish (or white) discharge that burns the mucous membranes. Some bouts of bacterial vaginal infections can be prevented by wiping from front to back after urination or defecation and by washing the hands after touching the anus.

Standard medical treatment for bacterial vaginal infections is either a hit-or-miss affair of prescribing antibiotics that kill a wide variety of bacteria or undergoing an agonizing wait for a day or two for the results of a test to determine which antibiotic is effective. Since many of the bacteria that can overgrow cannot live in air, most doctors' offices and clinics are not able to collect a living sample of the bacteria. Special equipment is needed to find these anaerobic bacteria. Thus the term that generally is used to describe a bacterial infection for which no organism can be found is "nonspecific vaginitis."

Self-treatment can begin as soon as a woman notices symptoms and is the same regardless of the type of bacteria found. As in the case of trichomoniasis, douching with various solutions once or twice a day for a few days or using a garlic suppository has been found helpful. Women are most familiar with a vinegar douche (one or two tablespoons of vinegar to a quart of water, to which can be added the oil of one clove of garlic), but a diluted or full-strength Betadine douche is becoming the preferred treatment. Herbal douches of the following herbs can also be used: Motherwort,

Uva Ursi, Bayberry bark, Chickweed, Pipsissewa, Prickly Ash bark, Yarrow, Witch Hazel bark, Fleabane, Sumac berries, and White Oak bark.

Chris Nelson, a self-helper from Chico, California, has included a couple of recipes for herbal douches in her book on home remedies (1977). One recipe is to steep a teaspoon of a mixture of Comfrey leaves, Goldenseal, and Sage for 20 minutes. Cool and strain. Another is to simmer one tablespoon of Slippery Elm bark for 20 mintues in one cup of water. Add two tablespoons of Plantain leaves and steep for 10 minutes. Cool and strain.

CONCLUSION

Vaginal infections have been the bane of many women's lives, and the sufferers have formed a dependable clientele for gynecologists. Today, women in Self-Help Clinics have found that safe and inexpensive alternative remedies seem to be far superior to the drugs normally prescribed. Self-help groups have formed to find ways to put an end to persistent infections. Dramatic breakthroughs have been made by changing certain aspects of life style and by building better health habits. Discussing all the contributory factors can help a woman to discover the specific things that may be causing her problems and the changes she can make that may help the situation.

Stress is often the main problem. Finding ways to change a stressful life situation is sometimes impossible, but adequate rest, vigorous regular exercise, and taking B-complex vitamins can help in dealing with stress.

A change in the method of birth control may be necessary. Some women are sensitive to spermidical jellies and some find condoms or diaphragms irritating. For many, going off the Pill or having an IUD removed is sometimes all that is needed to arrest the vicious cycle.

Self-diagnosis and self-treatment of vaginal infections are some of the spectacular improvements women have made in their own health care, but these are by no means the only ones. A woman can apply the same principles of learning about healthy functioning, sharing information with other women, and applying common sense, in approaching many aspects of her sexuality and reproduction.

REFERENCES

Billings, John J., *Natural Family Planning: The Ovulation Method*, 3rd ed. Collegeville, Minn.: Liturgical Press, 1975.

Federal of Feminist Women's Health Centers, *A New View of a Woman's Body*. New York: Simon & Schuster, 1981.

Fisher, Alexander A., "Allergic Reaction to Feminine Deodorant Spray," *Archives of Dermatology*, 108 (December 1973), 801–2.

Hopkins, Harold C., "Helping the Consumer Play Safe," *FDA Consumer*, May 1975, p. 15.

Nelson, Chris, *Self-Help Home Remedies*. Chico, Calif.: Feminist Women's Health Center, 1977.

1980 Physician's Desk Reference. Oradell, N.J.: Litton Publications, Inc., 1980.

Chapter Twenty-Six

SELF-DIAGNOSTIC TESTS

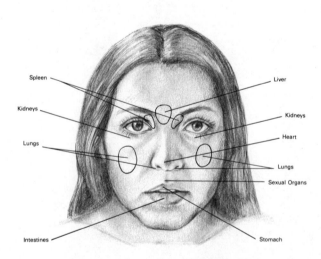

The above areas of the face are used for spotting problems in the organs concerned. Abnormal colors, changes in the texture of the skin, or surface eruptions or rashes are early signs of developing problems.

David Sobel

Self-diagnosis is not new. For centuries, the principal form of health care throughout the world has been self-diagnosis and self-treatment. And today people with access to health professionals have working diagnoses in mind before they see them.

Until recently, the public has had few diagnostic tools at its disposal other than a thermometer. Lately, however, increasing numbers of home diagnostic tests, from pregnancy kits to blood pressure cuffs, have been marketed. This transfer of technology from professionals to the public is both promising and problematic. These tests hold great potential for empowering people in their own health care, for aiding earlier, more accurate diagnoses, for improving home self-monitoring of chronic diseases, and for substituting cost-effective self-care for more expensive professional care. There are, however, problems with the safety and accuracy of some self-diagnostic tests. There is also the threat of commercial exploitation. Here is a critical but sympathetic look at some of the self-diagnostic tests now available.

HOME PREGNANCY TESTS

In ancient Egypt, women poured their urine on papyrus leaves. If the plant survived, they were pregnant. Today women can use new, more accurate home pregnancy tests which can be purchased over the counter in drugstores. These tests, similar to those used in laboratories, test urine for the hormone human chorionic gonadotropin (HCG). HCG is secreted by the developing placenta and excreted in the urine of pregnant women. It usually takes 10 to 14 days after a pregnant woman misses her period for the HCG to enter the urine in sufficient quantities to be detected by the test. Home

389

pregnancy tests are private, convenient and inexpensive, but are far from foolproof.

The instructions that come with do-it-yourself pregnancy tests are complicated and must be followed precisely. Ten to 14 days after missing her menstrual period a woman adds a few drops of her first morning urine to the reagents in the pregnancy test kit. A first morning urine specimen is the most concentrated; this favors detection of HCG. She lets the test tube sit undisturbed for two hours, then reads the result. A dark donut-shaped deposit at the bottom of the tube indicates pregnancy. If no donut-shaped deposit appears, a repeat test is recommended the following week. The test kits are not reusable.

A false-negative test may result if the urine it tested too soon after a missed period, if it is not a concentrated first morning specimen, or if the pregnancy is ectopic, that is, if the fetus attaches itself to a Fallopian tube instead of the uterine wall. Other inaccurate results may occur if the test is not read at the specified time, if there is a detergent residue on the urine-collecting container, or if the test is exposed to heat, sunlight, or vibration. In studies conducted by one manufacturer, the home test was 97 percent accurate when *positive*. If the test was *negative*, however, the chance was one in five that the woman was still pregnant—a 20 percent false-negative rate. That's why it's important to repeat a negative test.

Home pregnancy tests, though new, grossed $40 million in 1979 and sales are expected to double in 1980. Brand names such as e.p.t., Answer, Predictor, Acu-Test and Daisy 2 are available at most pharmacies. They cost from $9 to $14, and some contain two tests per kit to permit repeat testing.

While these tests are convenient, private and relatively inexpensive, they often cost more and provide somewhat less accurate results than pregnancy tests obtained at family planning clinics, doctors' offices or Planned Parenthood affiliates. It is encouraging, however, the women can now choose pregnancy testing at home.

HOME THROAT CULTURES

Every parent has experienced the hassle of dealing with a child's sore throat. The sick uncomfortable child must be carted off to the physician's office for the obligatory throat culture. Depending on the season, pediatricians take throat cultures in 20 to 40 percent of office visits. The reason is that the sore throat might be caused by a certain bacteria (beta-hemolytic streptococcus Group A) which, in a small proportion of cases, has the nasty tendency to cause rheumatic heart disease and kidney disease. To prevent these possible complications, and to prevent unnecessary use of antibiotics, pediatricians culture sore throats and treat strep-positive cases with antibiotics.

At the Columbia Health Plan in Maryland, parents were taught to perform throat cultures themselves. When the results of cultures taken by parents were compared with those taken by clinic assistants, they agreed in 136 out of 137 cases, demonstrating the accuracy and reliability of parent participation. Furthermore, when parents obtained the cultures at home, they took them more frequently than a doctor could and detected a higher rate of strep-positive throats. In addition, home throat culturing reduced pediatric office visits by an estimated 15 to 20 percent. The home cultures also appeared to have the advantages of greater parental participation in care, better understanding of the importance of treating strep throat, earlier diagnosis, decreased contagion due to exposure of other sick children in waiting rooms, and efficient strep screening for family members without symptoms in families where a child was diagnosed as having strep throat.

A present there is no reliable, convenient way for parents to grow and read throat cultures in their homes. Home throat culturing is only possible where doctors are willing to demonstrate the culture technique, provide the inexpensive throat swabs, and accept the swabs for laboratory culturing.

If the doctor is cooperative, it's quite simple to obtain a throat culture. The child is asked to open his or her mouth and say "Ahhh" while the parent swabs the tonsils and back of the throat with a sterile cotton applicator. The parent then returns the swab to its sterile container and sends it to the laboratory for culturing.

URINARY TRACT INFECTIONS

Urinary tract infections, also called bladder infections or cystitis, are very common in women. Two simple tests, the nitrite test and the urine culture, have been developed for professional use. They have also been found effective for self-diagnosis at home. Home urine testing provides a convenient and inexpensive alternative to frequent office visits for women with the recurrent infections, or those in high-risk situations (pregnancy or kidney stones), where these infections are more common and more serious. The tests are also a convenient way to check for bacteria in the urine, following antibiotic treatment for these infections.

More than 95 percent of urinary tract infections are caused by bacteria that do not absorb a specific stain developed by Dr. Gram, hence the term Gram-negative bacteria. These bacteria produce nitrite in the urine. The nitrite dip-stick is the simplest way to check for these bacteria in the urine, a condition called bacteriuria. A nitrite dip-stick is dipped into a urine specimen which has been allowed to incubate and concentrate in the bladder for at least four hours; a first morning urine sample is preferable because it is concentrated. The test is read 30 seconds after dipping. If the dip-stick turns pink, it means there is nitrite in the urine which indicates a likelihood of significant bacteriuria. A negative test should be repeated on three consecutive mornings for confirmation. Nearly 90 percent of urinary tract infections can be detected with the nitrite dip-strip used on three consecutive morning urine samples.

Urine can also be cultured at home by dipping a culture slide into it and incubating the slide for 18 to 24 hours in a warm part of the house. The appearance of small dots on the culture slide indicates bacterial colonies. A rough estmate of the concentration of bacteria can be made by comparing the density of the dots to a standard. This test detects bacteriuria with an accuracy greater than 90 percent.

Nitrite dip-sticks are stocked by many pharmacies and cost 20¢ to 30¢ each. Dip-culture slides cost approximately $1 and can be ordered through most pharmacies or obtained from clinics that use them. For comparison, laboratory urine analysis may cost $25.

DIABETIC SELF-MONITORING

One of the most widely used and accepted self-monitoring tests is home urine testing for blood sugar (glucose) by diabetics. Urine glucose tests, however, may not provide information about actual blood glucose levels precise enough for diabetics to adjust their insulin requirements accurately. Diabetics are often hospitalized to obtain precise blood glucose measurements and adjust their diet and insulin requirements, particularly in high-risk diabetics such as those who are pregnant. There are, however, marked advantages to self-administered blood glucose measurement at home. These include lower cost, greater convenience, and increased understanding of diabetes on the part of diabetics.

A portable blood glucose meter about the size of a portable tape recorder is now available for home use. The diabetic pricks his or her fingertip and transfers a drop of blood to a small reagent strip. This strip is then placed in the meter and an estimate of blood glucose is made from the color reaction on the reagent strip. This process takes only a few minutes.

Several studies have confirmed the reliability and accuracy of the home glucose meter. These studies also suggest enthusiastic acceptance by diabetics and better control of their diabetes as a result.

Home glucose meters cost approximately $500 and require wall current for operation. Smaller, battery-operated models are anticipated in the future which should increase self-testing among diabetics.

BOWEL CANCER SCREENING

Cancer of the colon and rectum is the most common cancer in the United States. More than 100,000 new cases occur each year. Because prevention of this cancer is not well understood, attention has focused on early detection when it is more curable. Colon/rectal cancers bleed easily. A simple test, Hemoccult-II, has been developed to detect blood in the stool even when it cannot be seen.

Roughage in the diet encourages early colon/rectal cancer lesions to bleed, so those being tested are advised to eat a high-fiber diet for two to three days before the test. They are also instructed to avoid red meats, which can give false-positive results, and high doses of vitamin C, which can inhibit the test reaction. Then, for three consecutive bowel movements, two small samples from different parts of the stool are taken with a small wooden spatula. These are smeared on Hemoccult-II fiber paper for a total of six specimens. A few drops of developing solution are added to the specimens within four days. A bluish discoloration of any of the six specimens is considered a positive result, and further evaluation is then necessary to determine the source of the bleeding. Because the incidence of bowel cancer increases sharply after age 45, it is generally recommended that this test be done annually for those 45 or older.

When performed properly the Hemoccult-II test appears to be both accurate and useful. In two large studies of more than 30,000 people, approximately one to two percent has positive tests for invisible or "occult" blood and of those, 10 to 12 percent had bowel cancer. In both groups, the cancers detected by screening for occult blood were more localized and more curable than the cancer lesions detected by other methods.

Hemoccult-II packets, with self-mailer, instructions, and wooden spatulas are available from most physicians or public health facilities. They cost about 50¢ to $1 per packet. The developing and reading of the test is possible at home, but the developing solution is expensive and difficult to obtain. Therefore, specimens are usually collected at home and returned by mail to a physician or laboratory.

HOME BLOOD PRESSURE MONITORING

High blood pressure, or hypertension, is an epidemic. One out of every five American adults has elevated blood pressure and many do not know they have this disease, often called "the silent killer." Careful control of blood pressure—by diet, exercise, relaxation, or medication—significantly reduces the risk of heart disease and stroke, two of today's leading causes of death. Home blood pressure monitoring can help maintain and adjust blood pressure control programs.

Several types of home blood pressure kits are available from about $25 and up, from mercury cuffs with stethoscopes to newer electronic devices. (*Consumer Reports* recently rated home blood pressure devices—see *Resources.*) Simple coin-operated, self-administered automatic blood pressure screening devices have also been developed for the general public. These devices are appearing in many public places.

Blood pressure devices have different instructions, and except for the automatic devices, their use requires some supervision and practice. No blood pressure device is absolutely accurate every time. However, with good equipment, correct instruction and practice, most people can learn to take reliable blood pressure measurements. Nonetheless, several cautions are in order. Blood pressure varies with age, time of day, drug use, stress, and other factors. A single measurement of elevated blood pressure does not constitute a diagnosis of high blood pressure. Abnormal measurements should be rechecked and confirmed. Home blood pressure monitoring is a good opportunity for doctor-patient partnership, but self-adjustment of antihypertensive medications without medical supervision is not recommended.

RESOURCES

Home Pregnancy Tests

"The e.p.t. Do-It-Yourself Early Pregnancy Test," *Medical Letter*, 20 (April 1978), 39–40.

"Home Tests for Pregnancy," *Newsweek*, September 3, 1979, p. 69.

Brigette Joran, "The Self-Diagnosis of Early Pregnancy: An Investigation of Lay Competence," *Medical Anthropology*, 1 (Spring 1977), 38.

Home Throat Cultures

Harvey P. Katz, and Robert R. Clancy, "Accuracy of a Home Throat Culture Program: A Study of Parent Participation in Health Care," *Pediatrics*, 53 (May 1974), 687–91.

"Mom and Dad Take Good Throat Swabs," *Medical World News*, December 12, 1977, p. 73.

D. Schwartz, H. Katz, and B. Starfield, "Patterns and Determinants of Usage in a Home Throat Culture Program: An Evaluation of Parental Involvement in Family Health Care," 19th Annual Meeting Ambulatory Pediatric Association, Atlanta, Georgia, April 1979.

Diabetes

Charles M. Peterson, "Take Care of Your Diabetes: A New Approach to Self-Management," St. Paul, Minn., 1979.

P. H. Sonksen, S. L. Judd, and C. Lowy, "Home Monitoring of Blood Glucose," *Lancet*, 1 (1978), 729–32.

S. Wallford, E. A. M. Gale, A. P. Allison, and R. B. Tattersall, "Self-Monitoring of Blood Glucose," *Lancet* 1 (1978), 732–36.

Information on blood glucose meters may be obtained from:

Eyetone/Dextrostix, Ames Company, Division of Miles Laboratories, Inc., Elkhart, Ind.

Urinary Tract Infections

Calvin M. Kunin and Jane E. DeGroot, "Self-Screening for Significant Bacteriuria," *Journal of the American Medical Association*, 231 (March 1975), 1349–53.

J.Y. Gillenwater et al., "Home Urine Cultures by the Dip-Strip Method: Results in 289 Cultures," *Pediatrics*, 58 (October 1976), 508–12.

"Home Testing for Recurrent Bacteriuria Using Nitrite Strips," *American Journal of Diseases of Children*, 132 (January 1978), 46–48.

Michael F. Miriovsky, "Office Analysis of Bacteriuria," *American Family Physician*, 19 (May 1979), 121–26.

Nitrite Dip-Strips may be obtained from:

Microstix Nitrite Reagent Strips, Ames Company, Division of Miles Laboratories, Inc., Elkhart, Ind.

Urine Culture slides may be obtained from:

Culturia, Clinical Convenience Products, Inc., Madison, Wis.

or

Bacturcult, Wampole Laboratories, Division of Carter-Wallace Inc., Cranbury, N.J.

Colon/Rectal Cancer

"Hemoccult-II," *Medical Letter*, 21 (April 1979), 36.

"Early Hemoccult Results 'Encouraging,' " *Journal of the American Medical Association*, 239 (1978), 1118.

S. J. Winawer et al., "Results of a Screening Program for the Detection of Early Colon Cancer Polyps Using Fecal Occult Blood Testing," *Gastroenterology*, 72 (1977), 1127–50.

Thomas W. Eldwood, Allan Erickson, and Seymour Lieberman, "Comparative Educational Approaches to Screening for Colorectal Cancer," *American Journal of Public Health*, 68 (February 1978), 135–38.

Home Blood Pressure Monitoring:

"Blood Pressure Kits," *Consumer Reports*, March 1979, pp. 142–46.

Keith W. Sehnert, and Howard Eisenberg, "Blood Pressure: Use of the Sphygmomanometer," in *How to Be Your Own Doctor (Sometimes)*. New York: Grosset and Dunlap, 1975.

D. M. Berkson, I. T. Whipple, L. Sherman et al., "Evaluation of an Automated Blood Pressure Device Intended for General Public Use," *American Journal of Public Health*, 69 (May 1979), 473–79.

SUGGESTED READINGS

Bates, Barbara, *A Guide to Physical Examination*. Philadelphia: J. B. Lippincott Company, 1974.

Evans, Glen, *The Family Circle Guide to Self-Help*. New York: Ballantine Books, Inc., 1979.

Ferguson, Tom, ed., *Medical Self-Care*. Inverness, Calif., 1980.

———, *Medical Self-Care: Access to Medical Tools*. New York: Summit Books, Inc., 1979.

Gartner, Alan, and Frank Riessman, *Self-Help in the Human Services*. San Francisco: Jossey-Bass, Inc., Publishers, 1977.

Grant, Richard H., "Family and Self-Help Education in Isolated Rural Communitites," *Health Education Monographs*, 5, no. (Summer 1977), 145–60.

Hassler, Herbert, and Raymond Harris, *The Bodywork Book: Medical Tests You Can Do in Your Home*. New York: Avon Books.

Homan, William E., and editors of *Consumer Guide, Caring for Your Child. A Complete Medical Guide*. New York: Harmony Books, 1979.

Kohlenberg, Robert K., *Migraine Relief: A Personal Treatment Program*. Seattle, Wash.: BSMC Publishing.

Levin, Arthur, *Talk Back to Your Doctor: How to Demand and Recognize High Quality Health Care*. New York: Doubleday & Co., Inc., 1975.

Levin, Lowell S., "Forces and Issues in the Revival of Interest in Self-Care," *Health Education Monographs*, 5, no. 2 (Summer 1977), 115–20.

Levin, Lowell S., Alfred H. Katz, and Erik Holst, *Self-Care Lay Initiatives in Health*. New York: Prodist Press, 1976.

Sehnert, Keith W., "A 'Doctor' in Every Home," in Eddie Miller, ed., *Help Yourself*. Chicago: Blue Cross Association, 1978.

Sehnert, Keith W., and Howard Eisenberg, *How to Be Your Own Doctor (Sometimes)*. New York: Grosset & Dunlap, Inc., 1975.

Travis, John, *Wellness Resource Kit for Helping Professionals*. Mill Valley, Calif.: Wellness Associates.

Chapter Twenty-Seven

THE ROLE OF PSYCHOACTIVE DRUGS IN MEDICAL SELF-HELP

Andrew T. Weil

In some parts of this chapter, the medical use of illegal drugs is described. However, this author does not advocate the use of illegal drugs to readers of this text. Rather, the purpose of this survey is to present current research information regarding the possible uses of nonpharmaceutical psychoactive drugs in their organic form for common disease ailments. Many of these drugs are already in use by consumers in a setting of inappropriate prescription, in ill-advised dosage, and by improper routes of administration. This article presents guidelines as to proper usage of such drugs in a nonclinical settting. Historically, psychoactive drugs, including those mentioned here, which subsequently attained illegal status, have been a part of the pharmacopeia of medical practitioners.

Psychoactive drugs have always been popular in medicine because they make patients feel different. Doctors like them because they often make patients go away satisfied that something has been done. Outside of medical situations, people may take the same drugs for recreational purposes: to get high or to enhance social interaction and pleasure. Prescribing of psychoactive drugs by doctors is legitimate use, but taking them for fun is considered drug abuse, a latter-day evil. Actually, these two patterns have much in common, and both can produce either good or bad results (Szasz 1974).

ADVANTAGES AND DISADVANTAGES OF PSYCHOACTIVE DRUGS

Human involvement with drugs that affect the mind is only one aspect of general human fascination with other states of consciousness (Weil 1972).

High states are reinforcing, even to very young children, who avidly experiment with methods of changing awareness. Children early discover such techniques as spinning and mutual choking and use these techniques frequently despite uncomfortable side effects (Weil 1980). Many of the activities to which grown-ups devote most of their time, energy, and money take us out of ourselves temporarily and make us feel at our best, at the peak of our powers, i.e., high. Athletics, music, dance, sex, falling in love, being in the wilderness, high speed, meditation, religious ecstasy, and many other activities are capable of making us high.

The advantage of drugs is that they work powerfully and immediately. Their disadvantage is that they reinforce a dangerous illusion about the nature of highs; that they come from outside of us. In fact, highs seem to be the result of latent capacities of the nervous system. The highs of drugs are not really different from the highs obtained without drugs (Weil 1980). Drugs work by making us feel different; they strongly affect our psychophysiology by their direct pharmacological actions. Feeling different, does not mean being high. People who get rewarding highs from drugs have learned to associate the direct effects of the drugs with inner experiences they seek. Until this association develops, they can take high doses of drugs and not feel high, and if they take the drugs too often, the association will often break down, again leaving them drugged but not high.

In terms of their ability to induce interesting changes in consciousness, psychoactive drugs are really *active placebos*, that is, they have real, intrinsic effects on the mind-body, but the desired states of consciousness that users report are indirect effects, linked to the drug effects by learned association.

Being high can be an effective technique for dealing with illness. If you have a headache, and all you can think about is the headache, it will get worse and worse, claiming all of your attention. However, if you have a headache and can get high in some way, you can shift your attention to the good feeling of the high, and often the headache will fade away into nothingness. By enabling people to take their minds off the discomfort of symptoms, psychoactive drugs can genuinely make people feel better, at least temporarily. Sometimes this break in the cycle of illness will even permit symptoms to subside for long periods, allowing real healing to occur.

The use of drugs to make people feel good when sick or injured certainly has its place, both in formal treatment by physicians and in self-care. It is also somewhat risky, however, because at root it is symptomatic treatment that does not go to the underlying cause of illness. If illness persists and use of the drug is continued regularly, the possibility of dependence is very real, whether the drug is one we commonly think of as addicting, like morphine, or one we commonly think of as not, like coffee or marijuana.

HISTORICAL USE OF DRUGS—PROMOTED BY MEDICAL PROFESSION

Historically, doctors have been the greatest promoters of drug abuse in the world, pushing psychoactive drugs shamelessly and creating widespread dependence through ignorance of the nature of these drugs. In the early nineteenth century, opium was the mainstay of medical treatment. Later, tincture of cannabis and alcohol came into widespread use. The isolation of morphine from opium and the invention of the hypodermic syringe in time for the American Civil War greatly increased the ability of physicians to make patients drug-dependent. At the end of the nineteenth century, the medical profession touted cocaine as a cure-all and especially recommended it as remedy for morphine addiction, which had become the leading iatrogenic disease (Grinspoon and Bakalar 1976).

The present century has seen a parade of new psychoactive drugs, each in turn achieving tremendous popularity with doctors, then falling into disrepute as consequences of overuse became apparent. All of the synthetic opiates, like Dilaudid, Demoral, and Talwin, were eagerly introduced as nonaddicting narcotics. In the 1950s and early 1960s, amphetamines were handed out like candy for all sorts of vague complaints. More recently, Valium and Librium have become the most widely prescribed of all drugs (Hughes and Brewin 1979).

DANGERS OF DRUG ADDICTION

The prominence of psychoactive drugs in clinical medicine reflects the need of doctors to do something for patients whose conditions are often not understandable or not treatable by conventional methods.

Critics of the practice of prescribing psychoactive drugs point out that women are the more frequent recipients. In the heyday of amphetamines (and related drugs like Ritalin), pharmaceutical company ads frequently pictured tired housewives as potential beneficiaries of these stimulants. More recently, Valium and Librium have become popular for mass usage (ibid.).

Whether male or female, patients should beware of long-term use of any psychoactive drug for symptomatic relief. It will not cure the disease and can easily lead to an unproductive drug habit, one that is difficult to break. This precaution applies whether the drug is obtained on the black market and self-administered, or whether it is received from a pharmacy on a doctor's orders. It is just not good medicine over time.

BENEFICIAL SHORT-TERM USE OF PSYCHOACTIVE DRUGS— FOR SPECIFIC SITUATIONS

Short-term use of psychoactive drugs is another matter. As noted earlier, a person who can use a drug to feel high may be able to break the vicious cycle by which symptoms claim attention. For the purpose of curing minor complaints in this way, drugs work best when used least frequently—that is, when they are saved for occasions that really count. Their use should be stopped as soon as the problem abates, and they should never be continued for more than a few days in a row.

Some examples of the profitable short-term self-help use of recreational drugs are having a hot toddy and going right to bed when coming down with a cold, or taking marijuana during labor to deal with the pain of contractions.

There is an enormous range of individual response to psychoactive drugs, making it difficult to say what conditions they are good for. For example, some people respond favorably to marijuana; they can get usefully high on it, then use the high to take their minds off various physical ailments. But remember marijuana treats individuals, not conditions. It is not a remedy for headaches, although individuals who respond to it may be able to use it for headaches, menstrual cramps, stomachaches, and other problems. This concept of a drug is very different from the "magic bullet" concept that prevails in conventional medicine. Doctors like strong drugs that treat specific diseases. They do not like panaceas, and they do not want to hear about individual variation.

INDICATIONS FOR THE USE OF COMMON PSYCHOACTIVE DRUGS

Psychoactive drugs, aside from their general action as triggers of high states, may also relieve certain specific problems by virtue of their direct pharmacological actions. For example, marijuana counteracts nausea and vomiting and has been used in conjunction with cancer chemotherapy to relieve those side effects. It also lowers intraocular pressure and may be helpful to victims of glaucoma. In addition, it relaxes bronchial smooth muscle during asthma attacks (but should be eaten rather than smoked for this purpose), and it alleviates muscle spasticity in such conditions as multiple sclerosis. It is worth trying marijuana for these medical problems because it is one of the least toxic drugs known, much safer than most pharmaceutical preparations. See also the appendix to this chapter for the section by Michael Castleman on marijuana.

Here are some other specific indications for the use of common psychoactive drugs:*

1. *Alcohol*. In moderate and occasional use, alcohol is a good relaxant. It may protect against heart attacks. Obstetricians also use it to stop premature onset of labor.

2. *Coffee*. Like amphetamines, coffee has a sedating effect on hyperactive children and may be a safer drug to use than other prescribed drugs. It is a strong stimulant and laxative for most people and should not be used continually lest dependency develop.

3. *Other caffeine sources*. Coffee is much stronger than other caffeine plants, probably because it contains oil-soluable drugs that synergize the caffeine. Coffee is a strong irritant of the stomach and of the urinary bladder, especially in women. Therefore women with urinary problems should avoid coffee and experiment with alternatives. One such possibility is guaraná, made from the seed of an Amazonian shrub and widely consumed in Brazil. It has more caffeine than coffee but is not as irritating. Guaraná can be obtained in pill or powder form at health food stores. Maté is another alternate to coffee. It is the national drink of Argentina, made from the leaf of a holly that contains caffeine. It is obtainable at health food stores and stores that sell imported teas. Both of these coffee substitutes serve the same functions as coffee.

4. *Cocaine*. Tampons soaked in a solution of cocaine can dramatically relieve menstrual cramps. The drug may also specificially alleviate rheumatoid arthritis and a variety of other musculoskeletal disorders. Cocaine has a significant potential for misuse and dependence, however, and should be taken with great caution.

5. *Coca leaf*. The natural source of cocaine, coca is much safer than the isolated alkaloid as well as more effective as a remedy (Weil 1981). It is a superior tonic, acting over time to normalize body functions and increase general vitality and resistance without causing undue stimula-

---

*Heroin is being used for the pain of terminal cancer at hospices in England. "Brompton's Mixture," containing heroin, morphine, cocaine, and alcohol was developed at Brompton Hospital in London. Dr. Elizabeth Kubler-Ross, whose life work is the care of the dying, has said that without Brompton's Mixture she could not do her work. It keeps the patients pain-free and alert and enables her to help them live until they die. When herion was first made by European chemists in the nineteenth century, its image was beneficient (from the word "hero"). Hospices in the United States are urging its legalization for terminal cancer patients. It is difficult to see what harm heroin can do to a dying patient, considering its known therapeutic properties. [Editor's note]

tion. Its abuse potential is low. Coca also seems to regulate carbohydrate metabolism and may treat hypoglycemia and diabetes. It can be a good aid to losing weight because it decreases appetite while providing vitamins, minerals, and oral gratification. It also treats laryngitis and vocal fatigue, making it useful to singers and public speakers. Finally, it is a good remedy for many disorders of the digestive system and for motion sickness. At present, coca leaf is unavailable in the United States, but researchers are working to document its medical effects, so that it may eventually become a prescription drug.

6. *Psychedelic drugs* (LSD, mescaline, peyote, psilocybin mushrooms, MDA, etc.). This group of substances can produce bad psychological reactions if not used carefully—that is, with experienced guides in good settings. By enabling people to get new perspectives on their bodies, minds, and external reality, psychedelic drugs have great potential to bring about medical cures, even of serious physical diseases. For example, in skilled hands they have catalyzed cures of alcoholism and cancer. They have also been used successfully in counseling dying patients and reconciling them to the imminence of their deaths. MDA has a striking antiallergic effect and could be used to train people how to live with allergens and not have attacks (Weil 1980). Unfortunately, all of these drugs are officially declared to have no therapeutic usefulness and are unavailable to doctors. Furthermore, research on their medical potential is virtually nonexistent (Grinspoon and Bakalar 1979).

7. *Opium*. Every household medicine chest used to have a bottle of tincture of opium ("laudanum"). That preparation is still available on prescription but is considered an old-fashioned drug. Yet opium is the single best remedy for severe intestinal cramps, muscle aches, and many other forms of acute pain. Its abuse potential is not high; large doses cause nausea, which encourages only moderate use, and most people learn to save opium for occasions when they really need it. Tincture of opium is also the best remedy for the diarrhea of travelers, especially when accompanied by cramps. It is much superior to Lo-Motil and other synthetics.

8. *Valerian*. A root with a strong smell that many people find unpleasant, valerian is one of the safest natural sedatives. It is best taken as a tincture, mixed with a little water before bedtime. Tinctures of valerian root are now available in health food stores or from herb companies. For people in need of daytime calming or help with sleep at night, valerian is an excellent alternative to Valium or other barbiturates.

SUGGESTIONS FOR HOME USE

If you decide to experiment with psychoactive drugs as home remedies, here are some suggestions to follow:

1. Save these substances for occasions when you need them. The more frequently you take them, the less effective they will be.

2. Natural forms of these drugs are safer and often better than isolated derivatives of them.

3. Take psychoactive drugs by mouth. Introduced into the bloodstream by more direct routes, such as smoking, snorting, or injecting, they become much more toxic and more productive of problems.

4. Take adequate doses but do not exceed them. Large doses of these drugs often become unpleasant.

5. Continue the drug only as long as necessary. If the problem responds to the treatment, stop taking the drug as soon as you feel better. Also stop taking it if the problem does not respond after a reasonable trial.

6. Remember that the effects of psychoactive drugs are exquisitely dependent on set and setting. Pay attention to the manner and circumstances in which you take them and your reasons for taking them.

CONCLUSION

Used intelligently, psychoactive drugs can be helpful additions to the repertory of techniques available for self-care. They have been around since the dawn of history and doubtless will be with us till history ends. Their potential is thoroughly ambivalent: they can be used creatively or destructively, and learning to handle them wisely requires knowledge and experience.

REFERENCES

Grinspoon, L., and J. B. Bakalar, *Cocaine: A Drug and Its Social Evolution*. New York: Basic Books, Inc., Publishers, 1976.

——, *Psychedelic Drugs Reconsidered*. New York: Basic Books, Inc., Publishers, 1979.

Hughes, R., and R. Brewin, *The Tranquilizing of America: Pill Popping and the American Way of Life*, New York: Harcourt Brace Jovanovich, Inc., 1979.

Szasz, T., *Ceremonial Chemistry: The Ritual Persecution of Drugs, Addicts, and Pushers*. Garden City, N.Y.: Anchor Books, 1974.

Weil, A. T., *The Natural Mind: A New Way of Looking at Drugs and the Higher Consciousness*. Boston: Houghton Mifflin Company, 1972.

——, *The Marriage of the Sun and Moon: A Quest for Unity in Consciousness*. Boston: Houghton Mifflin Company, 1980.

——, "The Therapeutic Value of Coca in Contemporary Medicine," *Journal of Ethnopharmacology*, vol. 3, nos. 2/3 (1981).

SUGGESTED READINGS

Grof, Stanislav, *LSD Psychotherapy*. Pomona, Calif.: Hunter House, 1978.

Kakar, Sudhir, *Shamans, Mystics and Doctors*. New York: Alfred Knopf, 1983.

Palmer, Cynthia and Michael Horowitz, *Shaman Woman, Mainline Lady: Women's Writings on the Drug Experience*. New York: William Morrow, 1983.

Stafford, Petter, *Psychedelics Encyclopedia*. Berkeley, Calif.: And/Or Press, 1980.

Young, Lawrence et al., *Recreational Drugs*. New York: Berkeley Books, 1977.

ADDRESSES

An organization researching the medical uses of marijuana is the:

Alliance for Cannabis Therapeutics
P.O. Box 23691
L'Enfant Plaza Station
Washington, D.C. 20024

An organization coordinating research on the therapeutic effects of coca is the:

Beneficial Plant Research
   Association
418 Mission Avenue
San Rafael, CA 94901

APPENDIX—RX MARIJUANA*

Queen Victoria's phsycian prescribed it for migraine headaches. The ancient Chinese used it as an anesthetic. The Vietnamese have used it for centuries to treat allergies, rheumatism, and tapeworm. Ukrainian folk healers prescribed it for toothaches. And until this century American doctors and pharmacists recommended "tincture of cannabis" for eye strain, upset stomach, depression, nervous tension, and epilepsy. In fact, marijuana was so routinely prescribed in this country that during the Congressional hearings that led to its prohibition in 1937, a spokesman for the conservative American Medical Association (AMA) urged that it *remain legal* for use as a prescription drug because of the "advantages to be derived from its medicinal use."

Today, health researchers are slowly rediscovering its therapeutic value. Its use as medicine is still fairly restricted, but one day your doctor might hand you a joint—or a THC pill—and say, "Take this and call me in the morning."

Marijuana has already proved so successful as a treatment for the severe nausea associated with cancer chemotherapy that recently, the Surgeon General announced that the National Cancer Institute would begin making THC pills available to the estimated 35,000 cancer patients with this problem.

*Written by Michael Casteman and published in *Medical Self-Care*, Iverness, Calif., 1980.

It remains to be seen, however, how quickly prescription THC will become available. In the meantime, many cancer patients will probably have to continue to obtain their THC "informally." Roger Roffman, an assistant professor of social work at the University of Washington who works with that state's pilot program to make marijuana available to cancer chemotherapy patients, has written a 48-page booklet, "Using Marijuana in the Reduction of Nausea Associated with Cancer Chemotherapy"—see Resources. Written for both physicians and patients, it discusses in everyday terms how marijuana works to alleviate nausea and how to acquire, prepare, and use the drug. For those who are reluctant to carry an easily recognized illegal substance, the booklet includes recipes for marijuana cookies and brownies.

In the future, marijuana may also be used to treat:

Asthma. Marijuana expands (dilates) the bronchioles of the lungs[1] and has been suggested as a treatment for their constriction in people with asthma. Marijuana should be eaten rather than smoked for this purpose.

Epilepsy. Animal studies show that THC is an anticonvulsant.[2] Although folk healers used marijuana for this purpose in the past, its value as an antiepileptic drug in humans remains to be investigated.

Glaucoma. Marijuana decreases fluid pressure in the eye[3] and has shown promise as a treatment for glaucoma. THC eyedrops have been used in patients who prefer to avoid the drug's psychoactive effects.

Depression. Because its euphoric effect is the major reason for its recreational use, marijuana has been tested as an antidepressant, so far with mixed results. One study[4] showed that it alleviated depression in cancer patients. Another,[5] however, detected no antidepressive effects.

In December 1979, the AMA House of Delegates, the organization's governing body, adopted a new position on the therapeutic potential of marijuana: "Marijuana, like any other drug, has potential for harm as well as for good. The traditional triad of dose size, duration of use and makeup of the user is a highly appropriate touchstone for evaluating its risks and benefits." NORML (National Organization for the Reform of Marijuana Laws) could not have said it any better.

RESOURCES

Roger Roffman, *Using Marijuana in the Reduction of Nausea Associated with Cancer Chemotherapy*. Seattle, Wash.: Murray Publishing Co., 1980.

REFERENCES

[1]Tashkin, D. P. et al., "Acute Pulmonary Physiologic Effects of Smoked Marijuana and Oral Delta-9-THC in Young Men," *New England Journal of Medicine*, 289 (1973), 336–41.

[2]Cohen, S., and R. C. Stillman, eds. *The Therapeutic Potential of Marijuana*. New York: Plenum Publishing Corporation, 1976.

[3]Hepler, R. S., and I. M. Frank, "Marijuana Smoking and Intraocular Pressure," *JAMA*, 217 (1971), 1392.

[4]Regelson, W. et al., "Delta-9-THC as an Effective Antidepressant and Appetite Stimulating Agent in Advanced Cancer Patients," in *Pharmacology of Marihuana*, edited by M. K. Braude and S. Szara, New York: Raven Press, 1976, pp. 763–77.

[5]Kotin, J. et al., "Tetrahydrocannabinol in Depressed Patients," *Archives of General Psychiatry*, 28 (1973), 345–48.

Appendix

SUGGESTED READINGS IN WOMEN'S HEALTH

Mara Klempner

Airola, Paavo, *Every Woman's Book: Dr. Airola's Practical Guide to Holistic Health*. Phoenix: Health Plus Publishers, 1979. This book contains some useful alternative treatments for specific female health problems; however, its positive aspects are overshadowed by the offensiveness of Dr. Airola's personal views on virtually every aspect of women's lives.

Annas, George, *The Rights of Hospital Patients*. New York: Avon Books, 1975. This is a useful guide for those wishing to know their legal rights concerning hospital matters. Some of the areas covered are: confidentiality, informed consent, the right to refuse treatment, and access to hospital records.

Ardell, Donald, *High Level Wellness: An Alternative to Doctors, Drugs and Disease*. Emmaus, Pa.: Rodale Press, 1977. The author emphasizes the importance of integrating physical fitness, nutrition, stress management, self-responsibility, and environmental factors in order to achieve "High Level Wellness." Includes a detailed health evaluation.

Arekart-Treichel, Joan, *Biotypes: The Critical Link between Your Personality and Your Health*. New York Times Books, 1981. Describes how certain personality factors affect specific organs in the body, causing disease.

Berkeley Holistic Health Center, *The Holistic Health Handbook: A Tool for Attaining Wholeness of Body, Mind, and Spirit*. Berkeley, Calif.: And/Or Press, 1978. This is a compilation of writings describing dozens of alternative healing modalities. There is a description and philosophy of each method, as well as specific ways it can be used.

Bermosk, Loretta, and Sarah Porter, *Women's Health and Human Wholeness*. New York: Appleton-Century-Crofts/Prentice-Hall, Inc., 1979. This is one of the few books that integrates health care and feminism with holistic principles. Includes chapters on the history of women's health care providers, sexism in women's health care, experiences of nurses in the health care system, and a blueprint for a "Woman's Healthing Model."

Bertherat, Therese, and Carol Bernstein, *The Body Has Its Reasons: Anti-Exercises and Self-Awareness*. New York: Avon Books, 1977. A fascinating personal account of the author's experiences when learning and teaching body awareness. includes examples of "preliminaries," special recipes for the body designed to unlock its inner wisdom and balance.

Bloomfield, Harold, and Robert Kory, *The Holistic Way to Health and Happiness: A New Approach to Complete Lifetime Wellness*. New York: Simon & Schuster, 1978. A good, "popular" book describing the philosophy and practice of holistic medicine, with an emphasis on the healing power of TM (Transcendental Meditation).

Boston Women's Health Book Collective. *Our Bodies, Ourselves: A Book by and for Women*. New York: Simon & Schuster, 1979. The original, and still one of the best books on self-help for women. Integrates personal accounts of women's experiences with relevant information on a variety of topics to create a comprehensive personal and political view of women's mental and physical health.

Campbell, Margaret, *Why Would a Girl Go into Medicine?* Old Westbury, N.Y.: The Feminist Press, 1974. This is an in-depth study of discrimination against women in major U.S. medical schools. An absorbing work, written by a woman physician.

Carlson, Rick, *The End of Medicine*. New York: Wiley-Interscience, 1975. The author expounds on the flaws of our current medical system and the need for a system that prevents disease and promotes health.

Carrol, David, *The Complete Book of Natural Medicines*. New York: Summit/Simon & Schuster, 1980. This is an excellent, practical guide to self-healing. Contains theory and usage of over a dozen natural therapies, as well as specific healing programs for common ailments.

Cooke, Cynthia, and Susan Sworkin, *The Ms. Guide to a Woman's Health*, revised ed. New York: Berkeley Books, 1981. An informative manual on women's health care, from puberty to old age. Includes chapters on well-woman care, infertility, sexual health, etc.

Coombs, Barbara et al., *An Invitation to Your Health: Your Personal Responsibility*. Menlo Park, Calif.: The Benjamin/Cummings Publishing Co., 1980. This textbook, written primarily for college-level health education classes, stresses self-care and preventive health. Includes flow charts for 42 common medical problems.

Corea, Gena, *The Hidden Malpractice: How American Medicine Mistreats Women*. New York: Jove Publications, 1977. This is a profound and saddening exposé of post and present discrimination against women by men in the medical field. Well-written and thoroughly documented, an excellent book.

Cowan, Belita, *Women's Health Care: Resources, Writings, Bibliographies*. Ann Arbor, Mich.: Anshen Publishing, 1978. A comprehensive, partially annotated guide to the literature published on the politics of women's health prior to 1978. Includes hundreds of books and articles covering such topics as Gynecological Self-Help, Sterilization Abuse, Malpractice, Women in the Health Professions, and Synthetic Estrogens.

The Diagram Group, *Woman's Body: An Owner's Manual*. New York: Bantam Books, Inc., 1977. Includes well-illustrated and informative but sometimes superficial descriptions of topics relating to women's health. Written from a primarily traditional point of view.

Dreifus, Claudia, ed., *Seizing Our Bodies: The Politics of Women's Health*. New York: Vintage Books/Random House, 1977. An excellent collection of articles written by activists in the women's health movement. Chapters cover a variety of health issues and are well documented: examples include: The Women's Health Movement (Marieskind), The Dangers of Oral Contraception (Seaman), What Medical Students Learn about Women (Weiss), and Vaginal Politics (Frankfort).

Ehrenreich, Barbara, and Deidre English, *Complaints and Disorders: The Sexual Politics of Sickness*. Old Westbury, N.Y.: The Feminist Press, 1973. Glass Mountain Pamphlet No. 2. The authors paint a vivid portrait of how class prejudice influenced doctors' care of women during the nineteenth and early twentieth centuries.

————, *For Her Own Good: 150 Years of Experts' Advice to Women*. Garden City, N.Y.: Anchor Press/Doubleday, 1978. This book traces the myths perpetrated by male professionals to keep women ignorant and powerless, particularly in regard to their own bodies.

Farquhar, John, *The American Way of Life Need Not Be Hazardous to Your Health*. New York: W. W. Norton & Co., Inc., 1978. As more women take on high pressure careers, their rate of heart attacks and strokes is rising. This book offers information and concrete suggestions for prevention of heart disease. Contains good, common-sense guidelines for anyone concerned about his or her health.

Federation of Feminist Women's Health Centers, *A New View of a Woman's Body*. New York: Simon & Schuster, 1981. An excellent self-help book written by women dedicated to helping other women take charge of their own bodies. It is fully illustrated and includes a unique section of color photographs depicting women's genitalia. Highly recommended.

Flynn, Patricia, and Anne Randolph, *Holistic Health: The Art and Science of Care*. Bowie, Md.: Robert J. Brady Co., 1980. A practical, well-researched guide offering a wide selection of exercises, tools, and up-to-date information the clinician can use in her practice. Emphasis is on whole person care.

Frankfort, Ellen, *Vaginal Politics*. New York: Quadrangle Books, 1972. A comprehensive overview of medical sexism and how it affects women's health care in such areas as abortion and cancer.

Grissum, Marlene, and Carol Spengler, *Womanpower and Health Care*. Boston: Little, Brown & Company, 1976. Describes the socialization process that prevents or inhibits women from taking a more equal role as providers in our health care system.

Grossinger, Richard, *Planet Medicine: From Stone Age Shamanism to Post-Industrial Healing*. New York: Anchor/Doubleday, 1980. The author describes ancient and modern healing modalities that are based on harmony between man and nature. Raises some important moral questions about our own allopathic system of health care.

Hastings, Arthur, ed., *Health for the Whole Person: The Complete Guide to Holistic Medicine*. Boulder, Colo.: Westview Press, 1980. A collection of 31 essays, many written by pioneers in the holistic health field. Some of the topics covered are: health in its social context, ageing, alternative medical models, and a look at the future of health care in the United States.

Hill, Ann, ed., *A Visual Encyclopedia of Unconventional Medicine*. New York: Crown Publishers, Inc., 1979. Probably the best guide to alternative therapies published to date. Contains excellent descriptions, photos, and illustrations of over 120 different healing modalities.

Huttman, Barbara, *The Patient's Advocate: The Complete Handbook of Patients' Rights*. New York: Penguin Books, 1981. This highly readable guide demystifies the hospital experience, giving the patient a chance at winning "the hospital game." Told from an "insider's" perspective.

Illich, Ivan, *Medical Nemesis: The Expropriation of Health*. New York: Pantheon Books/Random House, 1976. A stimulating and thoroughly documented critique of modern technological medicine. The author argues persuasively that our current medical system is itself a cause of more disease than it alleviates.

Isis and the Boston Women's Health Book Collective, *International Women's Health Resource Guide*. Preliminary draft edition, July 1980. An annotated guide to publications from all over the world on women's health issues. Each selection is translated into Spanish, French, Italian, and English. Informative, but cluttered and difficult to use.

Kaslof, Leslie, *Wholistic Dimensions in Healing: A Resource Guide*. New York: Doubleday & Co., Inc., 1978. Probably the most comprehensive list ever compiled of holistic and alternative healing organizations, schools, and centers found in the United States. Each section is introduced by a short description of a different healing modality. A good resource book, but will need some updating.

Lanson, Lucienne, *From Woman to Woman: A Gynecologist Answers Questions about You and Your Body*. New York: Alfred A. Knopf, Inc., 1981. An expanded version of Dr. Lanson's 1975 book. Includes up-to-date information on traditional gynecological care and pathology in a question-answer format. There is also a helpful glossary of gynecological terms.

Lauersen, Niels, and Steven Whitney, *It's Your Body: A Woman's Guide to Gynecology*. New York: Grosset & Dunlap, Inc., 1977. Although focused primarily on female reproductive pathology rather than health, this guide is well written and provides information that your own gynecologist may not have the time or inclination to provide.

Lettvin, Maggie, *Maggie's Woman's Book: Her Personal Plan for Health and Fitness for Women of Every Age*. Boston: Houghton Mifflin Company, 1980. A well-organized, easy to use book. The emphasis is on exercises that tone the entire body, but there is a lot of information on diet and self-treatment as well.

Madaras, Lynda, and Jane Patterson, *Womancare: A Gynecological Guide to Your Body*. New York: Avon Books, 1981. This is a good reference book on gynecology from an allopathic, "symptom-oriented" perspective. It includes symptoms, causes, diagnoses, and treatments for most gynecological problems.

Marieskind, Helen, *Women in the Health System: Patients, Providers, and Programs*. St. Louis: The C. V. Mosby Company, 1980. This textbook provides data from the National Center for Health Statistics on ambulatory health care, women and occupational health, the impact of technology on women's health care, women's health activism, and a myriad of other facts relating to women and the health care system.

Martin, Leonide, *Health Care of Women*. Philadelphia: J. B. Lippincott Company, 1978. A good textbook for providers of health services, as well as a useful resource for the health care needs of the average woman. Includes an excellent explanation of abnormal Pap smears.

Mattson, Phyllis, *Holistic Health in Perspective*. Palo Alto, Calif.: Mayfield Publishing Company, 1981. Describes the principles of holistic philosophy, and, using an anthropological perspective, compares these with the principles of other medical systems. Discusses the evolution of the holistic movement, the healing and diagnostic practices of holistic medicine, and the problems of evaluating holistic health practices.

Mendelsohn, Robert, *Male Practice: How Doctors Manipulate Women*. Chicago: Contempoary Books, 1981. The author of *Confessions of a Medical Heretic* rails at the medical profession and its mistreatment of women.

Millman, Marcia, *The Unkindest Cut: Life in the Backrooms of Medicine*. New York: Morrow Quill Paperbacks, 1978. The author records full scenes she had witnessed in surgery rooms, mortality review conferences, and meeting rooms that reveal the competition and discord that exists between physicians, as well as their attitudes toward women patients and co-workers.

National Women's Health Network, *National Women's Health Network Resource Guides*. Washington, D.C., 1980. This is a series of nine separate booklets on: Abortion, Birth Control, Breast Cancer, DES, Hysterectomy, Maternal Health and Childbirth, Self-Help, and Sterilization. The quality of the booklets varies, but each contains an excellent list of women's health centers, films, advocacy groups, etc.

Notman, Malkah, ed., and Carol Nadelson, *The Woman Patient: Medical and Psychological Interfaces*. New York: Plenum Publishing Corporation, 1977. Seeks to address those issues of concern to women patients that medical staff often has difficulty understanding; for example, the emotional impact of abortion or the trauma of mastectomy. Sensitively written.

Nierenberg, Judith, and Florence Janovic, *The Hospital Experience*. Indianapolis: The Bobbs-Merrill Co., Inc., 1978. Forewarned is forearmed; this is a well-organized "consumer's guide" to hospitals. The authors describe in detail commonly administered diagnostics tests, treatments, and operations.

Oyle, Irving., *The New American Medicine Show*. Santa Cruz, Calif.: Unity Press, 1979. The author questions the basic assumption underlying our current beliefs about health and reality.

Padus, Emrika, *The Woman's Encyclopedia of Health and Natural Healing*. Emmaus, Pa.: Rodale Press, 1981. A compilation of hundreds of traditional and nontraditional treatments for a broad spectrum of women's health problems. This is a monumental achievement by a senior editor of *Prevention* magazine.

Paxton, Mary Jean Wallace, *The Female Body in Control: How the Control Mechanisms in a Woman's Physiology Make Her Special*. Englewood Cliffs, N.J.: Prentice-Hall, Inc., 1981. A somewhat technical work on female anatomy, using graphs, charts, and diagrams to explain the delicate balance of a woman's endocrine system. Includes coverage of alcohol, diet, and exercise.

Pelletier, Kenneth, *Holistic Medicine: From Stress to Optimum Health*. New York: Delacorte Press, 1979. An attempt to define the perimeters of holistic health. Includes current scientific research and a comprehensive health questionnaire.

————, *Mind as Healer, Mind as Slayer: A Holistic Approach to Preventing Stress Disorders*. New York: Dell Publishing, Co., Inc., 1979. Provides an in-depth look at stress and the new concepts of psychosomatic illness. The author argues that there is a place for both allopathic and holistic medicine, but the ultimate responsibility for health lies with the individual.

Popenoe, Chris, *Wellness. The Yes! Bookshop Guide*. Washington, D.C.: Yes! Inc., 1977. This is a comprehensive annotated guide to hundreds of books covering a wide range of alternative healing modalities.

Rusek, Sheryl, *The Women's Health Movement: Feminist Alternatives to Medical Control*. New York: Praeger Publishers, Inc., 1978. The author has written an excellent, thoroughly documented study of the history and politics of women's health care, particularly the rise of the feminist self-help movement.

Rush, Ann Kent, *Getting Clear: Body Work for Women*. New York: Random House, 1973. Bay Area women therapists share their games, exercises, philsophies, and stories. This is an excellent experiential guide to self-discovery and growth.

Samuels, Mike, and Hal Bennett, *The Well-Body Book*. New York: Random House, Inc., 1973. Emphasizes education, self-help, and offers exercises designed to teach one about one's own body and its particular needs and healing messages.

An excellent, unique guide for those open to new approaches to self-healing and willing to take the time and effort necessary to fully utilize what it has to offer.

Scully, Diana, *Men Who Control Women's Health: The Miseducation of Obstetrician-Gynecologists*. Boston: Houghton Mifflin Company, 1980. Includes a history of gynecology and "Strategies for Change" as well as fascinating quotes from resident physicians on such topics as why they chose gynecology and their view of minority patients. Provides a clearer understanding of the forces that contribute to the paternalistic, chauvinistic medical system we have today.

Selye, Hans, *The Stress of Life*. New York: McGraw-Hill Book Company, 1956, 1976. Dr. Selye discusses the biological mechanism of stress and its impact on health and disease. This is the definitive text on stress, written by a medical maverick who laid the foundation for legitimate study of psychosomatic medicine.

17 Women Doctors, *Every Woman's Health: The Complete Guide to Body and Mind*. Garden City, N.Y.: Doubleday & Co., Inc., 1980. In addition to the usual information on women's reproductive health, this book includes chapters on nutrition, fitness, your mind and feelings, midlife transitions, etc. It is consistently well-written, factual, and sensitive. Primarily allopathic, but incorporates some holistic concepts.

Sloane, Ethel, *Biology of Women*. New York: John Wiley & Sons, Inc., 1980. This is a broad overview of how women's bodies work and what affects their health. Includes basic anatomy and physiology as well as information about health-care products, sexuality for the disabled woman, menstrual cramps, etc.

Sobel, David, ed., *Ways of Health: Holistic Approaches to Ancient and Contemporary Medicine*. New York: Harcourt Brace Jovanovich, Inc., 1979. A collection of essays that challenge our present concepts of health and disease by examining popular healing modes of other cultures.

Stellman, Jeanne, *Women's Work, Women's Health: Myths and Realities*. New York: Pantheon Books, Inc., 1977. This is a more "politicized" version of *Work Is Dangerous to Your Health*. Emphasizes "hidden" health hazards on the job (e.g., office air pollution), the politics of work, work and reproductive health.

Stellman, Jeanne, and Susan Daum, *Work Is Dangerous to Your Health: A Handbook of Health Hazards in the Workplace and What You Can Do about Them*. New York: Vintage Books, 1973. A definitive work on occupational disease. Explains how exposure to stress, noise, and toxic chemicals affects the body and discusses ways to prevent or minimize their effects. Includes an appendix that lists health hazards by occupation.

Stewart, Felicia et al., *My Body, My Health: The Concerned Woman's Guide to Gynecology*. Somerset, N.J.: Wiley Medical Publications, 1979. A fine edition to the growing list of books concerned with educating women about their reproductive health (and dishealth). The information is clear and easy to understand; a good home resource guide.

NAME AND SUBJECT INDEX

NAME INDEX

Aaland, Mikkel, 330
Adams, A., 4
Adler, Charles, 342
Adler, Sheila, 342
Aguilar, Nona, 20
Airola, Paavo, 213, 214, 217, 218, 219, 221, 222
Alfonso, D., 114, 115
Ali, S. M., 237
Amman, W., 236, 239
Anthony, Susan B., 151n
Appenzeller, Otto, 316
Applegate, William A., 148, 210
Aristotle, 16
Armitage, K., 89
Armstrong, B., 221
Aronson, Shepard G., 126
Arthure, H., 114
Assagioli, Roberto, 132
Austin, Harriet, 151
Avicenna (early woman physician), 248
Azizi, F., 72

Backster, Cleve, 267
Baggish, M. S., 114
Baird, Pamela, 134
Bakalar, J. B., 401, 404
Baker, J. R., 16
Ballentine, Rudolph, 215, 216, 218, 224
Balter, M. B., 88
Banta, David, 37
Barber, I., 372
Barker, M. G., 106
Baron, E., 106
Barr, Jean Scott, 252
Bart, P., 5
Bass, R. A., 89
Beard, Gertrude, 247, 252
Bedortha, N., 149
Beecham, E., 58
Beecher, Catherine, 150, 151n
Beechman, W. D., 114
Benigno, B., 70
Benson, Herbert, 274, 298, 354
Benson, R. C., 114, 115
Berlin, J., 105
Bernard, Claude, 131
Bernstein, G. S., 16
Besant, Annie, 14
Betrus, Patricia, 344

Bhargava, A. K., 237
Bibbo, M., 65, 72
Bieber, I., 106
Bieler, Henry G., 211, 212, 217, 219
Billings, E. L., 20
Billings, J. J., 20, 381
Binstock, W. A., 86
Black, Maurice, 25
Black, S., 368, 371
Blackie, Marjery, 200
Bloomfield, H., 352, 354, 357, 359
Bole, Giles, 27
Bonadonna, G. U., 97
Borgman, R. D., 90
Bourse, B. W., 103
Bowers, K., 371
Bowes, W. A., 115
Boyne, Gil, 368, 374
Brackbill, Y., 38
Brandt, Thure, 250
Brann, A., 43
Brazelton, T., 41
Brewer, Gail Forza, 215, 216
Brewer, T. H., 230
Brewer, Tom, 215, 216
Brewin, R., 87, 401
Brosse, T., 352, 355
Brozan, Nadine, 11
Bucholz, C. Herman, 250
Buchsbaum, H. J., 114
Budoff, Penny Wise, 55, 57, 58, 95, 96, 98
Budzynski, Thomas H., 340
Bullock, B., 72
Bunker, J. P., 103, 104
Burmeister, Mary, 272

Caldeyro-Barcia, R., 36, 37, 40, 43
Campbell, Arthur A., 10
Cannon, Joseph, 317
Caranasos, G. J., 84, 86
Carnahan, Clarence, 342
Carrington, E., 58
Carrington, P., 351, 353, 354, 357, 358, 359
Casal, U. A., 248
Castleman, Michael, 402, 406n
Chalmers, I., 117
Chan, Pedro, 271
Chang, Min-Chuch, 10, 23
Charpil, Milos, 15
Chauhan, C. S., 237
Cheraskin, E., 214

Chu, W. Y., 169n
Chuang, L. S., 169n
Clark, David, 90
Cleopatra, 16
Cluff, L. E., 86
Coady, D. J., 119
Cohen, W. R., 119
Cole, P., 67, 105
Collea, J. V., 119
Colletti, L., 41
Collison, D., 184, 371
Colton, Helen, 254
Connell-Tatum, Elizabeth, 12
Connelly, Patricia, 210
Cooper, J. R., 85
Cooper, Kenneth, 311, 312, 313
Cooperstock, R., 85, 86
Copeland, Paul, 296
Corea, Gena, 95, 98, 103, 107
Cornell, William M., 152
Cosgrove, M., 72
Cousins, Norman, 340
Cowan, G., 4
Craigin, E. B., 114
Creedon, J. J., 105
Cresson, Frank M., 323
Cutler, J. C., 17, 18

Dalton, Katherine, 56
Davis, Adelle, 213, 214, 216, 217, 219
Davis, Paulina Wright, 150, 151
Deikman, A., 354
de la Verge, Eliza, 151
de Langre, Jacques, 272
De Lee, J. B., 116
De Sa Souza, Juliet, 299
de Waard, F., 221
Delaney, B., 36
Despard, Louisa L., 251
Deutch, R. M., 290
Dewan, Edmund, 20
Dewhurst, C. J., 117
Dicke, Elizabeth, 264
Dicker, R. C., 106
Dieckman, W., 70
Dietvorst, Thomas F., 342
Dodds, Sir Charles, 25–26
Douglas, R. C., 113, 117
Downer, Carol, 20, 380
Downing, George, 247, 266
Drellich, M. G., 106
Drucker, P., 129
Dunea, G., 85

Dutton, D., 66
Dyck, F. J., 104, 105

Eckstein, P., 16
Elgin, D., 356
Elizabeth II, Queen, 200
Ellenberg, J., 41
Ellerbrook, Wallace, 140
Elliott, J., 83, 87
Emerson, R. S., 105
Erickson, Donald J., 253
Estee, Mrs. S. M., 151, 154
Evans, G., 223
Evrard, J. R., 114

Farmilant, Eunice, 54, 331
Fasal, E., 69
Favero, R. V., 89
Feneslau, Catherine, 242
Ferdman, T. D., 231
Ferin, J., 18n
Fidell, L. S., 84, 86, 88, 89, 90
Findley, P., 113
Finkel, M., 36
Finkle, W., 65, 67
Fisher, Alexander A., 381
Fitzgerald, Paul, 56, 57
Flynn, A., 37
Forbes, Thomas Rogers, 249
Forni, G., 241
Fowler, Lydia Folger, 150
Fox, R. Fortescue, 251
Frankel, T., 114
Frankl, Victor, 132
Fredericks, C., 211, 217, 218, 220, 223
Freeman, A., 184
French, D. J., 343
Freud, Sigmund, 250, 365–66, 375
Frost, D., 223
Fuchs, D., 369
Fujikawa, Y., 248
Fulton, John F., 150
Funderburk, James, 303

Gabbe, S., 36
Galliford, B. W., 114
Gallup, George, 295
Gardner, Augustus K., 151
Garret, Tom, 253
Gega, Osamu, 280
Gibbs, C. E., 117
Gibbs, R. S., 114
Gill, W., 72
Giller, Robert M., 273
Glazier, William, 130
Gleason, Rachel Brooks, 150
Goddard, James, 77
Godec, C., 370
Gold, E. M., 114
Goldenberg, R. L., 115
Goldstein, D., 72
Goldstein, S., 354
Goldzieher, J., 70
Goleman, D., 355, 356
Gonzalez, Elizabeth Rasche, 219
Gordon, T., 190

Goryachev, V. S., 238
Gospal, K. S., 297
Goyan, Jere, 38
Grad, Bernard, 267
Graedon, J., 85, 87
Graham, Douglas, 252
Graham, Sylvester, 148
Granworth, G., 330
Green, Alyce, 335, 336, 338, 339, 340, 345, 352, 355
Green, E. E., 335, 336, 338, 339, 340, 355
Greenblatt, R. B., 231
Greenspan, J. R., 103, 104, 106
Greenwald, P., 65, 67
Greenwood, Sanja Goldsmith, 341
Gregg, Robert, 344
Grimke, Angelina, 151n
Grinspon, L., 401, 404

Hack, M., 115
Haddad, H., 119
Hagen, D., 114
Hahnemann, Samuel, 197, 198
Haire, Doris, 35, 36, 38
Harmer, Ruth M., 163
Harrison, M., 107
Hart, Donn V., 251
Harvey, Philip, 18
Hasan, J. M., 325
Hasting, A., 359
Hastings, Mary Lydia, 251
Hatcher, R. A., 18
Hawkins, D., 16, 232
Heczey, Maria, 342
Heimlich, J., 197
Heinonen, O., 70
Herbst, 36, 65, 70, 71
Hertz, Roy, 64, 69–70, 74, 75
Hiatt, H. H., 85
Hibbard, L. T., 105, 114, 119
Himes, N. E., 16
Hippocrates, 197, 209, 326
Hirsch, Jean, 20
Hirsch, Lolly, 20
Hoch, Z., 369
Hoff, Hebbel E., 150
Hoffer, A., 229, 231
Hohnadel, David C., 326
Holsten, W., 63, 76, 77
Hooper, S., 114
Hopkins, Harold C., 381
Hoult, I., 37
Huber, S. C., 28
Hughes, Muriel Joy, 249
Hughes, R., 87, 401
Huka, B., 17
Hunt, Angenette A., 147
Hunt, Harriet, 150
Hunt, Valery, 288n
Hyodo, Massayoshi, 280

Ikram, M., 240
Illich, Ivan, 132, 135
Inkeles, Alex, 149
Iyengar, B. K., 295, 298, 299, 300, 305

Jackson, James C., 151
Jackson, L., 20
Jacobs, Miriam, 264
Jacobson, Edmund, 274
Jain, A. K., 22
Jain, S. P., 114
Janackovic-Milojevic, B., 241
Javert, C. T., 230, 231
Jeffreys, M., 52
Jennings, J., 29
Jensen, Kathryn, 253
Jex-Blake, Sophia, 248
Jick, H., 17, 83, 84, 86
Jocano, F. Landa, 251
Johnson, R., 372
Johnson, V., 53, 106, 107
Jonas, Eugene, 20
Jones, V., 63, 74
Jordan, Susan, 16
Judd, H., 67
Jung, C. G., 132

Kakelik, Jan, 240
Kamenetz, Herman L., 247, 250
Kao, F. F., 184
Kao, J. J., 184
Karnaky, H., 70
Karvonen, M. S., 325
Kaslow, Arthur L., 128
Kayne, R. C., 85
Kelly, P., 371
Klempner, Mara, 5
Koch, James, 14
Koch-Weser, J., 87
Koepsell, T., 104
Kononikhina, N. F., 238
Krieger, Dolores, 259
Kubler-Ross, Elizabeth, 403n
Kuchera, L., 63, 73
Kushi, Michio, 167
Kushner, Rose, 95, 97

Lacey, Louise, 20
Lahann, H., 231
Lanuman, Lyn, 24
Landon, Parsons, 99
Larned, D., 108
Larson, C. P., 190
Latven, Albert R., 242
Lao-tsu, 166, 176
Lauersen, Niels, 14, 220, 223
Laventurier, M. F., 84
Laver, Bryan A., 249
Lawson, D. H., 86
Leavitt, J., 146
Lee, Benjamin, 250n
Lee, P. R., 85, 87
Leeb, C. S., 343
Leeuwenhoek, A. V., 16
Lennard, L. L., 90
Lerner, Gerda, 150
Le Shan, Lawrence, 345, 354
Lesnikov, E. P., 240
Levine, J., 88
Levine, S., 354, 356
Lewis, C. E., 103, 104

Lewis, Oscar, 329
Lien-teh, Wu, 248
Lietti, A., 241
Ling, per Herrik, 250
London, Robert, 219
Lowe, J. A., 113, 114, 117
Lucas-Championnier, Just, 251
Luce, Clare Booth, 9
Lundy, L. E., 119
Luthe, Wolfgang, 274, 338, 343

MacDonald, Christina, 252
MacKay, Charles, 249
MacLean, P. D., 336
Maddox, Hilary, 341, 342
Madoyan, O. O., 239
Maginniss, C., 90
Mahan, C., 118
Mallory, A., 65
Mann, Felix, 164
Marieskind, H. I., 108, 114, 116, 117
Markush, R. E., 89
Maronde, R. F., 83, 86
Massey, Wayne, 288n
Masters, W., 53, 106, 107
Masunaga, Shizato, 272
Mathews-Simon, Stephanie, 345
Maugh, T., 66, 85
Mays, E., 65
McAllister, A., 63, 74
McCarthy, E. G., 104
McCauley, Carole Spearin, 219, 221
McDowell, K., 372
McKinley, J. M., 52
McLachlan, J., 72
McMahon, B., 67
McMillan, Mary, 251
McQueen, E., 64
Mechanic, D., 86, 90
Mehling, Betty, 272
Melder, Keith, 150
Mellinger, G. D., 84, 88
Mendelsohn, Robert S., 125
Mendelson, G., 184
Mennell, James, 250n
Merril, B. S., 117
Mesmer, Franz Anton, 365
Mezger, Johan Georg, 250
Michaels, David, 24
Mihajlov, Milena, 241
Miles, Richard B., 128
Miller, Elizabeth Smith, 151n
Miller, Peter, 329
Miller, Richard J., 184
Minkoff, H. L., 116, 118, 119, 120
Mitchell, S. Weir, 250
Moertel, G., 86
Molton, Lawrence, 77
Montagu, Ashley, 254
Moots, B., 22
Morgan, S., 106
Morris, Freda, 370, 374, 375
Morris, Louis, 27n
Muinova, S. S., 238
Mullaney, Daniel J., 340
Muller, P. F., 114

Munch, James C., 242
Murai, Jiro, 272
Murav'ev, I. A., 238
Myers, R., 43

Needleman, J., 354
Nelson, Chris, 385
Nelson, K., 41, 115
Neutra, R. R., 120
Newbold, R., 72
Newland, Kathleen, 345
Newton, N., 106
Nichols, Mary Gove, 147, 148, 149, 150, 152
Nichols, Thomas L., 149
Nissen, Hartvig, 249
Noble, Elizabeth, 290, 297
Nolan, G., 36
Nora, A., 64
Nora, J., 64
Norris, Patricia, 339, 340, 345
Numbers, R., 146
Nydegger, Corinne, 251
Nydegger, William F., 251

Oakie, Susan, 23
Obretenova, N., 242
Ohaski, Watura, 272
O'Malley, Becky, 23
Orme-Johnson, D. W., 355
Ornstein, Robert E., 128
Ory, H., 24
Osborne, David, 342
Osmond, H., 229
Oster, Gerald, 21
Oster, Selmarre, 21
Ostrander, S., 20

Paeschke, K. D., 231
Paffenbarger, Ralph, 25, 69, 313
Panos, M., 197
Papez, J. M., 336
Parnell, P., 85
Passwater, R. A., 223
Paul, R. H., 120
Pauling, Linus, 228–32
Paulshock, B. Z., 106
Pauzner, L. E., 238
Pearce, Chilton Joseph, 128
Pelletier, Kenneth, 345
Pendleton, Bonnie, 272
Peritz, E., 69
Pettiti, Diane, 11, 23, 62, 114
Phillips, D. L., 89
Pincus, Gregory, 23
Piotrow, P. T., 18n
Plate, W. P., 25
Playfair, William S., 250, 250n
Polishuk, W. Z., 114
Poskanzer, D., 70
Postic, B., 18
Potter, R. G., 18n
Prescott, James W., 254
Prestivich, R., 190
Preston, Ann, 147
Price, Monica, 209

Price, Weston A., 209, 210, 215, 216
Procope, Berndt-Johan, 327
Puronen, P., 325

Quatrefages, A. A., 16

Ralston, D., 36, 39
Ranney, B., 119
Rapola, J., 330
Rawson, Philip, 248n
Raymond, Aurelia, 149
Rechnitz, Kurt, 20
Reed, Theordore P., 11
Reibmayer, Albert, 250
Reiter, Susan, 253
Rhead, G. W., 223
Rice, Ruth, 261–63
Richards, B. C., 103
Richards, M., 117
Ringsdorf, W., 214
Risse, G., 146, 200
Robboy, S., 71
Roffman, Roger, 406
Rolf, Ida, 287, 288, 289, 290
Rosch, Paul J., 345
Rose, Jeanne, 237n
Rosenblatt, D., 41
Rosenblum, A., 20
Rosenfeld, A., 24
Roshan, Sara, 14
Ross, C., 18n
Ross, J. E., 114
Rothman, Lorraine, 20, 380
Rotman, Marvin, 97, 98
Rubin, G. L., 114
Rush, Anne K., 266n
Ryan, Dale S., 236, 238

Salter, A., 368
Samborskaya, E. P., 231
Sammons, James H., 105
Sampson, G. A., 56
Sanger, Margaret, 9, 10, 15
Saxen, L., 330
Schneider, S., 36, 39
Schneidermann, L. J., 89
Schrauzer, G., 223
Schrinsky, D. C., 114
Schroeder, L., 20
Schultz, J. H., 336
Schutz, Howard, 134
Schwartz, A., 58
Schwartz, L., 355, 356, 358
Schwarz, R. H., 116, 118, 119, 120
Scott, D., 86
Scully, D., 5, 108
Seaman, Barbara, 9, 10, 12, 14, 15, 16, 18, 22, 25, 28, 54, 64, 213, 214, 215, 217, 218
Seaman, Gideon, 14, 15, 16, 18, 22, 28, 54, 64, 213, 214, 215, 217, 218
Sedlacek, Keith, 342
Segal, B. E., 89
Seidenberg, R., 90
Seligman, Jean, 22

Selye, Hans, 274
Settiwar, R. M., 295, 305
Shader, R., 88
Shader, R. I., 86
Shamberger, Raymond, 222, 223
Shapiro, D., 351, 352, 355, 356, 357, 360
Shealy, Norman, 139, 274
Shearer, M., 114
Shearin, R. B., 22
Sherman, B., 65
Shew, Marie Louise, 147, 148–49
Shute, Evan, 214, 222
Silver, A., 39, 43
Silverman, Janet, 167
Silverman, M., 85, 87
Simonton, C., 107, 345
Simonton, S., 107, 345, 371
Singh, B., 17, 18
Singh, R. H., 295, 305
Sitreri, P., 67
Sloan, Aaron B., 242
Smith, Connie, 13
Smith, D., 65, 70, 75
Snow, Arnold, 251
Snow, Ellen M., 149
Snowden, P., 16
Snyder, Solomon H., 184
Soiva, K., 329, 330
Sommers, Sheila, 99
Soranus of Ephesus (early Greek physician), 248
Southam, A. L., 28
Soyka, Fred, 328
Stadel, Bruce, 27, 30, 67, 85, 222
Stafl, D., 71
Stander, H. J., 230, 231
Stanton, H., 370
Stewart, Felicia Hams, 344
Stewart, R. B., 86
Stichler, J., 114, 115
Stim, Edward, 13
Stone, Harold, 214
Stone, Lucy, 151n
Strenkovskaya, A. G., 242
Studd, J., 41
Subrahmanyan, V., 240
Sunderman, F. W., 326
Swan, Shana, 23
Swenson, N., 105
Synder, Donald, 326
Syvalahti, E., 327
Szasz, T., 399
Szent-Gyorgi, 230

Taladay, P., 242
Talley, R. B., 84
Tappan, Frances M., 264n
Tart, C., 354
Taslitz, Norman, 252
Tatum, Howard J., 12
Taylor, Madison, 253
Taylor, R. W., 56
Taylor, Ronald, 286
Teaguarden, Iona, 272

Tebbets, C., 368, 374
Teeri, N., 328
Thacker, S., 37
Thayer, William, 253
Theuer, Richard, 26
Tietze, C., 74
Tompkins, Peter, 267
Tooke, William, 322
Tower, Donald, 40
Treichel, J. A., 21
Trotula of Salerno (early woman physician), 248
Tubbs, Walter, 342
Tuskayev, A., 238, 242

Ucko, L., 42
Udupa, K. N., 295, 305
Ulfelder, H., 70
Utidjian, H., 17

Vaillant, George, 134
Vasterling, H. W., 231
Vaughan, F., 354, 359
Verdeal, Kathey, 236, 238
Veridiano, N., 71
Vessey, M. P., 22
Vihwejuuri, H. J., 322
Virtanen, John, 329
Von Rottauscher, Anna, 323

Walczak, Michael, 214
Waldron, I., 84
Wallace, R. K., 352, 355
Wallnofer, Heinrich, 271
Walsh, R., 352, 354, 355, 359
Walters, E. D., 335
Weg, R. B., 87
Weideger, Paula, 51
Weil, A. T., 399, 400, 403, 404
Weinstein, M. C., 107
Weiss, K., 62, 70, 73, 85
Weiss, N., 65
Weissman, M. M., 89
Welch, R., 71
Wen, W., 190
Wensel, Louise O., 183, 193
Widmer, G. W., 104
Wilber, K., 354, 356
Williams, R. Sanders, 134
Wilson, Colleen, 380
Wilson, J. R., 4–5, 58
Wolfe, Sidney, 53, 67, 85
Wolf-Willets, Vivian, 344
Wong, K. Chimin, 248
Wood, Elizabeth, 247, 252
Wood, Peter, 314
Woods, Nancy Fugate, 344
Wright, R. C., 105, 106

Yip, S. K., 280
Young, D., 118

Zabludowski, J. B., 251
Zelin, Chen, 167
Zhang, Jin-an, 166, 170

Ziel, H., 65, 67
Zigler, Z., 374
Zola, I., 90
Zuck, T. T., 18n
Zucker, T. A., 213
Zussman, L., 107

SUBJECT INDEX

Abortion
  mortality rate, 21
  rights, 23, 30, 108
  prevention, alternative approach, 231, 380
  spontaneous (miscarriage), 21, 36, 61, 65, 66, 70–74
    induction of, 61, 187, 237–38, 248
Abortives, natural, 236, 237, 238
Abstinence/natural birth control, 19, 30
Aches, 51, 55
  self-help therapy, 404
Acne, 62
  alternative approach, 213, 239, 315
Acupressure, 131, 159, 271–83
Acupuncture, 159, 167–76 passim, 177–80, 182–95, 263–64, 266
Addiction, drug, 193, 357–58, 399–402
Adenocarcinoma, 70, 71
Adenosis, vaginal, 70–71
Advertising, drugs/devices, 18, 45, 75, 381, 401
Aerobic exercise, 53, 55, 159, 310–18
Aesthetic reactions, to various contraceptives, 13, 15, 17
Aging, see Menopause
Alcohol, 56, 84, 88, 134, 215
Alcoholism, self-help therapy, 193, 358, 404
Allergy
  and homeostatis, 136–40
  self-help therapy, 184, 192, 359, 404, 406
  to contraceptive, 17
Allopathy/homeopathy, compared, 157–60, 198
Alternative approaches to women's health care, 5, 162–408
  history/philosophy, 125–60
Alternative Birth Center Open House, 127
Amenorrhea, self-help therapy, 170, 178, 187, 341–43
American Academy of Pediatrics, 36
American College of Surgeons, 96, 97
American Medical Association, 3, 66, 406, 407
American Public Health Association, 76
Amniocentesis, risks in, 36
Amniotomy, risks in, 36, 43
Amphetamines, 88, 216, 401, 403

Analgesic drugs, 85, 86, 115
    alternatives to, 190
Anaprox, 58
Anemia, 25, 26, 28, 64
    alternative treatment, 170, 212–13,
        216, 217
Anesthesia, 41, 42, 106, 114, 115
    alternative approach, 185, 190, 406
Antidepressants, 3, 84, 87, 407
Antibiotics, 85, 86, 216, 382
Anxiety
    alternative approach, 185, 191–02,
        341, 356–57
    menopausal, 53, 67
    premenstrual, 55, 58
Apgar score, infant, 37, 41
Arthritis, 25, 27
    self-help therapy, 134, 193, 276–
        77, 300–02, 321, 371, 403, 406
Aspirin, 58, 86, 198
Asthma, self-help therapy, 202, 359,
    371, 402, 407
Attitudes, and homeostasis, 134, 135,
    138–42, 370
Autoimmune system
    food allergies and, 137, 192
    vasectomy and, 11

Backlash
    against sterilization, 10
    to pill/IUD, 29
"band-aid" sterilization, 11, 12
Barbiturates, 85, 88, 404
Barrier contraception, 12–18, 27, 29
Basal body temperature method, of
    timing ovulation, 19–20
"Belly-button" sterilization, 11
Bendectin, 35–36
Billings method, of natural birth con-
    trol, 20, 381
Bioenergetics, 159
Biofeedback, 159, 274, 334–49, 352
Bioflavonids, 213, 231
Biotin, 217
Birth control
    using biofeedback, 343
    using heat, 327
    see also Contraception
Birth defects, from
    obstetrical intervention/drug use,
        35–48, 64, 65, 66, 68–69, 70–74
    spermicides, 16–18
Bleeding, menstrual, profuse, 51, 54,
    213
Bloating, see Edema
Blood clots/clotting, 23, 134, 170, 218
Blood pressure, high, 22–23, 57
    self-help therapy, 359
Brain damage, fetal, and obstetric
    drugs, 36, 41–42, 43–44
Breast disease
    benign, 24, 25, 64
    male, and estrogen handling, 24
    malignant, 3, 24–25, 52, 64, 66, 67,
        95–100

Breast surgery
    alternative procedures, 97–100
    current treatment, 37,
Bromocriptin, 56

Caesarean surgery, 41
    alternative approach, 185
    current practice, 113–23
Caffeine, 100, 215, 403
Calcitonin, 53
Calcium depletion, 53, 55, 67
    alternative approach, 213, 214–15,
        216, 219
Calendar method, natural birth con-
    trol, 18–19
Cancer
    breast, 3, 24–25, 52, 64, 66, 67,
        95–100
    cervical, 26, 64, 71–72, 103
    colon/rectal, 393
    endometrical, 25–26, 52–53, 66,
        67, 69–70
    liver, 66, 69
    ovarian, 25–26, 52, 64, 66
    pituitary, 26, 66, 69
    uterine, 25–26, 52–53, 63, 64, 67,
        69–70, 103, 107
    vaginal, 62, 66, 70–72
Cancer, alternative approaches, 134,
    185, 219–24, 326–28, 345, 371,
    393, 402, 403n, 404, 407
Cap, see Cervical cap
Cardiovascular disease, 22–23, 30
    alternative approach, 229, 313
Catholic Church, and Billings birth
    control method, 381
Center for Disease Control (CDC),
    11, 21, 24, 103, 104
Cervical
    cancer, 26, 64, 71–72, 103
    cap, 12, 13, 14–15, 17
    erosion, 64
    mucous method of natural birth
        control, 20
    problems, alternative treatment,
        173–74
    self-examination, as contracep-
        tive method, 20–21
Chemical (tubal) blockage, 11
Childbirth
    drug use/obstetrical intervention,
        current, 35–45, 85, 115
    holistic/orthodox views, com-
        pared, 140, 141
    self-help approach, 185, 190, 200–
        01, 215–17, 242–43, 261–62,
        329–30
China
    IUD use in, 28
    traditional Chinese medicine, 54,
        159, 163–95, 223, 265
Chiropractic medicine, 131, 159
Chromium, 216
Cigarette smoking, 134, 215–16
Coca leaf, 403, 404

Cocaine, 401, 403, 403n
Coffee, 221, 400, 403
Columbia, contraceptive use in, 14–15
Conception
    after sterilization, 11–12
    during contraceptive use, 11, 13–
        15, 28
    effect on, after IUD/Pill use, 21–23
Condom, 12, 13, 15, 17, 18
Consent, informed, 4, 38, 41, 45
Constipation, 55
    self-help therapy, 342
Consumer action, effects of, 5, 10, 16,
    27, 44, 58, 98
Contraception/contraceptive
    barrier, 12–18, 27, 29
    calendar method, 18–19
    cervical cap, 12, 13, 14–15, 17
    cervical   mucous   (Billings)
        method, 20, 381
    chemical, 12, 13, 14, 15, 16–18
    condom, 12, 13, 15, 17, 18
    "cosmic" method, 20
    diaphragm, 9, 12, 13–14, 15, 17
    disease transmission and, 18, 27,
        29
    foams, spermicidal, 12, 16–18
    health risks associated with, 21–30
    in other countries, 14–16, 28–29
    intrauterine device (IUD), 9–10,
        12, 13, 14, 15–16, 21, 27–29
    male, 10–11, 18
    massage (method), 248
    "mini" pill for, 27
    morning-after pill, 61, 62, 63, 68,
        73–74
    natural birth control, 18–21, 29–30
    oral, 9–10, 12, 13, 14, 20, 21–27,
        28–29, 30, 61, 63, 69–70
    rhythm method, 18–19, 29–30
    spermicides, 12, 13, 14–15, 16–18
    sponges, 12, 13, 14
    sterilization, 9, 10–12, 14, 21, 105
    suppository, 12, 17
    "universal," search for, 9, 15–16
    use, and health risks, 10–12, 21–30
    use, and mortality risks, 10–12, 17,
        21, 28–29
    see also Birth Control
Copper
    dietary, 214
    in IUD, 27
    sperm susceptibility to, 16
"Cosmic" birth control, 20
Couple to Couple League, 20
Cramps
    alternative treatment, 186, 202,
        203–04, 213, 316–17, 372, 404
    menstrual, 4, 51, 57–58
    premenstrual, 55
Cream, contraceptive, 18
Crime, committed during menstrual
    distress, 54–55
Crying spells, premenstrual, 55
Cuba, IUD use in, 28

Cyst, benign, 24, 25, 99
  alternative treatment, 171, 174–75, 219

Darvon, 86
Death, *see* Mortality
Delivery, *see* Labor/delivery
Demerol, 401
Demonic theory of disease origin, 128
Dependence, drug, 88–90, 357–58, 400
Depression
  after hysterectomy, 106–07
  alternative treatment, 185, 191, 217, 305, 341, 344, 357, 406, 407
  menopausal, 51, 53, 67
  Pill use, 64
  premenstrual, 51, 55
DES (diethylstilbestrol)
  adverse effects
    in daughters, 65, 66, 68–69, 70–74
    in mothers, 72
    in sons, 72
  for problem pregnancies, 24–25, 66, 70
  in cattle feed, 72–73
  in morning-after pill, 73–74
Developing countries, contraceptive methods adopted, 15–16, 27–28, 29
Dexedrine, 87
Diabetes, 116
  alternative treatment, 167, 185, 214, 220, 315, 392
Diagnosis, medical sex-stereotyped, 3– 5, 86–90
Diaphragm, 9, 12, 13–14, 15, 17
Diarrhea, 58
  self-help therapy, 342, 404
Diet, *see* nutrition
Dilaudid, 401
Disease
  acute/episodic, 160
    self-help therapy, 201–02, 203, 230
  chronic/episodic distinction, 138, 160, 202
  eliminating, approaches to, 130–33
  origin, theories of,
    alternative, holistic views, 128–45
    historical views, 128–29
  prevention/self-healing, 147–55
  sexually transmitted, 17, 18, 27, 29, 382–84
Diuretics, 56, 215
Divine theory of disease origin, 128
Dizziness, menstrual, 55
  self-help therapy, 170
Doctors, motives for traditional diagnosis/treatment
  economic, 96, 104, 107–08, 115, 116, 120
  malpractice suits, fear of, 118, 119, 120

Doctor, motives (*Contd.*)
  pharmaceutical industry, 58, 66, 74–77, 85–86, 87, 90, 401
  sex stereotyping, 3–5, 86–90, 341, 399
  technology, 3, 36, 118–119, 120
  training, 4–5, 57–58, 78, 89–90, 96, 108, 118, 119, 120, 126, 185, 252–53
Drug use in obstetrics, effect
  long-term effect, after birth, 41–45
  on fetus, 35–36, 85
  on infant during labor/birth, 37–43, 115
  on mother, 37
  on unborn infant, 37, 38–40
Drugs
  addictive, 193, 399–402
  adverse reactions to, 83–84
  alternative approach, 190, 191, 382–86
  misprescribing of, 3, 5, 35–45, 83–93, 126
  pregnancy/childbirth, use in, 35–45, 85
  psychoactive, 56
    nonpharmaceutical, 399–408
  psychotropic, 83–93
    sex-bias prescribing, 86—90
  recreational use of, 399, 402
Duphaston, 56
Dydrogesterone, 56
Dysmenorrhea, 57–58
  alternative treatment, 170, 178, 186, 341–43
Dysplasia, cervical, 71, 173–74

Ectopic pregnancy
  and mortality rate, 21
  after sterilization, 11
  in DES daughters, 72
  in IUD users, 28
  in Pill users, 25, 27
Edema, premenstrual, 55, 56
  alternative approaches to, 213, 217, 220, 239, 342
Elavil, 87
Emko Foam, 17
Emotional aspect in healing, 125–42 passim, 171
Encare Oval, 17
Endometrical cancer, 25–26, 52–53, 66, 67, 69–70
Endometriosis, 103, 105, 107
  alternative treatment, 185, 186
Envoid, 23
Environmental contamination, and hemeostasis, 132, 137
Epidural block, 41
Epilepsy, 185, 406, 407
Episiotomy, risks of, 37
Essentials of Chinese Acupuncture, 168, 171, 176
Estrogen
  cancer relationship, 63–74
  creams, 53

Estrogen (*Contd.*)
  decline during menopause, 52, 53–54, 61, 107
  DES, 24–25, 65, 66, 68–69, 70–74
  historical development, 61–62
  male risk, in physically handling, 24
  naturally appearing in herbs, 236, 238–39, 243
  Premarin, 24–25, 68–69, 75
  promotion of, economic/social/political factors in, 74–77
  "reselling" of, 23, 30
Estrogen, universal use for
  acne, 62
  breast engorgement, postpartum, 63
  lactation inhibitor, 62, 63
  miscarriage, threatened, 24–25, 36, 61, 65, 66 68–69, 70–74
  morning-after pill, 61, 62, 63, 68, 73–74
  oral contraceptive, 24–26, 30, 61, 63, 73–74
  osteoporosis, 53, 67
  postmenopause, 52–54, 61, 63, 65, 66–68, 85, 107
  thinning hair, 62, 64
Estrogen replacement (ER) therapy, 52–54, 61, 63, 65, 66–68, 107
  alternatives to, 191, 214–15, 219–20
Exercise
  aerobic, 53, 55, 159, 310–18
  and homeostasis, 134, 137–38
  osteoporosis and, 53, 67
  PMS and, 55, 238, 342

Fainting, premenstrual, 55
Fallopian tubes
  cutting/tying, 11
  removal of, 103
Fat, dietary, 220–22, 223
Fatigue, 51, 53
  alternative treatment, 214, 217, 305, 359
Federation of Feminist Women's Health, 379
Feminist Women's Health Center (L.A.) 20, 380
Fertility control, *see* Contraception
Fertilization, *see* Conception
Fetus, dangers to, 35–45, 70–72, 85
Fibroids, uterine, 26, 64, 103, 107, 219
First aid, self-help modes, 201–02
Flagyl (metronidazole), 383
Foams, spermicidal, 12, 16–18
Folic acid, 216, 217, 219
FDA (Food and Drug Administration)
  and estrogen sex hormone drugs, 61–78
  condom standards set by, 18
  estrogen replacement, 53
  FDA Drug Bulletin, 62, 66, 88
  labeling, package
    the Pill, 10, 23, 27
    IUD, 10, 29

FDA (*Contd.*)
  mercury removal from Koromex spermicide 16–17
  obstetric drugs/procedures, 34–45
Forceps delivery, risks in, 37, 41, 43

Gastrointestinal disease, 55, 64
Germ theory, of disease origin, 128
Ginsent, 53
Glaucoma, alternative approaches to, 402, 407
Gossypol, 10

Hair loss, 62, 64, 217
Hatha Yoga, 159, 294–309
HDL (high-density lipoprotein), 134, 314–15
Headache
  alternatives approaches, 193, 202, 276, 315, 316, 321, 342, 344, 359
  menopausal, 51, 52, 53
  menstrual, 51, 55
  migraine, 51, 55, 57, 64, 85
  premenstrual, 55
Health reform movement, 125–45, 156–60
  19th century, 147–55
  20th century, alternative approaches, 162–408
Heart attacks in Pill/estrogen users, 22–23, 30, 64
  alternative approaches, 134, 185, 223, 403
Heat therapy, 321–32
Herbal medicine, 159, 167, 169–76, 234–45
Herpes
  and Nonoxynol-9, 18
  alternative approach, 193, 199
  childbirth and, 116
"High" states, 88, 400, 402
Holistic health care, 107
  alternative healing modes, 162–408
  and orthodox medicine, compared, 125–60
  definition, 133
Homeopathy, 197–206
  /allopathy, compared, 157–60
  /homeostasis, 131–42
Homeostasis, 765–67
  /homeopathy, 131–42
Hormonal imbalance, 53, 54, 55, 56, 66
  alternative approach, 237–39, 336–46, 352
Hormones, *see* Estrogen; Oral contraceptives
Hormone-vitamin dependence, 219–23
Hot flashes, menopausal, 51, 52, 53–54, 66–67
  alternative treatment, 214, 316, 331, 343–44
Hypertension, in Pill/estrogen users, 22–23, 64, 99

Hypertension (*Contd.*)
  alternative approaches, 134, 185, 202, 359, 393–94
Hyperthermia, 326–28, 329–30
Hypnosis, 159, 250, 364–74
Hypnotic drugs, 84, 85, 87
Hypoglycemia, 216, 220, 404
Hypothalmus gland, 54, 331, 336–43 passim
Hypothermia, in newborn, 43
Hysterectomy
  after sterilization, 10
  alternatives to, 107, 108, 223
  current treatment, 103, 105–06, 107–08
  in Pill users, 26
  unnecessary, 3, 104–07

Iatrogenic disease, 84–85, 135, 401
Illness, infectious, 138, 160
Imoglry, *see* Visualization
Inderal, 57
Indocin, 58
Infertility/sterility
  after contraceptive use, 21–23, 64
  alternative treatment, 171–72, 187, 202, 217–18, 248, 369–70
  and basal body temperature, 19
Informed consent, 4, 38, 41, 45, 63, 77–78, 108
Injury
  acute/episodic, 160
  chronic, and self-help therapy, 201–02
  surgical, 10, 11, 12
  traumatic, 138, 160
Insomnia, 85
  alternative treatment, 170, 185, 193, 359
  menopausal, 53
  premenstrual, 55
International Childbirth Education Association, 118
Intuition, aspect in healing, 125–42 passim
Iodine, dietary, 210, 213, 215–16, 218, 219, 221, 222
Ionization, and heat therapy, 318
Irritability
  alternative approach, 241
  menopausal, 51, 53
  premenstrual, 51, 55
IUD's (Intrauterine devices), 9–10, 12, 13, 14, 15–16
  adverse effects of, 21–22, 27–29
  deaths associated with, 21, 28–29
  infertility and, 21, 22
  pregnancy in users, 28

Jelly, contraceptive, 17, 18
Judasim, Orthodox, contraceptive use, 15–16

Koromex, 16–17

Labeling, patient package, 10, 23, 27, 27n, 44–45

Labor/delivery
  alternative approaches, 187, 190, 248, 251–52, 280, 329–30, 344, 402
  current drug/procedure risks, 35–45
  drug use, risks in, 35–45
  obstetrical intervention, risks of, 35–45
Lactation, 62, 63
  alternative approach, 171, 215–16, 243, 248, 252, 281, 330
Law/legal action
  and package warning labels, 27n, 44–45
  and poststerilization pregnancy, 11
Lethargy, 55, 341
Librium, 84, 87, 401
Light manipulation, to control ovulation, 20
Limbic response, 336–43 passim
Lithium, 56
Liver disorders in Pill/estrogen users, 26, 64, 65, 69
  alternative treatment, 218, 221
Lupectomy, 97, 98, 99

Marijuana
  nonpharmaceutical users, 400, 402, 406–07
  use in PMS, 56
Massage, 159, 167, 247–57
  reflexology and, 258–268
Mastectomy
  radical, 3, 95–97, 98
  simple, 97
Mastitis, alternative treatment, 175–76, 218, 242, 281
Medical Letter, 383
Meditation, as therapy, 107, 159, 350–62
Megavitamin therapy, 149, 229–32
Menninger Foundation, 274, 338–45, 352
Menopause, problems/distress, 5, 51, 52–54
  alternative approaches, 185, 190–91, 202, 214–15, 219–20, 243, 316, 321–31, 330–31, 343–44, 358
  estrogen replacement therapy, 52–54, 61, 63, 65, 66–68, 85, 107
  medical/social attitudes, past/current, 3, 5, 52, 54–55
Macrobiotic diet, 159, 223
Magnesium deficiency, 55
  alternative treatment, 213, 219
Male
  breast cancer risk, handling estrogens, 24
  contraception
    biofeedback, using, 343
    condom, 12, 13, 15, 17, 18
    heat, using, 327
    oral, 10

Male (*Cont.*)
  vasectomy, 10, 11
Mammography, 95, 98, 99
Manganese deficiency, 215
Marcaine,4 2
Menstrual disorders
  alternative treatment, 171, 172, 177–78, 185, 186–87, 203–04, 211–14, 231, 237–39, 279–80, 300, 316, 330, 341–43, 372–73
  dysmenorrhea, 51, 55, 57–58
  effect of sterilization, 10
  medical/social attitudes, past/current, 5, 51, 54–58
Menstrual extraction, 380
Mercury
  in spermicides, 16–18
  vaginally absorbed, 16–18
Metabolic disorders in Pill users, 22–23
  alternative treatment, 217–18, 315
Miasmatic theory of disease origin, 128
Middle East, contraceptive use in, 15–16
Migraine headache, 51, 55, 57, 64, 85
  alternative treatment, 202, 315, 316, 342
Minerals, depletion, 22, 26, 53, 55, 56, 67
  alternative treatment, 214–24
"Mini" pill, 27
Miscarriage, spontaneous, 21, 36, 61, 65, 66, 70–74
  alternative approach, 171–72, 200, 242
  induction of, 61, 187, 237–38, 248
  misuse of estrogen to prevent, 36, 61, 65, 66, 72–74
  mortality rate, 21
Morning-after pill, 61, 62, 63, 68, 73–74
Morphine, 400, 401, 403*n*
Mortality risks, from
  abortion, 21
  anesthesia, 106, 114
  Caesarean section, 114
  contraceptive use, 10–12, 17, 21, 28–29
  hysterectomy, 105, 106
  osteoporosis, 53
  pregnancy, 21
  sterilization, 10, 11, 21
Moxibustion (heat), 167–76 passim
Multiple sclerosis, 193, 402

Naprosyn, 58
National Academy of Sciences, 75, 83
National Cancer Institute, 62, 64, 74, 98, 406
National Center for Health Statistics, 113, 116
National Institute of Child Care and Human Development, 117, 118
National Institute of Occupational Safety and Health, 24

National Institute on Drug Abuse, 87, 88
National Institutes of Health, 14, 95–96
  Center for Population Research, 74
National Women's Health Network, 15*n*, 16, 38
Natural birth control, 18–21, 29–30, 343
Natural food, 209–11
Nausea
  alternative treatment, 200, 217, 242, 280–81, 342, 402, 406–407
  in estrogen users, 64
  in pregnancy, and drug use risk, 35–36
Nembutal, 85
Network Against Psychiatric Assault, 126
Neurological dysfunction
  alternative therapy, 171
  menopausal, 52, 53
  newborn, 38–44
  premenstrual, 55
Neurotic, historical medical view of women as, 4–5
New Hampshire Feminist Health Center, 15*n*
New Scientist, 9, 14
Newborn, effect of obstetrical intervention on, 35–48, 115, 201
Nonoxynol-9, 17, 18
Norethindrone, 30
Nutrition
  and homeostasis, 134, 136
  as prevention and therapy, 107, 159, 191, 209–27
  deficiency in pill users, 26, 217
  infertility and, 22, 187
  osteoporosis and, 53

Obesity, 193, 370, 404
Obstetrical intervention, current, 35–45, 140, 141
  alternative treatment, 171, 185, 187, 190
Opiates, synthetic, 401, 402
Opium, 401, 404
Oral contraceptives, 9–10, 12, 13, 14, 20
  deaths associated with, 21, 28–29
  disease associated with, 21–30, 382
  health benefits, claimed/disputed, 24, 25–27
  male, 10
  Pill safety study, discredited, 23–27
  "reselling" of, 23, 30
  use in premenstrual syndrome, 55
Organizations, lists of, for
  acupuncture, 195
  biofeedback, 349
  health, 5–7
  herbology, 245

Organizations, lists of, for (*Contd.*)
  holistic health, 144–45
  homeopathy, 205–06
  hypnosis, 377
  massage, 257
  megavitamin therapy, 232
  nutrition, 227
  pregnancy/birth, 47–48
  premenstrual syndrome, 59
  psychoactive drugs, medical use, 406
  rolfing, 292
Orthodox medicine, 3–123
  alternative approaches/healing techniques, 162–408
  and holistic health, analyzed/compared, 125–60
Osteopathy, 159
Osteoporosis
  alternative treatment, 214–15
  menopausal, 51, 53, 66, 67, 107
Ovaries
  alternative approach to problems, 170
  cancer of, 25–26, 52, 64, 66
  cysts, 24, 25
  removal of, 103, 107
Ovulation, methods of timing, 18–21, 29–30, 343
Oxytocin, as labor inducer, misuse of, 36, 42
Oxytoxynol, chemical in spermicide, 17

Pain, relief of, 37
  alternative approach, 184–85, 248, 252, 264, 272, 404
Pap smear, 66, 103, 217
Parathyroid, 214, 219
Passivity, historical view of women's inevitable, 4–5
Pelvic inflammatory disease (PID), 103
  alternative approach, 240
  in IUD user, 27
  in Pill users, 25, 27
Pharmaceutical companies
  Ayerst, 68
  Eli Lily, 75
  G. D. Searle, 23, 24
  Holland-Rantos, 16–18
  Mead Johnson, 23
  Ortho, 23
  Parke Davis, 23, 85
  Syntex, 23
  Vorhauer Laboratories, 15
Pharmaceutical industry, 44–55, 58
  influence on physicians, 66, 74–77, 85–86, 87, 90, 401
Phosphorous, 213
Photography, Kirlian, 158, 199
Physicians' Desk Reference, 66, 383
Pill, contraceptive, *see* Oral contraceptives
Pituitary disorders, in Pill users, 26, 66, 69

Pituitary disorders, in Pill users (*Cont.*)
 alternative treatment, 219, 239, 330, 336–43 passim
Placebos, 55, 56, 86, 400
Planned Parenthood Federation of America, 10, 13, 24
Plug, tubal, 11
PMS, *see* premenstrual syndrome
Polarity therapy, 131, 159
Polyps, 103
Ponstel, 58
Population control, 9–10, 21, 74, 108
Population Council, 12, 28
Postpartum
 body realignment, 290–91
 depression, 201, 344
 yoga exercises, 299–300
Potassium depletion, 56
 alternative approach, 217
Practitioner/client relationship, 133, 160
Pregnancy
 after sterilization, 11–12
 childbirth, current treatment, 35–48, 85, 115
  alternative treatment, 171, 200–01, 215–17, 229–32, 242–43, 285–92, 297–300, 304, 317, 329–30, 344, 358, 389–90, 404
 during contraceptive use, 11, 13–15, 28
 ectopic, 11, 21
 in IUD users, 28
  in Pill users, 25, 27
 mortality rate, 21
 teenage, 18
Preludin, 87
Premarin, 24–25, 68–69, 75
Premenstrual syndrome (PMS), 51, 55–57
 alternative treatment, 239, 341–43
Prevention
 nutrition as, 208–27
 of disease, 148–54, 160
Progestasert, 28
Progesterone
 as test for pregnancy, 35
 deficiency, alternative treatment, 231, 237, 239, 243, 341
 in estrogen replacement therapy, 53, 68
 use in premenstrual syndrome, 56
Progestins
 and ectopic pregnancy, 27
 in the Pill, 24, 26, 27, 30
 use in premenstrual syndrome, 55, 56
Program for Women's Concerns, 87
Prolactin, 56
Propranilol, 57
Prostaglandins, 42, 58, 238
Provera, 35
Psychedelic drugs, 404
Psychoactive drugs, 56, 399–408
 alternative nonpharmaceutical approach, 399–408

Psychological effects/symptoms
 alternative approach, 343–44, 351, 355–56
 of menopause, 51, 52–54, 67
 of menstrual distress, 51, 54–55
 of premenstrual distress, 55
 of vasectomy, 11
Psychophysiology, female
 alternative approach, 335–46
 present erroneous medical view of, 4–5, 54–55, 57, 58,78
Psychotropic drugs, 83–91
 alternatives to, 401, 404

Radiation treatment, of breast cancer, 96, 97, 98, 99
Radiography, 99
Reagan Administration, and consumer labeling, 27n
Reflexology, 159, 258–68
 massage and, 167, 247–57
Reliability
 of contraceptives, 13–15, 18, 29
 of sterilization, 11–12
Research funding, needed for
 barrier contraceptives, 21, 29
 biochemical studies, 30
 breast cancer, 99–100
 cervical cap, 14
 chemical spermicides, 17, 18
 Chinese medicine, 176, 193
 fertility after IUD use, 22
 menopausal problems, 52, 54
 menstruation, 54–55
 natural birth control, 21, 30
 nonsurgical sterilization, 11
 ovum/sperm production control, 343
 Pill safety, 23, 74–75
 premenstrual syndrome (PMS), 55–57
 universal contraceptive, 10
Reserpine, 95, 99
Reversibility, of sterilization, 11
Rheumatism, 170, 406
"Rhythm" birth control, 18–19, 29–30
Ritalin, 401
Rolf Institute, 288n, 291
Rolfing, 284–92
Rutgers University, 24

Safety
 of contraceptives, 10–12, 16–18, 21–30
 of drugs, 35–45, 84–86, 115, 402
 of Pill, a study, 23–27
 of procedures/tests, 3–4
Sauna baths, 53, 321–31
Schizophrenia, 193, 229
Seconal, 85, 87
Second opinion, affect on surgery rate, 104–05
Sedatives, misprescribing, 83, 84–85, 87
 self-help therapy, 404

Seizures
 alternative treatment, 184
 premenstrual, 55
Selenium, dietary, 216, 217, 218, 219, 221, 223
Self-diagnostic tests
 cancer, colon/rectal, 393, 395
 diabetes, 392, 395
 hypertension, 393–94, 395–96
 pregnancy, 389–90, 394
 throat culture, 390–91, 394
 urinary tract infection, 391–92, 395
Self-examination, cervical, 20–21, 379–86, 389–96
Self-healing, 125–45
 19th century, 146–54
 20th century, 378–86
Self-Help Clinics, 381–85
Self-hypnosis, 159, 364–74
Self-regulation, body, 131–32, 134–42
Semicid, 17
Sex bias, in orthodox health care, 3–5, 54–55, 57–58, 78, 86–90, 341
Sexual dysfunction, menopausal, 53, 66, 96, 106–07
 alternative treatment, 185, 369
Sexually transmitted disease, 17, 18, 27, 29, 382–84
Shunning, of
 menopausal women, 52, 343
 menstruating women, 54
Skin problems, in estrogen/Pill users, 26, 64, 66
Sonography, risks of, 36
Sperm production, 10, 327, 343
Spermicides, 12, 13, 14–15, 16–18
Spiritual aspects in healing, 125–42 passim, 158, 159, 323–25, 351
 see also Homeopathy
Sponges, contraceptive, 12, 13, 14–15
Stanozolol, 53
Sterility, after IUD/Pill use, 21–23
Sterilization
 deaths associated with, 21
 female, 9, 10–12, 14, 105
 male, 10–11
 pregnancy after, 11–12
Stimulants, 84, 87, 88
Stress
 alternative approaches, 274, 313–14, 351, 355–57, 360
 and homeostasis, 134, 135–36, 138–42
Strokes, in Pill/estrogen users, 23, 191, 193
 alternative approaches, 134, 190–91, 193
Suffering, historical medical view of women as, 4–5
Suicide
 in drug users, 84, 88, 134
 in Pill users, 23
Suppository, contraceptive
 foaming, 12, 17
 nonfoaming, 17

Surgery, unnecessary, 3–5, 95–97, 104–07
Sweat bathing, 320–32

Tai Chi Chuan (a movement therapy), 159
Talwin, 401
Tampon, contraceptive, 16
Teenage pregnancy rate, and condom advertising, 18
Temperature method, of natural birth control, 19–20
Tension
    premenstrual, 51, 55
    self-help therapy, 239, 272, 276–78, 313–14, 406
Thailand, contraceptive use in, 15–16
Therapy, nutrition as, 208–27
Thermal regulation, 43, 52, 53–54, 321–31
Thermography, 99
Thorazine, 99
Thyroid problems, in Pill users, 26
    alternative approaches, 219, 222, 231, 303
Tranquilizers
    inappropriate prescribing of, 83, 84, 87, 88, 95, 341, 356–57
    use for menstrual cramps, 58
    use in PMS, 56
Tubal ligation, 11, 105, 108
Tuinal, 85
Tumors, 24, 25, 26, 99
    alternative treatment, 171, 174–75

Ultrasound, 99
U.S. Surgeon General's Report, 134
"Universal" contraceptive, search for, 9, 15–16
Urinary tract disorders, in Pill users, 26

Urinary tract disorder, (*Contd.*)
    alternative treatment, 171, 173, 241, 321–26, 370, 379–80, 391–92
Uterus
    cancer of, 25–26, 52–53, 63, 64, 67, 69–70, 103, 107
    fibroids in, 26, 103
    perforation of, by IUD, 29
    removal of, 103, 105, 107
    self-help therapy, 171

Vacuum aspiration, 380
Vaccum extraction of infant, risks of, 43
Vaginal
    absorption of drugs, 16–18
    adenosis, 71
    cancer, 62, 66, 70–72
    infections/estrogen use, 64
    menopausal changes, 51, 53
    problems, alternative treatment, 173, 179, 199, 214, 240, 369, 372, 378–86
Valium, 83, 84, 87, 88, 401
    alternatives to, 404
Vasectomy, 10–11
Vasodilation, in PMS, 57
Vasomotor fluctuation. *See* Hot flashes
Visualization, 107, 336, 340, 345, 371–72
    see also Biofeedback
Vitamin A (retinol), 213, 216, 221
Vitamin B$_2$ (riboflavin), 26
Vitamin B$_6$ (pyridoxine), 26, 56, 213, 216, 217, 219
Vitamin B$_{12}$ (cyanocobalamin), 213, 217
Vitamin B$_{17}$ (laetrile), 211

Vitamin C (ascorbic acid) deficiency, 26
    alternative approaches, 213, 216, 218, 219, 239
    and pregnancy, 229–32
Vitamin D (calciferol), 53, 213, 215, 216, 219
Vitamin depletion
    alternative approaches to, 159, 214–19, 229–32, 404
    in menopausal women, 53
    in Pill users, 22, 26
Vitamin E (tocopherol), 199, 213, 214, 216, 218, 219, 221, 222, 231
Vitamin K (phylloquinone), 231
Vomiting, in pregnancy, and drug use risk, 35–36
    alternative approach, 197–98, 402

Walnut Creek Report (Pill safety study), 23–27
Warning, printed, patient. *See* Labeling, package
Weakness, during menstruation, 58
Winstrol, 53
Women's health
    alternative approaches, 162–408
    orthodox, traditional approach, 3–123
Women's movement, and self-healing, 125–45
    19th century, 147–55
    20th century, 378–86
World Health Organization (WHO), 14

Yoga, 107, 159, 294–309

Zinc deficiency, 26
    alternative approach, 213, 214, 215, 216, 218